From Midwives to Medicine

From Midwives to Medicine

THE BIRTH OF AMERICAN GYNECOLOGY

DEBORAH KUHN MCGREGOR

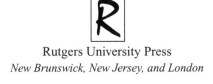

Rutgers University Press
New Brunswick, New Jersey, and London

Library of Congress Cataloging-in-Publication Data

McGregor, Deborah Kuhn.
    From midwives to medicine : the birth of American gynecology /
Deborah Kuhn McGregor.
      p.   cm.
    Includes bibliographical references and index.
    ISBN 0-8135-2571-3. — ISBN 0-8135-2572-1 (pbk.)
    1. Sims, J. Marion (James Marion), 1813–1883.   2. Gynecologists—
United States—Biography.   3. Generative organs, Female—Surgery—
United States—History—19th century.   4. Gynecology—United
States—History—19th century.   I. Title.
RG76.S5M367 1998
618.1'0092—dc21
[b]   98-6811
                                                            CIP

British Cataloging-in-Publication data for this book is available from the British Library

Manufactured in the United States of America

For Bob

CONTENTS

ILLUSTRATIONS AND TABLES

Illustrations

Tables

ACKNOWLEDGMENTS

I am grateful to Rutgers University Press for the opportunity to prepare a new and completely revised edition of my history of the origins of gynecology, *Sexual Surgery and the Origin of Gynecology: J. Marion Sims, His Hospital and His Patients*, published in 1989. Many years of library work, writing, and teaching have converged in this new effort. The Austin, Texas, gathering of the Midwives Alliance of North America in 1996 first gave me the idea and enthusiasm to update the book.

The University of Illinois at Springfield supported me in numerous ways, most especially with a sabbatical, giving me the time to think and conduct research. I am also indebted to my colleagues in the programs of history and women's studies who have offered stimulation and good conversation along the way. Carol Watson Lubrant helped immeasurably in the eleventh hour. Denise Green and the Brookens Library were invaluable sources. Judith Everson offered insight and support, and my students and their love of history kept me going.

Regina Morantz-Sanchez offered food for thought, a willingness to share knowledge, and an affirmation of the value of scholarly exchange. At Rutgers University Press, Doreen Valentine asked all the right questions. Alice Calaprice offered a wonderful way with words and an eagle eye. Robbie Davis-Floyd, Penfield Chester, and Marilyn Green gave the spark. Sarah Elbert, Bert Hansen, John Haller, and Todd Savitt read parts of the manuscript and offered valuable suggestions, and I am also indebted to Linda Keldermans. The Southern Illinois University School of Medicine has provided help in many ways; Barbara Mason, Lynn Cleverdon, and the Medical Library helped me in ways beyond my expectations. Phillip Davis has always offered interest and a willingness to help. I am indebted to many others, but the final product is of course my own responsibility.

Funding for research came in part from the SUNY-Binghamton Foundation, the National Endowment for the Humanities, and the History of Science Society. Funding for research and writing also came from the University of Illinois at Springfield, along with a subsidy for the full-color printing of the cover illustration.

I drew on the resources of several libraries in the course of my research: the Philadelphia College of Physicians and Surgeons and the Special Collections of the Jefferson Medical College in Philadelphia; the New York Academy of Medicine, the New York Public Library, the New York Historical Association, and the Bolling Medical Library Special Collections at St. Luke's Roosevelt Hospital in New York, where Nancy Panella and Joan Cardeval were very helpful; the Reynolds Library at the University of Alabama at Birmingham and the Alabama State Archives in Montgomery; the South Carolina Historical Society and the South Caroliniana Library; the Special Collections at the Hardin Health Sciences Library, University of Iowa; the Special Collections at the Health Sciences Library, Southern Illinois School of Medicine; and the many libraries of the University of Illinois in Champaign-Urbana. Cornell Medical Library Special Collections at New York Hospital and the archivist there, Adele Lerner, along with the Special Collections of Columbia University at the Augustus C. Long Health Sciences Library and its archivist, Barbara Paulson, offered rich resources. At the University of Alabama at Birmingham, Dr. Hugh Shingleton provided information on the location of artifacts and documents.

This book has grown, in part, out of the memory of Rick, Abby, and Sparrow, who died too young.

I am grateful to my family for their patience during the final days of the preparations of the manuscript. My mother, Agnes Kuhn, procured several valuable documents while providing moral support. My children, Molly, Leaf, Blue, Janna, and Bran, have all but one grown into majority over the course of preparation. Their interest and support is valuable beyond measure. Above all, I thank my spouse, Bob McGregor, an author in his own right, who gave editorial assistance, historical expertise, and ongoing assurances of successful completion. On this occasion he is truly The Midwife.

Prologue

———>●<———

In May 1857, a lady "possessed of ample means," as her physician, J. Marion Sims, recorded, visited him complaining of general disability and ill health.[1] Her high social status served to protect her anonymity; there is no record of her name or even an initial, nor is there testimony from her. The doctor's first evaluation determined that she suffered from an extreme nervous condition—he called it "deplorable."[2] Certainly this woman was confined and debilitated by her health, an "invalid," the physician said, for more than twenty years. Her greatest physical exertion was to walk across the room, which she did rarely, remaining mostly confined to her couch. The physician found the source of her problem to be in her reproductive organs.

Addressing other physicians, J. Marion Sims reported the case of this woman to exemplify a condition he called "vaginismus." For convenience, let us call her Patient X. Vaginismus left Patient X unable to bear any physical contact with her genitalia or to engage in sexual intercourse. Soon after her marriage, twenty-five years before her contact with Sims, a different physician had surgically removed a small nodule on her meatus urinarius (the duct where urine passes out of the body) and applied graduated bougies to coax her vagina open little by little. Bougies were a kind of plug that physicians of this era inserted into the vagina for a variety of female complaints, but for Patient X the treatment did not succeed. After visiting many different and well-known physicians in major American cities and in London, Paris, and other European urban centers, she came to Sims in New York City. At the time of her visit with Sims, he observed that forty-five-year-old Patient X had remained a virgin.

Ultimately Sims devised a surgical treatment for vaginismus, and this patient served as one of several original case studies. The first step the physician took was to try to examine Patient X vaginally. Visualize this as occurring in her home, on her couch. Such a procedure was not unusual, and in fact Sims followed the ways of his times. The image of such a personal examination being conducted in the heart of the home helps to emphasize how different the expectations and culture of the mid-nineteenth century were compared with today's. Because Patient X could not endure even the manual penetration of her vagina, the result of the examination was an immense, seemingly involuntary resistance marked by extreme vaginal contraction and overall disquiet. At first Sims could not proceed, but with the patient's insistence, he was able, to a limited degree, to examine her internally. The doctor said his patient begged him to go on so that he might find the source of her trouble and name her sickness for her.

After examining the patient, Sims went to several peers for assistance in observing her under anesthesia. He recruited four other physicians from various institutions in New York City to meet with the patient again in a private setting. Sims personally feared for the woman's well-being under anesthesia, so he asked two of the other doctors to anesthetize the patient. Under the effects of ether, the patient relaxed and the symptoms of spasmodic vaginal contractions ceased. While Sims was pleased with this result, he argued that the only permanent solution for cases of this type was a Y-shaped incision in the vaginal wall, though he refused to perform the surgery on this particular patient. "An untried process was not justifiable on one in her position in social life," he argued, "the Hospital being the legitimate field for experimental observation."[3]

Although we know nothing more about Patient X than what her physician ultimately reported in a published paper, her story embodies central themes in the history that follows on the origins, in the mid-1800s, of the medical specialty of gynecology. This field emerged through the medical practice of several nineteenth-century physicians, particularly that of J. Marion Sims. The institution he helped to establish and where he practiced intermittently for several years, the Woman's Hospital of the State of New York, also played a significant role.[4]

Several aspects of the case of Patient X resulted more from her position in social life than from her sickness. The use of anesthesia, for instance, was a response to her class, race, and gender. This medical encounter took place close to the time of the introduction of anesthesia, and the pattern of its use was just beginning to form. White upper-class women tended to be its main recipients.[5] Before and after this case, Sims practiced many surgeries using no anesthesia. Women who were subjects of gynecological practice in this period were often in far more need of anesthesia than Patient X had been, yet they never received it.

Central to this story are the diverse lives of the women who needed care.[6] While Patient X was a white woman of means, women of a wide variety of social strata and ethnicities played roles in the history of gynecology. They were victims as well as agents. They included slaves and Irish immigrants, Protestant women reformers, nurses and hospital matrons, European princesses, philanthropists, and prominent citizens and medical practitioners in the United States and Europe.

Male dominance of medical practice rested on the subordination of women and the objectification of their bodies. Though Sims refused to experiment on Patient X, he experimented freely on other women—patients or inmates, as they were known, of the hospital—often of a different class or race from Patient X. The designation of these women as hospital patients placed them in a lower class and/or race, women on whom doctors could experiment. Even though the Woman's Hospital of the State of New York also had patients of high social standing, they fell into a separate category and were less often the subject of untried surgeries.

Without access to these women's bodies, Sims could not have established himself in the medical world. Early gynecological surgery in the United States had already taken place earlier, during and after the Civil War. Sims was a Southerner by birth and began his career in the South. In his first private practice he treated slave patients. He began his career as a rural plantation physician, practicing in the Cotton Belt of frontier Alabama, eventually moving to New York City in the mid-1850s, when he was in his early forties. During these years, following peak immigration from the Irish potato famine, he founded a hospital with mostly Irish women as patients.[7] With the coming of the Civil War he moved to Europe and began a practice that included European royalty. The experimentation that pervaded his and his associates' early practice was enabled by historical events that allowed physicians to use patients according to their social status. Furthermore, as he suggested in his writing about Patient X, the institution of the hospital provided the necessary environment for medical experimentation.[8]

Religion was also an important part of the cultural context and played a definitive part in Sims's career and in the work of the New York City women hospital administrators and volunteers. Protestantism provided a common ground for them while working with Southerners during the heated years of the late 1850s. Religion also helped to form common ground among the physicians. Evangelical benevolence to some degree informed the relationship between the patients and those who governed the hospital. Common religious beliefs help to clarify the doctors' attitudes toward race and class, the shifts in the gender system, and the growing authority of science in the practice of medicine, which was transforming the field.[9]

With gynecology in the forefront of the professionalization and specialization in medicine, these profound changes were thoroughly interconnected with the history of gender and social relations.[10] How did the social and historical definition of womanhood and manhood during these years affect medical practice? In the development of gynecology and medical therapies for women, the physician, who was usually male, often took on the role of moral adviser and sought to make his female patient conform to the existing social expectations of womanhood, applying what were ultimately heralded as advanced techniques.[11]

Along with these medical therapies, premised on the subordination of women, came the determination of many women to become full participants in the public world of professional careers. Although some women successfully completed medical school and became doctors, many schools denied them access.[12] In the 1870s medical theory still posited that education was harmful for women. Those women who succeeded in becoming physicians often did so for the purpose of protecting what they saw as the privacy, frailties, and weaknesses of women.

In the case of Patient X, the physician became a kind of priest, yet the situation also led to his investigation of her most private areas. She apparently allowed Sims to proceed, and by implication would have allowed surgery. Patient X's experiences were typical for her time. Her aversion to heterosexual exchange follows the characterization of Victorian women as sexually repressed, sometimes "frigid," and even asexual.[13]

Since Patient X was close to the age of menopause, she was unlikely ever to bear a child. Indeed, this fact probably affected Sims's treatment of her. He saw that motherhood was improbable for her and, given her social class, decided that surgery was inappropriate. In his later works he revealed a strong inclination to view childbearing as the purpose of sexual intercourse and as the life goal for all women. The implication was that sexual exchange was no longer so important for Patient X because its purpose was vanishing. Yet in other women he used surgery to treat similar symptoms.

In approaching the history of women patients in the early years of gynecology, I attempt to include the patient as an active participant in her relationship with the physician.[14] Patient X probably approached Sims to find legitimation for her condition through a diagnosis of illness. At the same time, because of the tight boundaries under which upper-class women lived, the possibility exists that her invalidism was psychosomatic of her inability to find meaning in life. Being childless may well have been a burden for her, for motherhood was the essence of womanhood at this time.[15]

In the social history of medicine and women's health, ailments and conditions appear to change from one era to another. While vaginismus is still a recognized condition and bears the same name that Sims gave it, how medical professionals prioritize, define, and treat the disorder has changed greatly.[16] Therapies today assume the origins of vaginismus to be more psychological than physical. The social and cultural context of the middle decades of the 1800s helps to explain the professional recognition Sims received for treating vaginismus. His therapies and the priorities he exhibited in medical care fit with a culture that at once denied sexuality and yet saw it everywhere.[17] Vaginismus was one of several examples of the early gynecologists' focus on female reproduction and sexuality as the keys to health.

During the decades of the mid-nineteenth century, the roles and social expectations for women transmogrified. Historians characterize seventeenth- and eighteenth-century American women as childbearers, but due to the complexity of their lives, their participation in society went well beyond simply giving birth repeatedly. Furthermore, there were variations in the rate of childbirth according to locale and economic and social status.

In the late eighteenth century, with the advent of the American Revolution, families' emphasis began to shift from childbearing to child raising.[18] Rather than give birth roughly every two years until the end of fertility or death, women gradually created smaller families and were increasingly expected to dedicate themselves to the rearing of their children. By the end of the nineteenth century, following a slow but steady decrease in population growth, the average number of children in a white family was four, where it had been eight at the beginning of the nineteenth century. While these figures may not be accurate and mask variations in region, class, and ethnicity, they help to illustrate the significant demographic changes that occurred during the nineteenth century.[19] This "Demographic Transition" quantifies the significant redefinition of culture during this time.

Changes in medical practice mirrored the Demographic Transition. Many of the earliest surgeries in gynecology treated women who were either mothers of many children or were members of what society deemed "other" due to their class and/or ethnicity. Often, because of the material conditions of their lives, they fell outside the expectations the larger society had of them. The biology of female reproductivity joined women into one group, but culturally perceived differences of race and class often still separated them. Manipulating these elements of social fragmentation, doctors used the social standards for gender when treating their first gynecology patients and thereby won approval for its practices. Gynecological surgeries outside this focus met with criticism.

In the mid-nineteenth century, the practice of surgery, obstetrics, and midwifery led to gynecology and became an alternative to the healing practices associated with midwifery. Besides aiding in childbirth, midwifery included diverse medical therapies for female ailments and was the domain of women healers for centuries.[20] In the eighteenth century, William Hunter, an English physician, had outlined the physiological changes in a woman's body during the nine months of pregnancy. This knowledge, together with the availability of forceps, helped create the new practice of obstetrics.

Obstetric, as it was called then, or the Obstetrick Art, originally referred to the activities of the midwife; in the early nineteenth century the word became plural—obstetrics. [21] This new science of obstetrics included more than what was represented by midwifery. Medical training moved into the specific areas of women's health that deal with parturition. In nineteenth-century America, male medical practitioners made steady inroads into this once all-female heritage, supervising birth in greater numbers, establishing the specialty of obstetrics, and creating the practice of gynecology. Gynecology, a word that came into vogue in the mid-nineteenth century, meant the study of woman in terms of her functions and diseases.[22] Medical therapies were at this time focused on the individual and her environment and social situation. There was no concept of disease as largely microscopic or involving microorganisms such as viruses and bacteria.[23]

Childbirth in the mid-nineteenth century was markedly different from childbirth in the West today, and problems associated with pregnancy and birth influenced the early practice of gynecology. Among the first experimental surgeries for female disorders was an attempt to mend what were then known as "accidents of childbirth." A few years before the identification of vaginismus, Sims innovated and experimented with an operation that won him his status as the founder of gynecology—surgery for vesico-vaginal fistula, a condition of vaginal tears resulting from difficult childbirth. How did a significant professional specialty emerge from the treatment of a condition that is almost unknown today? We will find the answer later in this book.

Abortion and contraception were also included in the new specialty of women's reproduction.[24] Until now they were part of the practice of surgeons and general practitioners, or midwives and women healers. Most physicians did not specialize until after professionalization was well underway.

Contemporary scholars consider the practice of gynecology by Sims and his colleagues to be the hallmark that led to modern medicine. This modernity emerged from new medical techniques, especially in clinical medicine and surgery, as well as other factors, including economic, social, and political changes. It was the result of waves of immigration, the formation of the middle class, a newly defined working class, the growth of science and technology, reforms in religion, the rise of institutions, the growth and redefinition of individualism, the Civil War, and, eventually, the successful implementation of industrial capitalism.

Although J. Marion Sims is pivotal in the history of gynecology, he did not create it by himself. In the case of Patient X, Sims turned to and involved his peers in his early New York practice. By doing so, he gained legitimacy and identified a common ethical groundwork. In the article describing the case, a surgeon, Edmund R. Peaslee, who later became a colleague of Sims at the Woman's Hospital, urged moderation and caution in the surgeries suggested by Sims, but praised him for his identification of vaginismus and for his innovative surgical therapy. Sims was generally able to maintain the support of other surgeons both before and after the Civil War, but sometimes he failed. Practioners thus embarked on a course of conflict and consensus to establish professional standards in gynecological practice.

The chapters that follow chart the history of gynecology and gynecological surgery through the 1870s. The focus is on the lives of the patients, the participation of women philanthropists and volunteers who worked to establish the Woman's Hospital of the State of New York, the social history of the disorders and conditions identified as the subjects of gynecological practice, and the emergence of a group of men who established themselves as professionals in a medical specialty concerned with women.

CHAPTER 1

Peoples and Places

——————✦——————

*U*nderstanding the origins of Western modern medical practices requires a view of society as a whole. What we know as gynecology came out of medicine practiced in Europe as well as in the United States. Throughout much of the nineteenth century, many American physicians studied on the continent or in England or at least were aware of the scholarship coming out of the various countries there—depending on the time and their interest. Through the increased availability and publication of medical journals, practitioners increasingly became part of an international medical community.[1] Reciprocity went in several directions as European and British medical men drew more and more from medical practice in the United States.

A look at the late 1700s and early 1800s reveals an exchange between medical history and political, economic, and social systems. In fact, they were of one cloth, with a warp and woof of common threads and some shared patterns. The turn of the nineteenth century was a tremendously complex time during which new political systems emerged and individualism and republican government began to take form in the United States. Although it changed at various times and did not necessarily occur in a linear progression, industrial capitalism throughout the Western world, deeply woven into political systems, became the dominant economic system. In American history, Benjamin Rush literally exemplified this interplay. A physician, he was both a signer of the Declaration of Independence and a practitioner of what we now call heroic therapies in medicine.[2] He understood most sickness to be the result of physical overstimulation, and as a result, he used "depletion," most often bloodletting, to restore the body's equilibrium. He was a social activist and philosopher. Some of his medical treatments for insanity were part of an effort to move toward the creation of what he saw as a perfect society based on homogeneity and moral perfection—his vision for the republic. His idea was to guide individuals to practice self-government with an internalized sense of right and wrong; although each should act as an individual, the moral framework was to be held in common by all. As far as racial diversity was concerned, Rush thought skin pigments were changeable and in an ideal world all people would be white-skinned.[3] Stemming from early origins outside the United States, the medicine Rush practiced reflected a common medical approach in America through the middle of the century, and emphasized therapies based on purgation and depletion, especially through bleeding but also by use of large doses of mercury, calomel, and opium.[4]

Another representative figure of the period was the English philosopher Thomas Malthus, who in 1798 published his *Essay on the Principle of Population*. Scholars today recognize this piece as a classic and as a signifier of critical trends and perspectives for the early nineteenth century. Malthus, who studied to be a minister and was also one of the first to discuss political economy, intended to write a scientific examination of the population of England as it was in the throes of industrialization (being further along in the process than other countries, including the United States). His essay laid out a mathematical formula to show that the agricultural ability to produce food was increasing arithmetically while the population increased geometrically. Hence soon, he argued, there would be a great scarcity of food, and starvation and early death were inevitable for the excess population. In his essay Malthus went on to enumerate further "positive checks" on population, including famine, pestilence, and war. He argued that population imbalance and its greatest growth were a result of the high rate of reproduction, particularly among the poor or, as he knew them, the laboring classes. Leaving control in the hands of what was understood to be a natural order—much as Adam Smith, in *Causes of the Wealth of Nations* (1776), suggested that an invisible hand would govern under a laissez faire economy—in essence Malthus wrote that there was no way for humans to control overpopulation. According to Malthus, however, those with moral stamina, which to him meant having the proper values and a fairly high social status, would protect themselves by marrying later and thereby having fewer children. The sacrifice of the others through positive checks on population was simply part of the moral economy of the time: if government tried to assist those in poverty, once given food they would only reproduce at an even greater rate.[5]

Not surprisingly, Malthus did not see how the contemporary historical context influenced his writing, nor did he necessarily intend that his argument serve the class system that was emerging under industrial capitalism.

A present-day reading of his essay would disclose that he regarded class differences as fixed and that he embraced the social status quo. The essay clarifies how the bourgeois class depended on the sacrifices of the working class in the early industrial period in urban England. Influenced by the eighteenth-century mathematician and physicist Sir Isaac Newton, Malthus believed his own work represented a universal and hence timeless law of human behavior.

In the early nineteenth century, Malthus's essay generated a debate concerning the growth of human populations beyond the means of the earth to support it. The debate included the ethics and means of controlling fertility, a debate that still rages and will continue into the next millennium. The work also offers a view of life in the early nineteenth century, which helps us understand how medicine was practiced then.[6] Malthus's formula suggests the historical proximity of epidemics and famine at that time. Although the ravages of the plague a few centuries earlier had already taken their toll, there were ongoing epidemics throughout the century, including cholera and yellow fever, as well as the deadly presence of tuberculosis.[7] Recognizing the immanence of death and disease during this time helps to clarify how practitioners and patients related to each other and to their environment. Although they were not terribly successful at it, medical practitioners, unlike Malthus, sought to intervene and stop disease. All too often, however, desperate conditions led to desperate measures.

Malthus's writing introduced a transformative concept—population.[8] While the word represented people in numbers, "population" invited a sense of science and objectivity in the analysis of human life—even in one's own country. Influenced by the sixteenth- and seventeenth-century work of Francis Bacon, philosophers and scientists in Malthus's time cultivated the numerical record keeping of people and culture, of what some have called the "social body," and various measurements of individual bodies as well.[9] Malthus's *Essay on the Principle of Population*, together with Baconian "political arithmetic" or statistics, would later become the study of demographics.[10] He spoke about the death of infants and the aged, exhibiting neither emotion, prejudice, nor stereotype. He considered the high rate of infant mortality as a positive check of the population. The word "population" also allowed Malthus to talk about sexuality and desire. By placing sexual exchange and the birthrate in the center of his formula, he could refer to reproduction without talking directly about women as its critical agents.

Malthus's work is thus highly related to the rise of the middle class and bourgeois morality in Western society. Painted with broad strokes, his conceptualization suggests an important shift in social roles. Cultural values of the nineteenth century urged women to be domestic keepers of the home and the moral instructors of their children, at the same time urging them to bear fewer offspring.[11] While the gender system designated women as the keepers of morality, in Malthus's framework it was up to men to control fertility through moral restraint, and he argued that only the middle- and upper-class man was capable of doing this. Even though only women give birth, their influence was at best indirect. Although this newly emerging culture and economic system influenced nearly everyone, by the middle of the nineteenth century these values came to describe mostly middle- and upper-class women.

Class is as fundamental to Malthus's paradigm as sex. In the emerging order of industrial capitalism, class provided a pivotal sector. The working class, which performed wage labor, was the lowest social stratum, but to be successful the social system needed many laborers who were paid as little as possible—sometimes below subsistence level. Deeply implicated in the laboring tier were the social constructions of race and sex. Often class, race, and sex were interchangeable. Some segments of the population had to serve as outsiders, although they were categorized as "other." The biological basis for these categories is slippery and virtually nonextant.[12] Women provided one large category that transcended race but did not necessarily supersede it. Cultural or ethnic groups, such as the Irish, the Native American, and the African American, found their own designations. Malthus did not involve race or gender in his essay on population, but his reliance on a concept of a class of laborers is important to the historical experience of women and various ethnic groups as told in this book.

Various sources provided an adequate supply of labor to power the changes in the economic system. In the United States, slavery was becoming more and more entrenched in the economy of the country. Large cotton plantations in the Deep South, worked by slaves, provided the raw material that textile factories in the North needed. England had ended its slave trade in 1807 and emancipated slaves throughout the British Empire in 1833, but in the United States, after the end of the foreign slave trade in 1808, a domestic slave trade continued until the time of the Civil War. The political economy of the South included a growing slave population.

Related to the study of population was the rise of "race science."[13] Scientists and philosophers began to study peoples and the origins of the human species. Social science research—especially the ethnology of early anthropology—in the first half of the nineteenth century involved measuring skulls and people's heights and keeping extensive records of physical qualities of designated groups of people. As early as the Middle Ages, people had already established a culture of racial hierarchy, associating black and white with good and evil and making other assumptions that led to a tradition of social power built on racial prejudice.[14] In the early nineteenth century, consumed with defining race and establishing distinctions, many scholars built on the idea of a Great Chain of Being, which derived from the Enlightenment and created a visualization of racial hierarchy through a ladder of life. This ladder moved upwards from primates—apes, orangutans, and others—through various races of humans, then women, and finally arriving at the highest level: Caucasian men.[15] One effect of the Great Chain of Being was to forge a facetious but lasting link between African peoples and primates.[16]

Central to the story of race and science in this period was the debate over human origins. After Carolus Linnaeus, an eighteenth-century Swedish botanist, had developed a system of taxonomy that gave species a fixed definition—precluding evolution—scholars, scientists, and anthropologists argued whether humans were one species or many, based either on race or sex.[17] There were two schools of thought, monogeny and polygeny; the former argued that all humans had a common origin and were of one species, the latter that there were multiple species.[18] The implications of the argument were many and its scope was international. The argument also split over issues of religion, with those embracing the biblical story of human origins favoring monogeny, and the others believing in polygeny. There were also those who fell somewhere in between while holding on to their faith in Christianity.[19] Further complicating the scholarly dispute over single and multiple human origins was the emergence of the American School of Anthropology founded by Josiah Nott, an American physician, a Southerner, and an advocate of slavery; Samuel Morton, an American anthropologist; and Louis Agassiz, a Swiss naturalist who had immigrated to the United States. Although it was made up of more Northerners than Southerners and was mostly anti-slavery, the American School provided the scientific research used to defend slavery during the 1840s and 1850s. Also at issue were two debates: one over the authority of religion in a society that increasingly turned to science as a framework, and another over the future of colonized peoples throughout the world, including Native Americans in the United States and African slaves in several countries, including the United States.[20]

It is important to note that sex and race often went hand in hand in eighteenth- and nineteenth-century science.[21] Although the American School did not include women explicitly in its efforts to categorize humans by race, Samuel Morton's massive research on skull size provided significant data for the American School and included comparisons by sex as well as race. Demonstrating the imbrication of race and sex into this "race science," certain races on the low end of the spectrum were characterized as womanlike because of their smaller skull size. Research and experiments in craniometry (the science of skull measurement) failed for the most part to take into account the accompanying variations in body size.[22]

At the turn of the century, the keeping and analyzing of statistics on individuals and populations became a significant activity. It served many purposes, including governmental administration, research into human origins, and the practice of medicine. Pierre Louis, a nineteenth-century French physician, was influential in the keeping of case records and statistics on morbidity and mortality. While the gradual inclusion of Louis's Baconian emphasis on quantitative methods was not revolutionary in medical practice, such statistical and empirical bases did help to make medicine clinical.[23]

There were many changes and choices in the practice of medicine in the nineteenth century. In the United States, the rise of sectarian medicine accompanied the social leveling, transformations, and disorder associated with the presidency of Andrew Jackson from 1829 to 1837. The more standard, or allopathic, medicine adhered to a stratified social order by excluding women and groups designated by race, particularly African Americans, from medical schools.[24] During the Jacksonian period there was also a flurry of religious growth, including the Second Great Awakening and the associated development of numerous religious sects. Much of the change in the practice of medicine is highly complex and difficult to decipher because the meanings of medical and scientific terms have changed over time, and because there were differences among physicians across national and professional lines—especially, in the early decades, between physicians and surgeons.[25] "Empiricism," for instance, was a negative word among physicians and denoted quack medicine; to be an empiric was to be the lowest among practitioners.[26] Yet record keeping and the practice of clinical medicine (including pathological anatomy) managed to survive this connotation, and in the late nineteenth century joined with laboratory medicine to establish the foundations of modern medical practice.[27]

During the 1830s some American physicians began to stop using the depleting or heroic therapies. Heroic therapies had come from an abstract idea (rather than a nosology of many distinct diseases) or philosophy that considered the body to be out of balance when sick.[28] This was an eighteenth-century idea of the "body economy."[29] Bleeding, for instance, was used to counteract systemic overstimulation that resulted in sickness, often in fever and inflammation. Such a perspective is in sharp contrast to our current definitions of disease and sickness, which focus overwhelmingly on somatic or cellular, highly specific disease locations. Alternatives included treatments that addressed each individual in terms of race, environment, temperament, class, and sex. While this was a specificity of treatment, it was still radically different from our perspective today. Part of the transformation of medical therapies and healing in the nineteenth century stems from the influence of Descartes and the belief in the separation of mind from body. For centuries medicine had been more philosophical and systems-based than derived from observation and empirical research, but in the nineteenth century this changed and medicine became scientific in a whole new sense.[30]

Because the narrative events of the development of gynecology in this history happened in the United States, mostly in the South, my focus will be primarily on America. There were many different schools of thought and practices of healing here during the 1830s and 1840s, offering divergent therapies, from water to nutrition to botanicals. Some of these practices were within the confines of regular medicine as taught in medical schools. The very essence of regular medicine was challenged, however, since the Jacksonian period brought with it the abrogation of a national medical standard.[31] Medical licensing became erratic and medical education itself slowly metamorphosed throughout the century. Some healing regimens came from individuals outside of medicine, such as water cures, where women took an active role in maintaining alternative medical practices.[32] Thomsonian medicine, which was herbally based, was disseminated by individuals knocking on doors and selling their system. The idea was that each person could be his or her own physician. Although the premise of Thomsonian medicine was that medical schools were unnecessary, its practitioners eventually turned to a standard of regular medical education. Also popular were therapies focused on dietary measures, such as the use of whole wheat flour.[33]

Many physicians in the United States believed in the close relationship between the environment and health. Perhaps this is partly why individuals such as Benjamin Rush were responsive to Malthus's essay, understanding the concept of a sustainable population.[34] Still, the country was large, larger than anyone could really fathom in the first decades of the nineteenth century, and the environment seemed to make the United States exceptional; the challenge was to fill unsettled areas with people, especially those of European descent. The settlement of the frontier that took place over the next hundred years influenced and was influenced by a changing epidemiology. For example, climatology medicine emerged in the early nineteenth century, and American medical texts included charts that combined data from weather and sickness patterns to show their correlation, as in the work of physician Daniel Drake.[35]

With the passing of time, there was a growing political, social, and economic definition of the country by region—the West, the North, and the South. As the demographics of migration and settlement shifted, so did the social geography. Above all, the coming of the Civil War and the decades of conflict over slavery that preceded it contributed to an emphasis on environment or region as defining existence. Sectional divisions were strong and dynamic. The border states that fought with the Union during the war but maintained slavery until war's end are emblematic of this confusion.[36]

In the history of medicine, scholars have long debated the issue of "southern distinctiveness."[37] Partly because of arguments associated with the American School, we have come to think of medical practice in the antebellum South as "States' Rights Medicine,"[38] meaning that some Southern-sympathizing physicians wed their politics and medical therapies. Using the data from early anthropology and the work of Josiah Nott, George Glidden, Samuel Morton, and others, the American School argued that the Southern environment was unique and that the system of slavery suited the peoples who lived in the region. There were different sicknesses there, and people responded to diseases in different ways. This fundamental difference, they argued, separated slaves from their masters because of their different races or places of origin. Slaves were less prone to contract malaria than their masters, for instance, a phenomenon substantiated in the medical history of immunology.[39] The inherent prejudice of the American School, based on the perceived differences of race, led to the conclusion that slavery was the best living arrangement for African Americans, who suffered from what seemed to the members of the American School a lesser intelligence than whites.

The Education of J. Marion Sims

While this book is based on institutional history and the experiences of many individuals, the story begins with J. Marion Sims. The early nineteenth century provided the time, and the South provided the place, for Sims's youth, most of his education, and all of his early career. Sickness, death, slavery, early clinical medicine, and regional distinctiveness all played a part in his life and the choices he made.

J. Marion Sims was born in the back country South Carolina piedmont in 1813, where his Scotch-Irish ancestry was typical of the population of the time.[40] His mother, Mahala Mackey, whose red hair reaffirmed her ancestry, could trace her heritage to immigrants who had arrived in the eighteenth century. His father, Jack Sims, came from relatively poor people who had been farmers for several generations but had kept no record of their migration. During their life in the small town of Hanging Rock, Lancaster County, J. Marion Sims remembered his father hunting fox and playing billiards, and his mother's unhappiness about his father's choice of recreation. His father gave up the hounds but never the billiards.[41] Sims's father was uneducated and did not learn to read and write until his children went to school. His mother, in contrast, attended school in her childhood and had learned to read and write early. Jack Sims's education was cut short by his participation in the War of 1812, during which he was promoted from captain to colonel. Afterwards he returned to Hanging Rock to manage a small farm and store, and eventually to acquire a small number of slaves.

In 1824 the Sims family moved to the town of Lancaster, where Jack Sims ran a tavern and, in 1827, served as sheriff and Commissioner of Public Buildings.[42] Mahala Mackey Sims helped with the support of her family by tending the many boarders who stayed at their lodging place, the only inn in town. Thus J. Marion Sims came from a family of plain folk in the Southern social structure, a family not so much dependent on the labor of slaves as on the Southern political economy of slavery. Sims's father and mother used various strategies, including long-standing indebtedness to one of the wealthier families in the county, to maintain a separate household and to support their children.[43]

Despite Sims's protestations that slaves played only a small part in his life, particularly in the maintenance of his family of origin, he recorded a few memories that suggest otherwise. The overriding emotion appears to be fear and disgust, with a touch of curiosity and admiration for slave culture. Sims recalled the "two great bugbears of my young life . . . mad dogs and runaway niggers, with which the minds of the young were so often demoralized by negro stories."[44] When the family moved to Lancaster village in 1824, Sims (who was about eleven) and his younger brother stayed behind at the first home in Hanging Rock in order to continue attending school. The boys were left with Jack's slaves and an unidentified manager who was in charge of them. "Here we were very much neglected," Sims recalled, "and white children living among negroes . . . were sure to become lousy."[45] Lice, Sims insisted, were always present in a slave population. A different memory surfaced with Sims's portrait of a slave who visited the house to tell stories every Saturday night about animals, told in the African tradition. The storyteller, Cudjo, had been a prince in Africa and was only four feet tall. He had a striking appearance, with tattoos on his face. He told the stories with drama to impress Sims and the other children, succeeding in terrifying them as well. Sims saved his pennies every week, as did the other children, to hear the stories Cudjo had to tell.[46] It is possible that Cudjo practiced some form of conjuring, part of the healing tradition of Africa.[47] Perhaps he influenced Sims by introducing him to a storytelling tradition.

J. Marion Sims's memory of fear of runaway slaves may have resulted from the Denmark Vesey slave revolt in Charleston in 1822. Although he was quite young at the time, the intensity with which adults responded to resistance must have made a strong impression on him. In 1831 Nat Turner led a group of slaves to rebellion in Southhampton County, Virginia. Because fifty-five or more whites were killed during this revolt, the repercussions were extreme throughout the region. Many slaves were falsely accused, and eventually slave codes were tightened.

Sims moved into young adulthood as the tension over slavery mounted. Giving education a priority it had not known in his own life, Jack Sims sent J. Marion Sims, his first-born son, to boarding school at the Franklin Academy in Lancaster, and then to South Carolina College, seventy miles south of Lancaster in Columbia, where he received his bachelor's degree in 1832. That same year, a few months before Sims graduated from South Carolina College, his mother died at the age of forty from what was termed "bilious remittent fever," possibly typhoid fever combined with malaria.[48] Sims recalled ruefully that she might have been blessed to miss his maturity, since she dreamed that he might become a divinity student and later a Presbyterian minister.[49] Perhaps, on the other hand, her early death motivated him to pursue a medical career.

While Sims was at South Carolina College in Columbia, a momentous showdown occurred between the state government and the federal government headed by Andrew Jackson. This was the Nullification Crisis of 1831, orchestrated through the ideas of John C. Calhoun and strongly advocated by many citizens of South Carolina.[50] Sims never wrote about these events in his memoir, *The Story of My Life*, which was published after his death in 1886, and he appears to have been uninvolved politically.[51] He chose rather to tell stories of his grandmother during the American Revolution and his father during the War of 1812. Recalling these stories later in life helped to cement his ties to the nation as a whole rather than to reinforce the divisions he experienced during the Civil War. Still, the heated atmosphere must have made a fundamental impression on a young man coming of age.

One of the most frequently quoted passages from Sims's memoir is his father's response to Sims's announcement that he intended to study medicine. The language reflects Sims's memory of the time many decades before he recorded it. He narrated his memories and stories to a young woman patient in the early 1880s as part of her therapy. A stenographer then wrote the stories down, and Sims's son edited and published the manuscript along with an appendix that included several letters written by Sims.[52] By then Sims had become a world-renowned surgeon recalling the circumstances of his humble origins.

> *J. Marion Sims:* If I must study a profession, there is nothing left for me to do but to study medicine.
>
> *His father:* Well, I suppose that I can not [*sic*] control you; but it is a profession for which I have the utmost contempt. There is no science in it. There is no honor to be achieved in it; no reputation to be made, and to think that *my* son should be going around from house to house through this country, with a box of pills in one hand and a squirt in the other, to ameliorate human suffering, is a thought I never supposed I should have to contemplate.[53]

The language and references to the practice of medicine make a mockery of medical practice in the 1820s. They provide a caricature of the traditional absurd image of medical education and practice prevalent during Sims's youth.

Sims was probably ambivalent about the accuracy or appropriateness of the image. The original manuscript was edited to say "a lancet and a syringe," and "a box of pills and a squirt" was crossed out—by whom or for what reason is not known.[54] The images of "a box of pills and a squirt" uphold the almost stereotypical view we have of medicine in the 1830s when Sims set about to become a physician. Heroic therapies with massive dosages of mercury, calomel, opium, and later quinine and with extensive use of bleeding—cupping and leeching—did not evoke confidence among lay people. Jack Sims's contempt was for therapies such as these, and a memory of these practices as wholly inadequate persists to this day. Nonetheless, the final image is of the physician addressing suffering, hardly a condemnation of the profession.

Although aspiring physicians with sufficient economic support could venture to Europe to seek in-depth training, others sought local schooling where admission required very little background and the requirements for a medical degree were minimal. When Sims went to medical school, many changes were taking place in medical education, particularly in the study of the anatomy of morbid pathology. Although there was no uniform standard nor national regulation of medicine in the United States—indeed, experiences of medical students varied from country to country—there was some common ground, especially by the time Sims began his studies in the 1830s. Influenced by Theophile Laennec and Xavier Bichat, medical professionals began to reconceptualize sickness as disease, often with a local origin, moving closer to the pathology we know today.[55] Medical students faced intense lectures and in the course of working on a medical degree learned a great deal more about human physiology and medicine than the image of a "box of pills and a squirt" might suggest. However, ongoing medical disagreements and uneven acceptance of pathological anatomy and clinical teaching, as well as regional differences, made the education of aspiring physicians irregular.[56]

When Sims embarked on his medical education, he did not know if he would become a physician or a surgeon, the two specializations at the time. He undertook to become a physician and realized only slowly, and only after he was practicing on his own, that he would primarily become a surgeon. His interest in both surgery and medicine made him particularly aware of the shifting body of medical knowledge in morbid anatomy. Both medical schools he attended exposed him to the debates and emerging medical knowledge from France, Germany and Great Britain.[57] He began his studies at a recently established (1827) South Carolina college, the Medical College of the State of South Carolina, in Charleston, in 1833, and later went north to Philadelphia to another new medical school, Jefferson Medical College, where he studied from 1834 until the spring of 1835, when he was graduated with a medical degree.

At that time, medical education in the United States consisted of lectures for one or two terms at a medical college or university, with apprenticeships independently arranged by the student. Apprenticeships often provided students with the only hands-on experience they had. Clinical experience in medical school was very difficult for students to obtain, particularly in outlying areas. In 1834, in between his education in Charleston and Philadelphia, Sims was apprenticed to a physician in Lancaster.

The term during which Sims entered South Carolina College was the school's first session after it had undergone a reorganization. The college began as an affiliate of the school in Columbia where Sims had done his undergraduate work. Extensive scandals and controversies had raged at the first institution, so a second one was created in Charleston. A regionally self-conscious effort to establish Southern medical schools had led to the establishment of South Carolina's Medical College, the second to be built in the Old South.[58] The institution boasted of its access to cadavers, but there was no clinical experience with live patients.[59] Sims later recalled dissecting corpses as a student in the deadhouse, where he was alone with ten or twelve bodies, with only one candle for light. He vividly recalled that the candle fell over, leaving him in the dark surrounded by corpses; he had to feel his way out.[60]

Autopsy, dissection, and hours in the deadhouse helped medical students like Sims during this period when medical education was preponderantly theoretical. Sims was lucky to have had the use of human specimens. Such opportunities for medical students and professionals were greatly limited by the social stigma regarding autopsies and the common refusal to donate bodies for medical students.[61] In the South the slave population was providing autopsy material for many medical students.[62] This is not because slaves had no traditions about death and burial, but because they often had no choice in the matter.[63]

At the College of Charleston, Sims went through the newly established curricular requirements for license—a three-month term of lectures and a faculty review at the end. Although he was situated in a newly established college with political legitimation still in progress, the education he received there was fairly typical for the time.[64]

Apparently Sims felt the need for further education outside his home state. After a few months of apprenticeship in his hometown, he set off, in October 1834, for Jefferson Medical College in Philadelphia. In the eighteenth century, Southern medical students often went to Scotland or England for their education, but now Philadelphia had also become a hub of medical education. Like the Medical College of South Carolina, Jefferson College was a relatively new school, and one fraught with conflict. Physician and surgeon George McClellan had obtained a charter for Jefferson College in 1825, after four years of struggle and competition with the University of Pennsylvania. McClellan, the father of General George McClellan, was an immensely fiery and independent individual. He fought continually with the trustees of the school until his resignation in 1838.[65] There was, however, a "boldness, novelty and success of McClellan's surgical operations."[66] In the 1840s his colleague M. E. Darrach remarked that McClellan spent many hours in the Philadelphia almshouse, which held material for dissection and pathological study: "Each corpse in the deadhouse was marked by his autopsy and surgical operations."[67]

Certainly McClellan provided a strong example for Sims. Primarily he was a role model whom Sims chose to emulate. He also manifested the same bravado of style that Sims would later evince in his own surgical practice.

Sims too came to possess a reputation for high-tempered exchanges with administrators. He recalled in his autobiography that McClellan noticed him and encouraged him to pursue bold and innovative operations, giving him hands-on experience in the operating room.

Sims recalled the atmosphere of one such operation in which he assisted:

> It was a case in which he exsected a portion of necrosed rib, without injury to the plural cavity. He talked to the patient all the time of the operation, for it was before the days of anaesthetics, and when it required great nerve to be a good surgeon. He would gouge and chisel and work away, and say to the man, "Courage my brave fellow, courage; we wound but to heal; it will soon be over. Courage, my dear fellow; it will soon be over."[68]

"We wound but to heal" must have been a chorus in Sims's mind during the fifteen-plus years he practiced surgery without the help of anesthesia. With the work of McClellan, his colleagues, and their successors—including J. Marion Sims—Jefferson Medical College contributed to Philadelphia's reputation as a center of medical education and practice. Several other important physicians of the nineteenth century, including S. Weir Mitchell and Samuel D. Gross, were students at the college. Several renowned teachers also taught at the college, with Charles Meigs perhaps one of the most eminent. By the middle of the nineteenth century, Jefferson College was highly regarded for its instruction in surgery.[69]

In addition to McClellan, Sims also expressed great admiration for his anatomy professor, Granville Sharp Pattison. After teaching clinical medicine in London, Pattison was especially skilled as the teacher of surgical anatomy and morbid pathology, and thus contributed to Sims's later successes.[70]

During Sims's years at college he encountered influences from outside the realm of pathological anatomy and his regular medical education that were also central to his later career. Sims's acquaintances, teachers, and peers were part of the intellectual and social milieu in these early antebellum years. Their perspective and his relationship with them provides a framework for understanding the pivotal first fifteen years of his medical practice.

One of Sims's acquaintances, and likely a role model, was Josiah Nott, who was nine years his senior. During his college days as an undergraduate, Sims witnessed several duels, and in one of them Josiah C. Nott served as the attending physician—the same man who later gained attention as a founder of the American School.[71] At this time Nott was on his way to prominence as a Southern surgeon and physician practicing in Columbia. Nott's younger brother was in Sims's class at Columbia; Rufus Nott was one of Josiah Nott's four brothers, and all five of them became physicians. Unlike Sims's own family, the Nott family was wealthy and Josiah Nott's father encouraged his sons to pursue medical careers because he regretted he himself had not become a physician. As part of an aristocracy, the Nott family viewed the study of medicine as an elite career. By the time Sims knew him, Josiah Nott was the personal physician of Wade Hampton, the wealthiest plantation owner in South Carolina. Sims's undergraduate education opened his eyes to the possibilities medicine might offer. The rise of medical education in the 1830s thus offered opportunities to individuals regardless of class.[72]

This was the beginning of a long acquaintance, possibly a friendship, between Sims and Josiah Nott. While Nott's interests in ethnography and the issues of early anthropology were only incipient, he and Sims undoubtedly talked about the relationship of religion to science and medicine. The atmosphere at South Carolina College was supercharged with this topic. As the reader will recall, Nott became adamantly anti-Christian as he developed his argument for a polygenic origin of humans. Nott came to believe that the dogma of those who accepted Mosaic law stood in the way of comprehending what he saw as the true multiple origins of peoples.

Of a similar stripe, Thomas Cooper, the president of South Carolina College at Columbia when Sims studied there, created quite a stir as he advocated the pursuit of scientific practice from an anticlerical stance. In a time when religious belief was strong, Cooper used his lecture podium as a professor of geology to argue against the validity of Genesis.[73] Cooper was ousted from his presidency at the College in the early 1830s. Although Cooper's appointment at the college was evidence of the increasing academic and intellectual significance attached to the study of science, his ouster demonstrated the public's refusal openly to question Christianity. Sims personally agreed with this position as he looked back on these years. He remembered Cooper as "a greater infidel" than "Darwin and Tyndall and Huxley."[74] The question for some was whether science and religion were compatible or at war.

For Sims and for others there was a way to resolve the tension between science and religion, and this was a rational orthodoxy. Linked to the Scottish Common Sense School of Philosophy of the eighteenth century, this perspective argued that science was a way of knowing God through the powers of reason. Religion through science offered faith and an explanation of the world.[75] A key intellectual figure who articulated this theology was a peer of Sims as an undergraduate and came to figure as a prominent friend, relative, and religious inspiration. That person was James Henley Thornwell.

Thornwell, like Sims, spent his undergraduate years at South Carolina College somewhat uncertain about his career. Even then he was known to be an intellectual genius and exceptionally articulate. Physically he must have resembled Sims himself, since, like Sims, he was small in stature and weighed only one hundred pounds. Because of the power of his oratory, Sims felt sure he would become a lawyer and politician. In 1832, however, Thornwell converted to Presbyterianism and went to a seminary to study for the ministry. In fact, Thornwell started as a minister for the new Presbyterian Church in Lancaster, South Carolina, which had never before had a Presbyterian church.[76]

After finishing at Jefferson Medical School, Sims returned to Lancaster to set up a practice with the help, once again, of his preceptor, Churchill Jones. Jones was the brother of the Sims family's late creditor, Bartlett Jones. Jack Sims had been in debt to Bartlett—also a physician and surgeon—for many years. Jones, in fact, had helped Jack Sims to win the appointment as a commissioner in the village. The Jones family, like the Notts, provided for Sims the model of a wealthy family of physicians across generations. Jack Sims's son now not only sought a medical career like that of the Jones brothers, but also pined for the hand of Bartlett's daughter, Theresa.

In the early 1830s, a marriage between Marion and Theresa was only a remote possibility. They kept their relationship secret for many years to avoid the wrath of Theresa's wealthy mother, who heartily disapproved of Marion Sims as a potential son-in-law, probably because of his lower economic and social status. Sims's struggle to win Theresa Jones's hand was complicated by the tension between the culture of betrothal and marriage in which the fathers of both parties were the chief decision makers and the central determinant was economic status, not love or affection. These two were in love and wanted to marry, but complications arose for them as well as their parents.[77] Marion's letters to Theresa suggest that once the marriage had become a possibility, after he moved to the Deep South to set up a practice and to prepare for their lives together, he became impatient for her to stay in touch and to offer regular support for their relationship. "MY DEAR, DEAR THERESA: Why in the world don't you write to me?"[78] Apparently she got cold feet from time to time or was pressured by her mother to withdraw from the relationship.

Here Thornwell came to play a particularly important and somewhat traditional role as a minister arranging a marriage. The Joneses had become members in the new Presbyterian church. Sims went to Thornwell for help in winning Theresa's hand in marriage. At the same time, Thornwell sought the hand of Betsy Witherspoon, Theresa's close friend and a cousin through marriage. Thornwell became a go-between and urged Sims to become a member of his church, which, because of Sims's background and natural affinity for Presbyterianism, was relatively easy for him, and he became a profoundly religious man. Yet Sims agonized when Thornwell wed Betsy Witherspoon before his and Theresa's betrothal occurred. Finally, in 1836, they were wed, making Thornwell not only a friend and colleague but also a relative.

Thornwell later returned to South Carolina College, where he taught moral philosophy and became president of the college in 1840. In 1855 he wrote *Discourses on Truth*. In the latter half of the nineteenth century he became well known as a leading intellectual figure and theologian.

After his medical studies in Philadelphia and his apprenticeship in Lancaster, Sims had married his childhood sweetheart and was ready to embark on a career.

The Early Practice of J. Marion Sims

After coming of age in the antebellum Old South and receiving part of his medical education there, Sims was ready to hang his shingle and start to practice his craft. His sorry lack of clinical experience meant that he would have to test much of his technique on his patients as he encountered them. His interest was in surgery but he was identified as a general-practice physician. His background had acquainted him with anatomy, the theoretical aspects of medicine, and the system of slavery. He also had firsthand knowledge of life in Philadelphia as well as the hill country of South Carolina and exposure to antebellum politics as tensions mounted between the North and the South. Still on his own, Sims embarked on his journey with an entrepreneurial frame of mind, with the need first and foremost to make a living.

After a difficult first few months as a physician in Lancaster, Sims set off in the fall of 1835 for rural Alabama, where he became a plantation physician. There he grew more deeply involved with slavery. In Montgomery County, at Mt. Meigs, where Sims took up residence, slaves accounted for 50.8 percent of the total population in 1830. By 1840, there were 15,486 slaves in the county, representing 63 percent of the population.[79] Life in rural Alabama during the 1830s and 1840s focused on the growth of cotton on large plantations. The use of the cotton gin and the growing manufacture of textiles made cotton production pivotal in the American economy, and slaves provided the labor for a demanding crop.

In the 1830s Alabama was still largely a frontier, having just become a

state in 1819. Soon after his arrival in south-central Alabama in 1836, Sims
fought briefly in a war with the Creek Indians.[80] In a letter to Theresa he called
the Native Americans "ruthless savages" and "infuriated hot-blooded animals."[81] This was a period of high migration of diverse populations. In Alabama alone, European Americans came with hundreds of thousands of slaves,
and 70,000 Native Americans were driven out.[82] The social system surrounding Sims's early medical career promoted a clearly visible hierarchy of human worth according to race.

Sims's move to Alabama had a profound effect upon his health. Before December 1836, he was stricken with malaria. He was weakened by
the disease over and over again and was frequently brought to death's door.
Sims was not alone in his illness. He traveled to Lowndes County several
times with the idea of settling there, only to find that the entire population,
slaves and masters alike, were stricken with malaria. Those living in the Deep
South at the time repeatedly encountered malaria, cholera, and yellow fever
epidemics. The North endured illnesses as well, but the Southern marshlands
were especially conducive to malaria, with the attendant suffering and frequent death.[83]

Medical therapies for malaria were only purgatives in Sims's time. In
treating himself he resisted the practice of bleeding and seemed to recover
with doses of the popular drug quinine, extracted from cinchona bark in the
early nineteenth century. Southern medical practitioners especially used this
prescription, but the pharmaceutical worked only if taken over a long period
of time.[84] Sims's own physical vulnerability developed into a chronic dysentery, which eventually drove him out of the South.[85]

Sims's close escape from death surely influenced his religion and medicine. Not long before they were to be married, he wrote Theresa in South
Carolina:

> When the body is emaciated, worn down by disease, and covered with
> a cold, clammy perspiration, with a mind correspondingly prostrated;
> then is the time that death appears in all its terrors to the mind of
> him who feels conscious that his course of life has not been in con-
> sistence with all the just principles of moral and religious rectitude.[86]

While he was doctored back to health, he also continued to serve as a physician to heal others.[87] To some degree, Sims's doctoring was an expression of
his religious beliefs. He wrote to Theresa, "I have the glorious consolation
of knowing (to a certainty) that, by a very simple operation, I have saved
one man's life who was left by older physicians to die."[88] He was also

competitive. While the culture of the plantation South strongly influenced Sims's life, he was also motivated by urban life, entrepreneurship, and the capitalistic economy. His education in the North and experience in cities were central factors in his life.

Even as Sims saw epidemics around him, his expertise in medicine addressed different pathologies. Often they were life threatening, but rarely did he deal with malaria, cholera, yellow fever, or dysentery. As he developed his skills as a surgeon, he turned to the treatment of eyes, jaws, and feet. His specialties came to include remedies for crossed eyes, harelips, and club feet, as well as tumors on the jaw.

In 1841, after several years of practicing as a rural plantation doctor and after each member of his family had endured a severe bout of malaria, Sims moved to Montgomery with his wife and children. In 1846 it became the capital of Alabama and was second only to Mobile as a trade center and cotton market for farmers. Both the railroad and the steamboat provided transportation in and out of the city.[89] It was here where Sims gained his expertise in clinical practice.

Sims prospered in Montgomery, and his family grew. He became the half-owner of a drugstore. Dr. Baldwin, a colleague in Montgomery, later recalled another of Sims's acquisitions, a four-wheeled cart and pony:

> [Sims's] buggy was indeed a queer and notable looking little land craft and by the way was the first fourwheeled vehicle ever used in Montgomery for the purpose of practicing medicine. . . . Thus seated in his buggy, with his little negro boy by his side, and panoplied with a medicine box and case of surgical instruments at his feet.[90]

Sims etched a memorable image for Baldwin. The possession of a buggy and slave indicated that Sims made a healthy living during many of his more than ten years in Montgomery.

Once he was settled in the city, Sims intensified his medical practice. At first his clientele were free blacks, but, as he later recalled, medical success soon attracted the most wealthy citizens, including the Jewish population.[91] He also began to operate in the presence of several doctors; his confidence in his surgical ability clearly grew. The move to Montgomery did not end his practice on plantations or on slave patients, however. He broadened the types of surgery he performed and brought in slave patients from plantations of the surrounding counties. Throughout his years of practice in antebellum Montgomery, slaves comprised a significant proportion of Sims's practice.

Anxious to establish his professional reputation, Sims quickly began writing up and publishing his cases. His first article described surgery for a woman with a harelip. In his publication Sims described her as a single white woman who was so disfigured that she always wore a veil. In 1844 Sims teamed up with a dentist to repair the worst of her defects. She was able for the first time to drink with some ease. Whether she gave up the veil after the corrective surgeries is not known. The procedure was published in the *Journal of Dental Surgery* in 1845.[92]

In his publications, Sims also described operations on the jaws of three male slaves. These are his only publications where he freely identifies the patients as slaves. All suffered from tumors, which Sims described as cancer. The youngest of the three, age nineteen, endured extreme surgical intervention and pain; he died after two operations. In his case, the techniques had been insufferable by today's standards. The technique involved removal of bone and extensive cutting of the jaw, for which Sims cited the influence of the French clinical surgeon Velpeau. In describing the surgery, Sims stressed the errors he made: a sponge left in the patient's mouth that nearly suffocated him, and a failure to stop the bleeding from the carotid artery. The wording suggests that he found the error and its effect to be of greater importance to readers of *The Journal of the American Medical Sciences* than the youth's actual death. With these reports on his jaw patients, Marion Sims found his voice on the printed page.[93]

Another group of patients was prominent in Sims's early practice: infants. In fact, his first two cases had been babies in Lancaster, South Carolina, before he moved to Alabama. In *The Story of My Life*, Sims recalled them in detail, including his inability to diagnose their sickness and the haphazard method of prescribing medication. However, his melodramatic tone in the entire volume may be a sign that he was prone to exaggeration and may have bent the facts to tell his tale more effectively.

Sims's pride and confidence in the correctness and innovation of his medical therapies now led him to mock his earlier medical practice. The stark contrast between the early failures and the later successes bolstered his perceptions on the significance of his innovations in surgery.

Nonetheless, the bare bones of Sims's recollections reveal a fairly accurate picture of the quality of medical practice in the antebellum South. For instance, before he took on plantation medicine and the treatment of slaves or free blacks, the history of his first two patients had been instructive. He handled the two young patients on his own in Lancaster after Churchill Jones had left the area. His first case was the eighteen-month-old son of the former mayor of Lancaster.

When I arrived I found a child about eighteen months old, very much emaciated, who had what we would call the summer complaint, or chronic diarrhoea. I examined the child minutely from head to foot. I looked at its gums, and as I always carried a lancet with me and had surgical propensities, as soon as I saw some swelling of the gums I at once took out my lancet and cut the gums down to the teeth. This was good so far as it went. But, when it came time to making up a prescription, I had no more idea of what ailed the child, or what to do for it, than if I had never studied medicine.[94]

To arrive at a possible prescription for the sick infant, Sims returned to his office and studied his medical text on childhood diseases, including prescriptions, by John Eberle. During Sims's tenure at Jefferson Medical School, John Eberle had been a professor there. He was remembered for his eclectic approach to medicine, drawing from various schools of contemporary thought (from François Broussais, for instance, who relied heavily on the use of leeches and bleeding) and structuring his text around the description of fever in various forms.[95] Eberle's texts comprised Sims's entire library, so he tried each prescription (a variety of compounds, according to his recollections), one by one. Unfortunately for both the patient and the practitioner, the symptoms persisted, and after a few days, the infant died.

Contrary to our understanding today, "teething" was considered a disease at this time.[96] Sims responded to the condition with a therapy that only worsened it. Such was the nature of Sims's clinical experience as he began to *practice* medicine. Young children, slaves, and women were often his patients in these early years.

Sims's second case, another infant with similar symptoms, received the same treatment, with the identical result. So-called summer complaint was a common cause of infant death in the nineteenth century, a period when the rate of both infant and child mortality was high. Children and babies were unable to survive extensive bouts of diarrhea, and at that time medical treatment did not include rehydration and the introduction of potassium.

After he gained his practical experience in the 1830s and 1840s in Alabama, Sims treated what he called "trismus nascentium"—similar to neonatal tetanus in present-day medicine and another example of what he encountered in infants.[97] He treated the condition mostly in slave babies, but not exclusively. These babies, often newborns, were usually stricken suddenly by the disease. They would cease sucking, begin to starve, and simultaneously suffer with seizures and fever. Sims explained the poor economic status as the underlying environmental cause of lockjaw:

> Wherever there are poverty, and filth, and laziness, or wherever the intellectual capacity is cramped, the moral and social feelings blunted, there it will be oftener found. Wealth, a cultivated intellect, a refined mind, an affectionate heart, are comparatively exempt from the ravages of this unmercifully fatal malady. But expose this class to the same *physical* causes, and they become equal sufferers with the first.[98] [Sims's emphasis]

To some degree, Sims perceived the same situation that many historians of slavery have noted—that a remarkably high proportion of slave infants died soon after birth.[99] Indeed, Sims practiced medicine in Alabama during a period of peak infant mortality among slaves.[100] Sims's argument went much further, though, and implied that the high rate of infant mortality was the result of moral weakness among blacks—their "filth," their "laziness," their "cramped intellectual capacity" and "blunted moral and social feelings," rather than to the system of slavery itself. He did mention poverty as an incriminating causal factor, but presumably the "filth" and "laziness" of blacks are what kept them poverty stricken. He never suggested a need to improve upon living conditions in order to treat the disease.

Today this illness is known as neonatal tetanus. Practices following birth in those years, particularly the wrapping of the vestigial umbilical cord on the newborn with unclean cloth, caused infection and ultimately death. Thus the mortality can be linked to midwife practices. Because tetanus originates in horse manure, it is possible that the proximity of horse stables to slave quarters was a direct cause of the high rate of tetanus and trismus nascentium among slave newborns.[101] In his first of three articles on the condition, Sims distinguished trismus nascentium from tetanus, making it more inclusive and sometimes including infantile paralysis under the designation.

The occurrence of infant death from trismus nascentium was not confined to slaves, or to conditions of poverty, however. In his articles Sims described different therapies and an occasional recovery. Recovery seems impossible in the context of the present-day definition of the disease, which is always fatal unless the victim has been inoculated. For instance, Sims described an instance of trismus nascentium in one of his own children, and cases among other whites as well.[102] He reported that happily his child recovered following the use of his devised technique, which consisted of laying

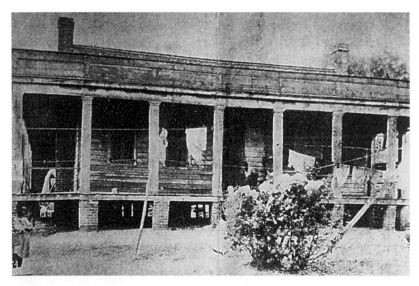

FIGURE 1. Home of Sims's first patients in Montgomery, Alabama. Taken by Edward Souchon, 1895. *(Courtesy of the Reynolds Historical Library, University of Alabama at Birmingham.)*

a child on its side, not on the back, in a cradle. Having made this discovery, Sims doubted the importance of treating the umbilicus of the newborn. Instead, he urged laying the child on its side as a way of relieving pressure on the back of the head, arguing that the parietal bones would wedge into the occiput and place direct pressure on the brain itself. Sims blamed nurses and mothers especially for holding their children in the crooks of their arms— perhaps during the night, perhaps while nursing. Cradles, too, were a bane. He found them to be narrow and hard, often lined with rags in slave quarters, permitting infants to sleep only on their backs.[103] He discovered his relatively simple and noninterventionist solution of placing the ailing child in a special position while he was examining a patient.

Unfortunately, many of Sims's patients died. Because some of them recovered following his remedy, he was inspired to publish his medical therapy as an innovation. In his first publication, dated 1846, he attributed the condition in part to an accident of childbirth. He argued that movement of the skull bones during a protracted birth contributed to the condition of trismus. In his follow-up article, dated 1848, he corrected his original essay by noting that flexibility of skull bones is normal in an infant undergoing birth, which is now understood to be true. Sims also gradually abandoned arguments that the spinal column of affected infants hemorrhaged during the disease.[104] Experience with treating patients definitely influenced the doctor's way of thinking about sickness and his understanding of the origins of diseases.

Finally, Sims turned to the baby's refusal to suck as the critical sign that it suffered from trismus and as a way to define the condition. This symptomology is more in concurrence with the condition of tetanus known today: "So well understood is this amongst the negroes, who have lost children with this disease, that they recognize it at once; they look for this *difficulty of sucking* with the greatest solicitude, and when it occurs, they give up the child as irretrievably lost" (Sims's emphasis).[105]

Even though this quoted passage shows some empathy for those who lost infants to the disease, Sims had exceptional freedom to experiment with the condition because the victims were slaves. This also gave him access to the bodies of those who died, to use for autopsies. With these tiny patients, Sims took an increasingly mechanical view of their condition, adding a surgical maneuver to the lateral side position for the sleeping baby. Taking responsibility and custody of a suffering slave infant overnight, Sims experimented with a crooked awl, prying the occiput and parietal bones into proper alignment. Here he demonstrated the *craft* that surgery once was. The success he met in treatment of this particular infant led him to recommend the therapy in extreme cases. In these instances he prescribed that it be repeated occasionally over several months, and predicted a happy outcome. In the treatment of his own patient, he found

> these contractions [from the disease] all gradually gave way, but were something like two months in doing so. During this time, I would occasionally puncture the scalp over the lambdoidal suture, with the point of a crooked awl, and prize [*sic*] out the edges of the parietal bones, and always, with the effect of greatly modifying the rigid flexures of the extremities. The operation, being simple and safe, was frequently performed, without the loss of a drop of blood, and invariably with the direct . . . effect above desired.[106]

Sims's published treatment of trismus nascentium met skepticism in some quarters, and appreciation in others.

Fatal diseases suffered by nineteenth-century infants, including slave children, must remain a mystery to some degree. Any analysis of the condition treated by J. Marion Sims contains an element of speculation: without knowing what the sickness really was, there is no way of evaluating the quality of Sims's therapy. If, in fact, the infants suffered from tetanus as it is defined today, Sims exhibited great skill as a surgeon in saving some of the victims. His success was inconsistent, however, and his diagnosis undoubtedly included more than modern symptoms of tetanus, leaving many questions unanswered about the health of Southern infants in the nineteenth century.

Sims failed to describe the condition of the patient except during the period immediately after he attended the patient. In the published cases of trismus nascentium, he clearly designated patients and families by class and race. The experimental surgery with a shoemaker's awl was practiced on slave infants only, according to these articles. In treating these same patients, he frequently described an autopsy done immediately after death. Sims blamed slave mothers and nurses for infant suffering, especially through their "ignorance." When describing infants who were under the charge of a plantation mistress or her own offspring, Sims would also criticize her way of caring for the infants, which included laying them improperly into their cradles.

In the mid-1840s, Sims was maturing as a surgeon and had become bold and innovative like his teacher, George McClellan. He was committed now to building on his already growing reputation as a physician. He used his dexterity to experiment with new operations and then sought immediate recognition for his efforts. The fact that he had published in the *American Journal of the Medical Sciences* suggests his interest in having a nationally recognized rather than a locally known career.

Sims also had come to rely heavily on the political economy of slavery to further his medical career. Repeating a pattern of innovative and experimental surgery practiced on well-defined populations, as exemplified by his first published cases, Sims began to treat women patients for a condition linked to childbirth. In December 1850, the federal census attributed seventeen slaves to J. Marion Sims—twelve females and five males. Eight were under the age of twelve.[107] In Montgomery, Sims had established a clinic where some of these slaves resided, both as patients and as assistants to Sims in his work. It was here that the original surgery occurred that would figure large in the origins of gynecology.

CHAPTER 2

Anarcha, Betsey, and Lucy

One of the most striking aspects of the story of the origins of gynecology in the nineteenth century is its connection with a female disorder called "vesico-vaginal fistula." How and why the focus on these rends that occur at childbirth became so important illuminates the once unfamiliar history of women and medicine.

Considered a medical condition in the nineteenth century, vesico-vaginal fistula consists of internal tears in the vaginal wall leading to urinary and sometimes also fecal incontinence. There was no known remedy for the condition, nor was its etiology understood other than in its immediate origins in childbirth. Often, during prolonged labor in the second stage as the cervix dilated, the infant's head would press upon the bony pelvic floor for many hours and sometimes days on end, cutting off all circulation to the soft vaginal tissues that cover the area, thereby eventually robbing them of necessary oxygen. A few days after delivery of the infant finally occurred, the affected and sometimes gangrenous tissue sloughed away and tears appeared in the septum separating the vagina from the bladder. These tears (vesico-vaginal fistulas) found any number of locations along this wall of tissue. Afflicted women suffered with a continual dribble of urine into the vagina. Sometimes tears extended to the rectum to create further damage, known as recto-vaginal fistula.

Despite the fact that, for hundreds of years, the symptoms of vesico-vaginal fistula appeared as a female disorder in medical texts, only in the mid-nineteenth century did medicine name the affliction.[1] Vesico-vaginal fistula meant something unique at this time. Although parturient women throughout much of history faced the possibility of incurring vaginal tears from childbirth and subsequent incontinence, and many still do today, when medicine became clinical and began to concentrate on female diseases vesico-vaginal fistulas became a focus. This preoccupation indicated that there was a higher incidence of the condition than occurs today, at least in many parts of the world. While today in the Southern Hemisphere there is a presence of fistulas similar to those treated in the nineteenth century, physicians in the northern hemisphere are familiar with vesico-vaginal fistulas more commonly as iatrogenic and a result of surgery for disorders and diseases of the bladder. Only rarely did vesico-vaginal fistulas like these occur in the mid-nineteenth century. For instance, at that time, a pessary (a device worn in the vagina to support the uterus) too long in place sometimes destroyed vaginal tissue with the same result. Then physicians often resorted to using pessaries and sponges for various female complaints. Sometimes women even used the products for contraception.[2] The nineteenth-century perception of vesico-vaginal fistulas also arose from a cultural context and from definitions of masculinity and femininity, situated in a class structure.

Dr. Johann Dieffenbach, a nineteenth-century surgeon from Heidelberg who was often quoted on the subject, described the condition this way: "There is not a more pitiable condition than that of a woman suffering from vesico-vaginal fistula. The urine constantly flowing into the vagina, and partially retained there, and heated, runs down the labia, perineum, and over the nates and thighs, producing a most intolerable stench. . . . The husband has an aversion for his own wife; a tender mother is exiled from the circle of her own children."[3] Such incontinence represented misery, but it could not have been the worst possible illness. During this time, for instance, many women *died* of puerperal fever following childbirth. Men, women, and children succumbed to various epidemic diseases, as we saw in the last chapter. There was an extraordinarily high rate of infant and child mortality.

In Dieffenbach's image, we gain a sense of the influence of middle-class culture on the definition of the condition. His words showed the centrality of the privatized nuclear family with the circle of children, a husband and "his own" wife, as the leitmotif. However, women across all lines of race and class suffered from vesico-vaginal fistula, some without the ability or perhaps desire to marry legally—as slaves, for instance—and others for various reasons without the comfort of children and a hearth as the center of their lives. Mid-nineteenth century culture revered motherhood; physicians who treated vesico-vaginal fistula became protectors of it.

For middle- and upper-class Europeans and European-Americans of this era, notions of femininity and masculinity led to defining woman as "the sex," with her identity deriving from her uterus. In the eighteenth and early nineteenth centuries, the scientific and anatomical definition of the uterus changed from being merely an inverted penis, to being different from male anatomy. Women became "other."[4] By the middle of the nineteenth century, these ideas meshed with definitions of women that were primarily constructed through motherhood. Thus gender moved toward an idea, perhaps an ideology, of a complementarity that excluded the possibility of equality between men and women.

Vesico-vaginal fistulas joined with childbearing to create an image of "suffering womanhood." As a specifically defined condition, "vesico-vaginal fistula" gained meaning through the relations between male physicians and their women patients.[5] These broad strokes create an image of a universal femininity, but in actuality the historical experience varied. A patient's treatment, for instance, was based on his or her social status determined by perceived differences based on cultural perceptions of race, class, and/or ethnicity.[6] Because vesico-vaginal fistulas were a relatively minor condition, medical practitioners experimented with different therapies. Patients considered to be of lower social status became likely targets of these practices.

By medical standards, vesico-vaginal fistulas were a physiological disorder demanding intervention by a surgeon. At the same time, medical recognition of vesico-vaginal fistula as a significant disorder directed the attention of physicians to childbirth as the seat of its pathology. Before the nineteenth century, childbirth was not considered a sickness; for the most part, physicians did not attend an uncomplicated birth until the late eighteenth century and then only under certain circumstances, provided the woman in labor or the midwife invited him. Now physicians were competing with midwives to supervise childbirth. Such attendance was useful in building a professional reputation, and unlike the physicians' inability to explain or stop the childbed fever that ravaged hospital wards and spiked maternal mortality rates, they could treat vesico-vaginal fistula without the threat of a tarnished reputation from a lost life.

To learn the significance of vesico-vaginal fistula as a female disorder (which was also fundamental to the professionalization of gynecology) requires understanding how the condition affected the lives of women. Why did women suffer from debilitating aftereffects of childbirth? What was the birth experience and what factors in the environment contributed to the creation of fistulas? As we encounter different groups of patients and women who were involved in institutionalizing medical therapies for vesico-vaginal fistulas, we will find different answers rooted in the diversity of those who suffered. We must start, however, with the historical experience of childbirth.

Childbirth involves a ritual and cultural heritage as well as variations

in pain, the history of bodies, and the possible inclusion of medical intervention.[7] In the United States today, where we live in a technocracy in which
birth is almost universally governed by fetal and neonatal technology during
labor as well as before and after childbirth, we may have difficulty understanding how different the life cycle was in the nineteenth century, when the
culture of childbirth was diverse and some women had to choose between
midwives and doctors.[8] In the modern Western world, there are variations in
childbirth, and there is limited variation within the United States itself. In
the nineteenth century, the high number of first-generation immigrants in the
United States and the variation in lifestyle on the frontier and on the Eastern
seaboard meant there were differences in the rite of childbirth as well. Furthermore, medicine itself was sharply divided in its practice, with some patients relying only on what they had at hand, to others receiving ether from
doctors by 1847 and then chloroform as anesthesia in childbirth. On the frontier, for instance, there were very few physicians so patients had no other
choice besides finding someone to assist them. In fact, most of the information on what happened during birth is not in the historical record. Only by
gathering pieces of what was once a whole picture can images be recovered.
For this we rely on medical records, texts, periodicals, statistics, journals, letters, and stories told across generations.

While physicians in the United States had begun to come to the urban
homes of upper-class women by the end of the eighteenth century, there was
still a cacophony of discord for decades concerning who should be in charge
or who should attend childbirth. Midwives had had a tradition of assisting
for hundreds of years and brought with them spiritual guidance, experience,
and knowledge handed down orally across generations. These became rituals and frameworks for the birthing mother. The therapies were often botani-
cal, from teas and infusions to ergot, and included recommending certain
positions for birth and using tools such as a birthing stool.

In the eighteenth century, William Hunter made enormous contributions
to the creation of a "new obstetrics," a science of childbirth premised on
Hunter's precise portrayal of the gravid uterus in the process of human gestation. This knowledge aided William Smellie's retooling of the forceps. Eventually the practice of obstetrics excluded women who were not asked about
knowledge they gained from their practice as midwives.

While the tension over who may supervise births was long lasting and
though the process took more than one hundred years to evolve into the
modern-day hospital birth, midwives continued to practice. In the unlikely
but possible case of a woman's labor that stopped or incurred problems, mid-

wives had no instrumental or surgical alternatives and went to physicians for help. At this time, Caesarian sections were not an alternative for a difficult birth. Although Caesarian sections had been around for centuries, both mythologically and in actual practice, cutting open a living woman to deliver a child directly out of the uterus and through the abdomen did not really become possible until the 1870s, and then the method was rarely used.[9] It is possible that during medieval times midwives and women surgeons as well as male surgeons performed what we know as C-sections. These procedures were largely performed on dead women, however. Until medical practitioners began to use antiseptic measures and anesthesia during surgery around the late nineteenth century, cutting open the abdominal cavity was virtually certain to result in infection and death. Midwives were often forced into some kind of surgery or intervention and had ways successfully to deliver a breech birth or twins. After forceps became available in the late 1700s, childbirth became easier. Even though it took decades for physicians to acquire the experience to use them, forceps provided physicians with a new authority at childbirth.

Throughout the nineteenth century, debates took place about whether midwives should be admitted to medical schools to study obstetrics so they could continue their tradition of attendance at birth, or whether male physicians should be the attendants.[10] Even after physicians had established themselves in childbirth, it was well into the twentieth century before experience and clinical education became part of obstetrical training for medical students. Although the issue of midwives versus doctors persisted, the conflict was couched always in terms of either one or the other. Medicine now challenged the centuries-old practice of midwifery and female-governed childbirth.

People often think that before the days of hospitalized birth, there was a high rate of death in childbirth. Indeed, more women died in childbirth then than now among the affluent, and among most of those in industrialized countries. However, there is no evidence linking the historical practice of midwifery with a high incidence of maternal mortality. Martha Ballard, a midwife in Maine at the turn of the century, and Patty Sessions, a Mormon midwife on the trail and in Utah, each lost very few women to death out of the thousands they attended.[11] Trying to determine exactly what the maternal mortality rate was across the population of the United States throughout the nineteenth century is virtually impossible. Records are far too unreliable to derive such a data set. There are many regional variations, and changes by decade and season. Other factors such as the presence of epidemics and other diseases also make such a determination difficult. Even birth records do not always tell the full story until well into the nineteenth century.[12]

Reading women's words makes it clear, however, that at the heart of the childbirth ritual during this time was the pregnant woman's knowledge of the possibility of death during childbirth. Sometimes there was more fear of death than actual death. Nonetheless, knowing that physicians carried instruments that might prevent the death of a woman and her child in birth seemed to motivate change, causing some women to call for medical help.

One region that did suffer a high maternal mortality rate was the South. Evidence suggests that the higher birthrate among white women influenced the rate of death. In the census of 1850, white women giving birth in the South died at a rate double that of women in New England and in the Mid-Atlantic states.[13] Southern women began to have smaller numbers of children after midcentury, following the Demographic Transition, following the trend of middle-class families in the northern states.[14]

There are no statistics on slave-women mortality during childbirth. We do know that the slave population in the nineteenth century had a high fertility rate. One rough estimate puts the rate of birth among these women at more than fifty per thousand. This would mean that 20 percent of those between the ages of fifteen and forty-four were pregnant every year.[15] In the Deep South, including Alabama, the birthrate was somewhat lower. Certainly the situation—heavy labor and emphasis on cotton production, and particularly the unhealthy environment—must have contributed to the difference. The high fertility rate may well be an underestimation given the incomplete records and the frequent failure to document infant and maternal deaths.

Midwives practiced on plantations and throughout the South, because the ratio of physicians to patients was too low for physicians to supervise all births. African American midwives were undoubtedly numerous, especially in areas with large slave populations. There is a strong likelihood that they delivered babies throughout the population, for whites as well as slaves, and they probably also worked in urban areas and among the free blacks there. Southern physicians therefore did not spend a great deal of time in obstetrical care.

The African tradition of midwifery and the practice of granny midwives—as the African American practitioners came to be known—has been passed down orally. Spiritual rituals, the use of herbs, and other long-standing traditions are similar to the practice of midwifery among the eighteenth-century European American colonists. Scholars have recently recognized that African American midwifery is a distinct tradition with a very different periodicity from that of many other midwives in the American past, and they are seeking to record some of its key elements,[16] though unfortunately the practice has nearly died out. While many tribes with different languages and cultures were brought into slavery in the United States, some common core aspects of midwifery typified the practice, often because of the blending of cultures into one. African American midwives interviewed in the twentieth century, for instance, generally feel they were chosen by God to practice their craft, what one midwife, Onnie Logan, called "mother-wit." While European history reveals the persecution of midwives, particularly in witch hunts, African history shows a greater reverence for midwives as healers. They were given high social status and authority in the community because of their expertise. In the slave community there was often a hierarchy that honored midwives and resembled a matrilineal West African cultural heritage.[17] Just as Southern physicians were at the core of their social web, practicing medicine among many different segments of society, so too did midwives, attending both their mistresses and field hands.[18]

Because Alabama's economy rested squarely on cotton in the 1830s and 1840s, there were many large plantations. The ratio of blacks to whites was very high—sometimes an advantage for slaves. There must have been many black midwives because granny midwives held a prominent place in childbirth in the "black belt" until the early 1970s. In the early decades of the 1900s in areas such as Alabama, 90 percent of births of African Americans were attended by midwives, mostly of African American origin.[19] The Tuskegee Institute in Macon County, where Marion Sims first practiced and where his network of plantation patients rested, established one of the two schools for midwives in the 1940s.

Although many details of the cultural and historical practices of childbirth are lost, comparing the ritual of birth with the medical practice of the times demonstrates how healing, spiritual and religious values, and medical practice were profoundly woven into day-to-day life. We can consider the lives of slave women who left no written record and only imagine what their lives were like, what their expectations and choices were.

Slavery itself has ended, but the patterns and traditions established under more than two hundred years of slavery continue to jeopardize the lives of black Americans. It is the African American women who carry the burden to this day.[20] Under slavery, women were pivotal in its very definition. Slavery was perpetuated through the status of the mother: if she was a slave, not only was she in slavery for her life, but so were her children. Harriet Jacobs, a woman who escaped slavery in the late 1850s, wrote powerfully about her life and her feelings as a mother and as one who lived in slavery: "When they told me my newborn babe was a girl, my heart was heavier than it had ever been before. Slavery is terrible for men; but it is far more terrible for women. Superadded to the burden common to all, *they* have wrongs, and sufferings, and mortifications peculiarly their own."[21] For Harriet Jacobs, the birth of a daughter meant even more suffering and the perpetuation of slavery, conditions she already knew too well.

As slavery changed, so did the slaves' roles. By the early nineteenth century, slave women were clearly recognized as so-called breeders. Their ability to reproduce became central to their worth as property to the master. Given that experiences varied widely by time, by region, by size of plantation, by personalities and a host of factors, it is safe to say that the culture and political economy of slavery imposed a role on them defined by their ability to reproduce. The implications for health were deleterious and related to the effects of multiple pregnancies, repeated at frequent intervals and under conditions that did not offer nurturance or support for the physical demands of the condition. Little allowance for pregnancy was made in terms of an enhanced diet or a lower work load. Any benefits given the pregnant woman came only in her last trimester. For some, whippings also continued well into pregnancy.[22]

In addition to the master's emphasis on reproduction, he would also make frequent sexual demands of his own on slave women. Such sexual exchange figured into the rate of reproduction, with the slave woman's status determining once again the status of the child. Not only did a slave make more slaves, she was often the object of aggressive sexual demands from those with power over her. On the one hand, there was her cultural heritage that measured the happiness and success of a woman by her fertility; on the other hand there was a political and economic system which abused the woman's ability to reproduce, which punished her offspring for their connection with her, and which often violated her intimacy that sometimes led to reproduction.

It is important to recognize that the slave community was able to withstand the violence and degradation of slavery through support among themselves. The midwife had a central role in a situation where pregnancy and childbirth were so common. The heritage of West African culture added to the women's centrality a tradition that placed high value on their fertility and reproductivity. While the midwives were held in high regard within the slave community, those outside, either slave masters or physicians and others in various positions of power, did not grant them the same respect.

Despite the pressures of the powerful masters, slaves did show resistance, often through infanticide, abortion, or refusal to get pregnant.[23] To provide herbal medicines that served as abortifacients as well as in childbirth, midwives worked out of a local knowledge of plants and the environment. In the first years of settlement, acclimation to the region was necessary before healers could practice.

Those who failed to see the burdens of slavery on slave women and the ill-effects of the harsh environment blamed the African American midwife for both the high mortality among the infants and the difficulties among parturient women. Thomas Affleck declared that among the slave infants, "a vast proportion die under nine or ten days, from the most unskillful management of negro midwives."[24] Dr. Marsh of Louisiana reported:

> It is a very common thing, very surprising to a professional man of experience at the north, to meet with cases so frequently of procidentia [prolapse] of the most aggravated character and long standing on most of our southern plantations. The reason for this, is the ignorance and obtrusive interference of our plantation accoucheurs and nigger midwives. . . . At the south almost every plantation has its midwife for laborers, who does not know any more of anatomy and obstetrics than of *law* and *theology*—and when they get a case instead of assisting nature, they try to usurp her place by positive violence; and the consequence is, that then the child is *hauled* forth, the most irremediable prolapsus is the consequence. (Emphasis is Marsh's)[25]

The unfortunate N-word appears in many sources such as these, used just as freely and prejudiciously by J. Marion Sims as by others. Despite the emphasis and hue in his words, Marsh remarkably joined the practice of the midwives to "plantation accoucheurs," who were in fact physicians who attended births and were probably much more likely to interfere in them.[26] On the other hand, midwives may have contributed to the incidence of neonatal tetanus by unwittingly continuing traditional treatments of the umbilicus in an environment that carried diseases they had never known.[27]

Surprisingly, Southern physicians sometimes expressed a preference for female supervision of childbirth, albeit a more educated version of what was being practiced. For example, Dr. R. H. Day of Pattersonville, Louisiana, argued: "If such cases must be put in the charge of women—to which I yield in hearty assent—let public opinion and the laws of our State require of all such a proper study and due qualification for their important responsible avocation."[28]

Without a doubt, slave women occasionally suffered great hardships during childbirth. The surprising use of Caesarians on slave women in the antebellum South is but one further example of the historical occurrence of prolonged labor, the desperation for treatment, and the willingness of physicians to experiment surgically on slave women before the introduction of anesthesia. The potential for death accompanying abdominal surgery such as a Caesarian operation was inordinately high—in fact, almost certain.

Nonetheless, fifteen successful cases of Caesarian sections were reported in Louisiana alone.[29] There were others in Virginia.[30] Otherwise, Caesarian sections were virtually unknown and scarcely practiced until the twentieth century. A French-trained surgeon, François Prevost (1771–1842), introduced the operation in Louisiana. He had fled Haiti following the successful slave insurrection led by Toussaint l'Ouverture in the early nineteenth century. In Louisiana, he proceeded to operate only on slave women, during a period from 1820 to 1825. In the following quote, medical historian John Duffy described the situation governing the use of Caesarian sections before the Civil War, which revealed the nexus of race and gender in antebellum Southern medicine:

> The fear of abdominal incisions was so great that it was generally considered much safer to destroy the child than sacrifice the life of the mother. The high risk involved in any abdominal surgery makes it more than a coincidence that so many early patients were slaves, and clearly indicates that southern surgeons and physicians were far more willing to try new procedures upon slaves than upon other women.[31]

Part of the historical experience of slave women in pregnancy and birth derived from their own physical well-being and the choices dictated by the reality of their health.[32] On the one hand, there was a rite of passage and a heritage of the practice of midwifery; on the other hand, there was the incidence of difficult delivery and potential ill-health of the infant, not to mention the infant's future as a slave. Adding to key factors shaping the lives of those in bondage was the absolute authority over them held by the slave master.[33]

Reasons for prolonged labor among black women were probably closely related to nutritional deficiencies in the typical slave diet. Lactose intolerance likely combined with deficiencies in their diet to cause serious problems.[34] For some people, including a relatively high percentage of African Americans, dairy products not only fail to yield calcium in digestion, but also cause sickness. Although scientific knowledge of enzymes, vitamins, and metabolism defines the condition of lactose intolerance today, no one recognized the central role of nutrition in quite this way in the nineteenth century.[35] The resultant calcium deficiency during childhood and adolescence often resulted in rickets. Even when slave owners did all they could to protect the health of their slaves, they could not address these special needs.

Although the condition was neither fatal nor completely debilitating, among other things, rickets did cause deformities of the pelvis, known then as a contracted pelvis. For some slave women, a contracted or misshapen pelvis no doubt contributed to a prolonged delivery. Lingering labor in turn led directly to the appearance of fistulas. Because rickets is not a fatal disease, there is little quantitative evidence for the extent of its historical presence. Many agree, however, that rickets was a fairly common condition in the nineteenth century and that it had a disproportionate presence among slaves.

Vesico-vaginal fistulas were among the minor or non-life-threatening effects of slavery that were rarely recorded. Although the damage caused by vesico-vaginal fistulas was not life-threatening, many women suffered prolonged labor because of them and this compromised their health. In these instances, midwives often called physicians for help. Ailments from poor diet to respiratory disease and injuries of reproductive organs plagued many women as well. The latter included prolapsed uteri and difficult childbirth. One scholar noted that "uterine troubles were of common occurrence among slave women."[36] The presence of vesico-vaginal fistulas among slave women was a clue to their health and the quality of their birthing experiences.

The Montgomery Experiments

In 1961, an illustrated history of medicine included a portrait of three slave women with J. Marion Sims and two apprenticed medical students in a roughly hewn building. This picture gives one version of a pivotal and freighted story in the history of gynecology—four years of repeated surgical experimentation on a core group of women patients who stayed for the duration of the surgeries. With the background of a draped white curtain and a table covered by a white sheet (much more indicative of contemporary medicine than nineteenth-century Montgomery, Alabama), here is a sanitized examination or operating room with a supplicant and timid woman, Lucy, listening to the doctor, J. Marion Sims, explain the procedure. She and the two others, Anarcha and Betsey, who peer around the curtain, are barefoot— the only evidence in the picture suggesting they might want for anything. Being barefoot as portrayed does not include an image of the wear and tear on feet caused by being shoeless. Lucy is on her knees in preparation for an

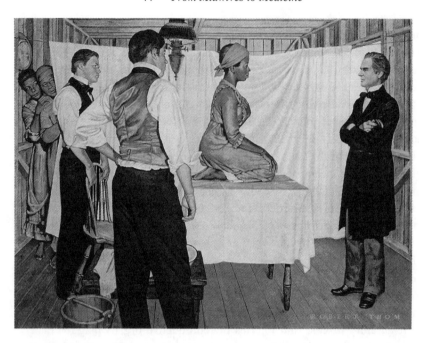

FIGURE 2. J. Marion Sims with Anarcha, Betsey, and Lucy and two physician part-
ners (illustration by Robert Thom), "J. Marion Sims: Gynecologic Surgeon." In George
A. Bender with Artist Robert A. Thom, *History of Medicine in Pictures* (Parke Davis,
1961). (*Permission for reproduction from Warner Lambert. Courtesy Southern Illinois University School of Medicine, Pearson Museum.*)

examination of her vagina that will require her to have a hands and knees
position. As an artistic rendering, Lucy is fully clothed, watching the doctor
with his instrument in hand—in fact a roughly fashioned speculum. Betsey
and Anarcha seem to share Lucy's childlike accommodation and mild curiosity in the events at hand. What the real nature of the relationship is among
the individuals portrayed can only be derived from imagination and from consideration of the setting. Certainly the picture portrays the authority the physician came to have and in fact reveals the underlying message of the medical
history, that the progress of medicine by the mid-twentieth century, when the
picture was made, represented a gift to women. There is also no visual rendering of the ailment the women suffered, not to mention the several years
of experimental surgery that followed Lucy's initial examination. While the
picture certainly reveals a great deal about how the artist and the medical
world of the early 1960s remembered Sims surgeries, the painting is also use-

ful because it helps to remind us of the past presence of these women as patients and of the need to try to reconstruct who they were and what happened to them. What the picture demonstrates is that the social historical context in which race relations find definition has a great deal to do with interpretations of medicine and healing. The artist's rendering was derived from the stories told by J. Marion Sims and from those told about him by medical peers and colleagues, not by the patients. The picture raises questions about the posture of the women and the nature of their participation.

By 1845 Anarcha, Betsey, and Lucy were gathered with eleven or twelve other slaves as residents in a Montgomery, Alabama, hospital established by Sims. Mostly, these women came from different plantations, sent by their masters, to be treated for vesico-vaginal fistulas. Lucy, Betsey, and Anarcha stayed with Marion Sims for four years or more and became memorialized by Sims in his book, *The Story of My Life*. What their personal wishes were is not written anywhere except through the interpretation of Sims. Anarcha, Betsey, and Lucy, and others as well, underwent numerous surgeries before finally finding some relief from their unfortunate disorders.

Anarcha had the first vesico-vaginal fistula Sims reported to have ever seen. At the age of seventeen, in June 1845, she encountered a difficult labor for her first birth. She labored three days without delivering. For assistance, Dr. Henry, who supervised the birth, went to Sims and brought him to Anarcha's quarters at the Westcott plantation, where she lived with seventy-five other slaves, only a mile out of Montgomery.[37]

After Anarcha's seventy-two hours of labor, which had virtually come to a standstill by the time of his arrival, Marion Sims offered help by applying forceps to the impacted head of the fetus. He recalled that he had little experience using the instrument. Once the child was born (probably a stillbirth), the young woman seemed to recover quite well, according to Sims's recollection. Five days after the birth, however, as was typical of vesico-vaginal fistula cases, the vaginal wall sloughed tissue and Anarcha, who had a particularly complicated case, lost her ability to control either urination or bowel function. She suffered extensive tissue damage, a recto-vaginal fistula. Only later did her master bring her to Sims in the hope he might repair the condition.

There was no mention of a midwife. Likely the midwife called for a physician's help after the labor failed to progress. Once trouble became associated with the birth, Anarcha was thrust into the hands of the doctors who practiced a very different method of therapy from that of the midwife.

For his part, Sims denied an interest in childbirth and generally ignored the presence of midwives. Although his cases of trismus nascentium were often infants he had delivered, he shunned an association with childbirth and turned to surgery as his specialty. When Sims wrote about vesico-vaginal fistula for the first time, he tied the incidence of fistulas to the use of forceps as an issue of medical intervention, calling for more ready use of forceps to avoid the tissue destruction such as Anarcha suffered. While he admitted that inexperience with instruments might itself cause tissue damage, he felt strongly that intervention might be very beneficial to the patient.

Unfortunately, forceps failed to prevent fistulas in Anarcha's case and may have helped to cause them. Looking at the wider picture, slavery provided context for her too-soon childbearing and the likely origin of a contracted pelvis produced by rickets. In 1852 Sims argued for a more complete and earlier use of forceps and had no further interest in the etiology of the condition.

Betsey and Lucy, like Anarcha, were young women who recently had delivered their first babies and suffered the unfortunate consequence of vesico-vaginal fistulas. Neither their deliveries nor the condition of their infants are ever described. If the babies lived, the chances are good the women breastfed them. Keeping them by their sides for the first months would have made sense.[38] Either the babies did not make it, or they stayed behind at the plantations. The stay at the Sims hospital also might have taken place a good while—even years—after these women gave birth.

Sims described Anarcha's condition when her master brought her to his hospital in Montgomery:

> [Anarcha] had not only an enormous fistula in the base of the bladder, but there was an extensive destruction of the posterior wall of the vagina, opening in to the rectum. . . . The urine was running day and night, saturating the bedding and clothing, and producing an inflammation of the external parts wherever it came in contact with the person, almost similar to confluent smallpox, with constant pain and burning. The odor from this saturation permeated everything . . . ; and, of course, her life was one of suffering and disgust.[39]

Note his language and reference to her as repugnant. Here also, in his article, the patient's condition is compared to smallpox—a terrible and deadly disease. In reality, while she was doubtless miserable and very uncomfortable, she was not dying. Nowhere is there mention of the circle of children nor the symbols of family called up by Dieffenbach in association with vesico-vaginal fistula, as quoted earlier.

Marion Sims's decision in the summer of 1845 to treat the fistulas of Anarcha, Betsey, Lucy, and others originated in a fortunate experiment of patient position in an analogous but dissimilar case. The discoveries he made in the technique and mechanics of gynecology in that case inspired the hope that he might treat the other women. Otherwise, Sims recalled having no therapy with which to treat the condition. As one of Sims's contemporaries, the renowned Samuel D. Gross, put it, these discoveries represented, "the thought that enabled him to lay the foundation of gynecology."[40]

A local white woman, Mrs. Merrill, who had been thrown from a pony, called Sims to treat her for pain in her back and pelvic region.[41] A member of the laboring class, this patient was a washer woman whose husband was in many respects completely unreliable, according to Sims. Nonetheless, Sims addressed her by her married name because he remembered her and treated her with full attention. After all, Sims treated patients from all parts of the social stratum and although his medical standards of treatment varied, he considered each a patient worthy of consideration. Drawing from his memories of a medical school lecture, Sims managed to relieve Mrs. Merrill by placing her on her hands and knees, a position that introduced atmospheric pressure into her vagina, dilated the vaginal canal, and greatly expanded his ability to examine her internally. He then used a crudely crafted speculum to examine her. Mrs. Merrill's relief was immediate, since the change in air pressure successfully relocated her uterus to its proper position.

In his "Silver Sutures" honorary address, in celebration of his achievements with vesico-vaginal fistula surgery, Sims described the clinical moment that brought relief to Mrs. Merrill as a moment of rebirth—emotional as well as rational or scientific.

> I cannot, nor is it needful to describe, my emotions when the air rushed in and dilated the vagina to its greatest capacity whereby its whole surface was seen at one view, for the first time by any mortal man. With this sudden flash of light, with the fistulous opening seen in its proper relations, seemingly without any appreciable process of ratiocination, all the principles of the operation were presented to my mind.[42]

The case of Mrs. Merrill convinced Sims that a surgical remedy for the tears of childbirth, vesico-vaginal fistulas, was possible. By simply designating the hands-and-knees position and inserting a speculum, Sims was sure many new medical therapies were possible.

Sims's innovations with vesico-vaginal fistulas paralleled in many ways the techniques he proposed for the treatment of trismus nascentium. Not employing theoretical concepts such as those involved in morbid pathology, he drew from a mechanical view of physiology, focused on what he understood to be the locus and source of the condition, and used craftlike means to address the sickness. His breakthroughs for vesico-vaginal fistulas came from his own panache and willingness to break cultural barriers, particularly in the treatment of female disorders, but his skill and success originated in a mechanical innovation that he saw as a technological victory.

Sims was among a very limited number of European doctors who began to practice what would be known as gynecology in the early nineteenth century. The denotation "gynecology" first appeared in 1847 to describe a medical department treating diseases and disorders peculiar to women.[43] Medical histories by early gynecologists cited French physician Joseph-Claude-Anselme Récamier's development and use of a speculum (a metroscope) and a curette in the 1820s as an important prelude to the successful specialization of gynecology.[44] There was a great deal of controversy about the benefit and propriety of the speculum. Many argued that for a physician, particularly male, to peer inside a female's vagina with the use of Récamier's metroscope was a kind of sexual violation. Hence, in this time whenever a practitioner recommended its use, the suggestion was qualified and carefully rationalized. Sims's experience with his version of the tool, however, motivated him to gather those cases of vesico-vaginal fistula that he had refused earlier because he could not treat them. He added a floor to his hospital, making room for sixteen beds, which included lodging for servants and gathered-in patients. Over the next three and one-half years, between January 1846 and June 1849, he experimented surgically on as many as eleven patients residing at a time, using various techniques involving suturing and repair of the tears as well as exploring ways to make the postoperative healing successful.[45]

Before the mid-nineteenth century, there was no known remedy for vesico-vaginal fistula. Drs. George Hayward, John Mettauer, and Joseph Pancoast all approximated Sims's technique in work they did, very close to the time of Sims's published account (1852) of his therapies for vesico-vaginal fistula. In Europe, the French surgeon A. J. Jobert de Lamballe experimented with plastic surgery in treating the condition. Sims, however, essentially was unaware of the strides made by others and proceeded to invent his own procedure. He added the use of a bent pewter spoon, a rough speculum, so that he could examine the vaginal walls, even high up near the cervix where some of the most difficult tears appear.[46] With the help of a Montgomery jeweler,

Sims later polished and refined this tool to become what is still well-known as Sims's duckbilled speculum.

This speculum was an immensely important instrument in the emerging specialty of gynecology and in aiding Sims's success in treating female disorders. Many physicians in the Victorian period shunned the impropriety of visually examining a woman internally. They found the use of touch far more genteel than intruding visually and instrumentally into a female's genitals. Sims felt no such sanctions, and rejoiced at the breadth of his field of vision, "I saw everything, as no man had seen before."[47]

Eager to devote the rest of his life to vesico-vaginal fistula, J. Marion Sims sent for as many cases as he could find. A few years later he remembered, "From this moment, my high resolve was taken. . . . I thought only of relieving the loveliest of all God's creations of one of the most loathsome maladies."[48] This passage provides an example of the moral drama and passion that Sims ascribed to his early endeavors with vesico-vaginal fistula patients. These thoughts did not fit with the lives of Anarcha, Betsey, and Lucy, nor with Sims's relationship with them. The words demonstrate that even as he operated on African American women, he was not thinking of them, but rather of middle- and upper-class white women.

In spite of his glowing phrases, the path to success was arduous. In corresponding with Samuel D. Gross, Sims noted: "When I began this work I was thirty-three years old, full of life, energy, endurance, and enthusiasm. I was so sure that I could cure any case in a few months that I proposed to the masters of these unfortunate young women to keep them at my own expense if they would clothe them and pay their taxes, and promised not to do anything that would endanger their lives or render their condition worse."[49]

Sims complained later that "as a matter of course this was an enormous [expense] for a young doctor in country practice."[50] The experiments unfortunately did take much longer than Sims expected.

During the first few months of experimentation in 1846, many Montgomery physicians attended the operations. As the number of operations grew, after a period of time had passed, Sims found himself operating alone, relying on the assistance of servants and of the hospitalized patients themselves.

In the first weeks and months of the original surgeries on the slave women, J. Marion Sims invited his medical colleagues to witness the operations. To include a large number of spectators was not uncommon, and to some degree, echoed medical activity throughout the antebellum South and the rest of rural America. "Especially in small towns, where the local doctor was about to perform an unusual or delicate operation," one scholar noted, "the entire population knew of it, and prominent citizens often observed, along with the physician's apprentices."[51]

Race, gender, and class entered the decision to invite spectators, however, since the surgery concerned female nakedness and exposure of genitals. The public nature of his experimental operations demonstrated his pride in his skill and his certainty about the moral rectitude of his medical practices.

There must have been moments of uncertainty, however. The discomfort felt by the women who submitted to numerous surgeries without success was accompanied by lean times for the Sims family. A partnership in a drugstore helped to augment his income, as did the few other cases he handled. After a few years of repeated surgeries and failed efforts, Sims, looking back, remembered that Theresa's brother, Dr. Rush Jones, in nearby Lowndes County, Alabama, demanded, to no avail, that Sims cease the experimental surgery on the slave women.

Over the four years, Sims claimed that the surgery for vesico-vaginal fistula was "not painful enough to justify the trouble [of anesthetic] and risk attending the administration."[52] Sims was not alone in his reluctance to use anesthetics for surgery deemed "minor" by most medical practitioners of the time.[53] In the late 1840s, physicians and surgeons alike were newly acquainted with the use of anesthetics, and as a rule they relied on such a chemically induced numbness for only a limited number of cases.

Looking back on the history of the introduction of anesthesia provides a glimpse of the role of technological innovation in medicine and surgery as well as in the wider society of the nineteenth century. Once the utility of anesthesia was clear, there was a fierce competition to discover who had used it first. William Morton, a Boston dentist, demonstrated the use of ether during surgery in 1846. In 1847, Sir James Y. Simpson of Scotland made the first use of anesthetic during childbirth. There was a prolonged debate across the Atlantic about who was the one who discovered anesthetic.[54] The Mexican War also provided a situation for limited use of chloroform and ether. Years went by before the use of anesthesia became standardized and efficient. Medical practitioners in the United States had difficulty securing patents for various application devices for ether in the intervening years. Ensuing debate over enforcement of the patents ended up on the floor of the U.S. Senate. Only after the Civil War did the surgical use of anesthesia become widespread and even then, cultural values intervened in its acceptance.

Gender, race, and class each contributed to medical notions determining the utility of anesthesia. In the case of the slave women, Sims apparently subscribed to a commonly held theory that blacks had a specific physiological tolerance for pain, unknown by whites.[55] He never felt the need to anesthetize his black patients in Montgomery. White women with vesico-vaginal fistulas who came to Sims in 1849, to have what finally had become viable surgical therapy, were unable to withstand the same operation without anesthesia.[56] Throughout his medical career Sims maintained a class-bound prescription for the use of anesthesia with an unspoken premise that those women in the wealthy tier were by far the most vulnerable to pain.

In his article on vesico-vaginal fistulas Sims recalled an upper-class white woman he had known, before his development of surgery for the condition, who died because she could not bear the thought of a lifetime affliction of vesico-vaginal fistula. Although her death was not from pain itself as we understand pain today, the story showed the connection between the ascribed high degree of sensitivity and personal mortification at being afflicted with such a lowly condition felt by a member of the upper social stratum.

In sharp contrast, Sims claimed that the slave women involved in his original experiments begged him to proceed with further surgery after a lapse of six weeks occurred between surgeries. "They were clamorous," Sims insisted.[57] These women also assisted him in surgery on other patients even after their own repeated operations.[58] Perhaps Sims's use of opium, administered only after surgery, motivated them at least in part. Opium did diminish pain, but addiction would result from long-term use. Since the patients were required to stay horizontal for nearly two weeks to enhance the process of healing, Sims gave them the narcotic medication for at least that long, often longer. He also found the complete constipation that accompanies the use of opium a necessity in the aftermath of surgery.[59] As a consequence, Lucy, Anarcha, and Betsey were undoubtedly habituated to opium, at least to some degree. Its presence in their bodies represented some relief for their condition and was likely preferable to an unfortunate existence on a plantation. Sims underscored the necessity of giving the patient minimal fluid and food during the recovery. He suggested that this postoperative treatment maximized healing of the fistula. He added position to this part of the recovery and insisted that the patient stay on her back for a fortnight. Seemingly, then, the opium satisfied all concerned. "Old fistula cases are generally used to opium," Sims said, "and where they are not they soon learn its beneficial effects."[60] Sims urged the use of the largest tolerable dose of opium, arguing that the pleasantness of the patient's dreamlife helped keep them flat in bed for two weeks.[61]

However, pain was not unknown in Sims's hospital. Although Sims published extensive descriptions of the same surgery, he rarely described the suffering involved in his experiments. Occasionally he alluded to the severity of discomfort, however. A close examination of his accounts opens a small window on the patients' experience in Sims's little hospital in the corner of his yard. At one point, Lucy nearly died. Sims described her brush with death and the extent of her suffering in an article he wrote.

In his first major article on vesico-vaginal fistulas of 1852, Sims emphasized the importance of developing a successful method to drain urine during healing and the subsequent creation of scar tissue (where sutures had been applied). He wrote about his efforts to find a way to keep the healing openings free from urine after an operation on Lucy: "With me, as with others, this has been the most serious obstacle to the success of the operation: for, if a single drop of urine finds its way through the fistulous orifice . . . a failure to some extent is almost inevitable."[62]

In Sims's early procedure he used a sponge, which became rigid after a few days and "perfectly saturated with calculous deposits, rendering its removal painful, difficult, and even dangerous."[63] "Lucy's agony was extreme," Sims reported in his autobiography.[64] These were strong words for one who rarely acknowledged the presence of pain among his patients in Montgomery. "She was much prostrated, and I thought she was going to die."[65] Lucy did recover, only to undergo many more operations.

In a separate passage, Sims described difficulties from a patient suffering during surgery. He reported difficulty from the "bearing down, sobbing, straining, or even voluntary resistance of the patient."[66] Pain and discomfort went hand in hand with the first years of unsuccessful and repeated operations, sometimes "even *voluntary resistance of the patient*" (emphasis mine).[67] Not only is this evidence of at least an occasional refusal to cooperate with the physician, but the message includes the likely event of *involuntary* resistance, which Sims must certainly have encountered from time to time.

After his failure with the use of the sponge following surgery, Sims devised a new tool, the sigmoid catheter. This was a small S-shaped tool, perforated, with an outlet at one end to drain off urine. This instrument added significantly to the physician's armamentarium because only with immediate and complete removal of the urine could the surgical wounds heal and the fistulas close.[68] With the sigmoid catheter, if a fistula failed to unite completely, a steady stream of urine no longer washed over the healing sutures. Previously, even the tiniest hole left unsutured had allowed the escape of urine. Also, the catheter had the advantage of keeping the patient from straining to urinate in the days following surgery, which would place undue pressure on the surgical wounds. This innovation was not still enough to declare success, however.

Sims remembered a loss of support among the local medical community as he continued with the surgeries, unable to close the tears permanently. He worked closely with jewelers and druggists as he pursued the experiments. One individual, William Wright, advertised himself as "machinist to Dr. Sims of this City."[69] In particular, Wright prided himself in the area of trusses, supporters, and aids for clubfoot. The jeweler, mentioned in Sims's autobiography, probably offered the most assistance in the perfection of the vesico-vaginal fistula operation.

Sims met failure after failure in his experiments. When he returned to the patient following surgery, the sutures would be festering with pus. These sutures had to remain in the tissues for several days to ensure closure of the fistula, but the duration only caused suppuration of the wound, with the result of certain failure for surgeon and patient. According to Sims, as he theorized after having found a workable method, the festering resulted from the sutures themselves—either silk or catgut, which absorbed bodily fluid and caused inflammation, ultimately promoting infection.

He reviewed techniques used by other physicians, especially John Mettauer of Virginia. Mettauer used leaden sutures, as opposed to silk, and found metallic ingredients important in operating successfully. Sims, however, was unhappy with lead. He went to his jeweler, a man named Swan, and asked for fine silver wire with which to suture wounds. Swan obliged his request. These silver sutures caused no inflammation.[70]

Sims sensed the near perfection of his surgical technique and applied his attention to devising more effective suturing methods. After much deliberation, he turned to the use of perforated shot to anchor sutures high up on the vaginal wall. He employed the same piece of lead shot he used in fishing. While Sims was unaware of the potential of lead poisoning, he did remove the anchor or clamplike apparatus after about a week of healing.

These various technological innovations, combined with Sims's dexterity and skill as a surgeon, culminated, finally, in the closing of one of Anarcha's fistulas at the base of her bladder, one of the larger tears that would admit the tip of Sims's little finger.[71] Her thirtieth surgery, in June 1849, marked the end of three and one-half years of surgical experimentation. After several days, the tear healed shut and at last the sutures could be removed without leaving damaging infection and small holes behind. Sims never recorded if he was able to close her remaining tears.

J. Marion Sims was convinced by his success with Anarcha that silver sutures were the key to his ability to mend vesico-vaginal fistulas. As he understood the technique then, and as he believed for several years after, the silver kept the wound from festering, allowed it to heal, and promoted the union of tissues. To this day, physicians debate the type of suture to use in the operation; to this day, the surgery is a difficult procedure, best pursued by the skilled surgeon, experienced in repairing vesico-vaginal fistulas.[72]

Unfortunately, there is no written testimony from Lucy or any of the slave women themselves to tell the story of their physical affliction or the treatment offered by Sims's early surgical gynecology. Thirty-two years later, Nathan Bozeman, a physician who was first Sims's apprentice, later his partner (in 1852), but ultimately his archrival, lamented the lack of records Sims kept on Anarcha, Betsey, and Lucy.[73] The sole records of these original operations are his reminiscences in *The Story of My Life* and very scattered descriptions of his original patients. There is no alternative but to take the patients' very participation as at least a modicum of willingness in their subjection to Sims's procedures, albeit with the resistance recorded by Sims. Nonetheless, these women did not own their bodies (in a very literal sense), could not leave at will, and could not seek medical treatment, such as Sims offered, independently of their owners. There is a possibility that staying with him in the hospital for nearly four years was a better choice than being on the plantation and working as slaves. For their masters perhaps, the slave women's incontinence compromised at best their ability to reproduce and probably to work as well. Within the more personal and perhaps more positive circle of the slave community, their lives too lost meaning when they were unable to bring forth children. Being habituated to opium is one further explanation for their acceptance of the situation.

The Ethics and Success of the First Gynecologic Surgeries

Medical specialization in gynecology gained a foothold here with Sims's several years of experimentation on slave women. In America, Northern medical practice, as well as Southern, depended upon a servile class for medical specimens, a group of people often defined as less and as other by virtue of perceived differences by race and sex and sometimes class. How did Sims gain the prominence he did in the North as well as the South, in Europe as well as America, with scarcely any attention paid to the origins of his experience—the initial experimental surgery that made his success possible?

During the early and mid-nineteenth century, increasing attention was given to what was to be the practice of gynecology. In 1849 Charles Meigs published a translation of French physician Marc Columbat's text, *A Treatise on the Diseases and Special Hygiene of Females*. This text treated various aspects of women's health with a focus on reproduction. There was an extensive discussion of vesico-vaginal fistulas and how to treat them from cautery to surgery. Columbat noted that there was essentially no cure. After describing the work of fellow French physician M. J. Jobert de Lamballe's surgery, Columbat stated, "almost all the surgical means for treatment of vagino-vesical fistula failed."[74] Soon after Sims's experiments in Montgomery and on the heels of the publication of his article on vesico-vaginal fistulas, other medical writings on surgical gynecology appeared. In England, Sir Spencer Wells had successfully operated for an ovarian tumor for the first time in 1853.[75] In 1854 I. Baker Brown, another British physician, published a text of operations on women, *On Some Diseases Admitting of Surgical Treatment*, and several other texts were published in this period. They typically bridged obstetrics and gynecology. Fleetwood Churchill's *On the Diseases of Women Including Those of Pregnancy and Childbed*, published for the first time in America in 1852, exemplifies the focus on women's health with an emphasis on reproduction.[76] The modern practice of gynecology began in the area of surgery, and the early publications and practice of the Scottish physician Sir James Y. Simpson contributed significantly. Sims's work was part of a somewhat collective medical inclination toward the specialty of gynecology. Other practitioners recognized his work, and soon after he had demonstrated his technique and published his article he gained widespread notice in the medical world. Accompanying the early growth of surgical gynecology, especially the practice of ovariotomy, as it was called—i.e., ovarian surgeries— was very intense criticism. Charles Meigs, the Philadelphia obstetrician, remarked vehemently upon such surgery in the treatment of ovarian disease, "A surgical operation being necessary in any case, is a reproach to medicine."[77] Once they held some promise of beneficial outcome, operations for vesico-vaginal fistulas were more acceptable than ovarian surgeries.

One of the signposts of the transition to scientific medicine was a demand for clinical experience, in the form of cadavers and particularly live subjects. In a coldly logical sense, the bodies of bondswomen, such as those used in Sims's surgical experimentation, fulfilled needs shared (following a common Southern interpretation) by the slave, the physician, the physician's assistants, and medical science in general. "Thus the young Southern physician found in slavery a means to an early start"; one scholar suggested, "while at the same time, the slaves found in the system a sort of health insurance."[78] Benefits for slaves, however, were offset by their invisibility as subjects of experiment. Practitioners often denied the slaves' objectification while slaves were completely dependent on their masters for determining what happened to their bodies.[79] Healing practices of African grandparents and the old ways as passed down across generations of slaves stood in stark contrast to the medicine offered the Southern black population in the nineteenth century by medical practitioners such as Sims.

Today there are many examples of similar experiments done on various groups socially defined as other. Often decades pass before the details of the episodes are publicly revealed. One recently recognized example from the twentieth century is the Tuskegee Study of syphilis sponsored by the United States Public Health Service. The experiment was conceived as a way to monitor the destruction of the final stage of the disease and did not involve any treatment. Quite the opposite in fact, the Tuskegee Study represented the administration of no treatment, even though treatments were known. The subjects included 399 syphilitic African American males from Macon County, Alabama. Not only is this further evidence of medical experimentation with race as a defining factor, but the forty years of experiment occurred in Macon County, Alabama, in the same area where the subjects of Sims's experiments had lived.[80] Sims practiced on plantations in that county before he moved to nearby Montgomery. The Tuskegee experiments were among the worst in the length of time, deceptive practices on unknowing patients, the complicity and support of the federal government, and the long-term denial by all responsible.

James Jones, who has written extensively about the Tuskegee Study, suggests the experiments and their history represent "A Moral Astigmatism," for those who were responsible.[81] Further examples of experimentation with radiation, use of prison populations and the mentally ill and developmentally disabled, and of Native Americans and African Americans in particular are well documented. Medical experimentation on African Americans reflected the beliefs of Southern whites in the antebellum years—emblematic of a social, political, and economic hierarchy denoting human worth by race. While Northerners were less directly involved, they easily overlooked the use of surgical experimentation on slaves. Social and cultural categories measuring human worth by race continue today at the ethical expense of all concerned.[82]

While there are parallels in ethical issues of experimentation, the nineteenth-century practice of medicine differed in important ways from medical practice today. The American Medical Association was formed only in 1847, just as Sims conducted his experimental surgeries in Alabama, and a national code of medical ethics evolved slowly and circuitously. Sims's generation of medical practitioners was largely self-governing, dependent on an internal code of honor and regulation.

An ethical probing of Sims's career and those of his Southern colleagues necessitates sensitivity regarding the complexities of the past, depth of racial and class biases in nineteenth-century surgical practice, and historical implications of those biases. There is no need to affix the adjective "racist," a term that belongs to the present.[83] Sims's medical activities clearly expose the profound integration of social values and morality with the shape of science itself.[84] He utilized unquestioned ideas about race and social hierarchy to facilitate surgical experimentation.

Unlike Josiah Nott, Samuel Cartwright, Thomas Affleck, and other Southern physicians whose medical practice was deeply saturated with perceptions of racial differences, Sims ignored race as a central factor in medical therapies. For instance, following his examination of Mrs. Merrill, who was white, he moved quickly to the possibility that he could cure slave women using the same techniques. Sims assumed that female anatomy was homologous between whites and blacks. Although the American School raised questions about physiological racial similarities, many practicing physicians made the same assumption as Sims. After all, in order to accept the use of slaves for demonstrative and experimental surgery, of African American cadavers for anatomy lessons, medical practitioners had to accept physiological parallels.

Having completed his vesico-vaginal fistula experiments before the American School existed, perhaps Sims accepted parallels between African Americans and Caucasians because he lacked either a scientific or theoretical basis for expecting differences. In the practice of delivering babies or in treating disorders of female reproductive organs, he noted no observable racial distinction. His concern was to establish the general applicability of technique.

By chance, J. Marion Sims left the South just as physicians of the American School became vocal. He was aware of their positions on medical issues however, having been friends with J. C. Nott. He toyed with the idea of moving to New Orleans, where much of the work of these physicians was being done. Although his own health interfered with continuing his life in the South and forced him to move north, and although he did not share allegiance to a so-called scientific basis for racial biological and medical distinctions, he maintained a belief in the moral correctness of the plantation system and held a strong allegiance to the South throughout his life.

In his letters Sims often voiced support for the system of slavery. Never did he express moral uncertainty because he had kept several women of bondage

over a period of three and one-half years expressly for the purpose of operating on them repeatedly. Nor did he seem to view bondage as being unfa-
vorably confining for his patients.

Not only was Sims free of moral compunctions regarding his experi-
mentations, but he remembered the four years in Montgomery as a response
to the entreaties of others. In the last years of his life, when he recalled his
first years of treating vesico-vaginal fistula patients in Montgomery, he described slave owners as pleading with him to operate on the women.

In his autobiography Sims re-created a dialogue with Lucy's owner, Tom
Zimmerman of Macon County. This reported conversation occurred before
Sims experienced his breakthrough in the case of Mrs. Merrill. Zimmerman
apparently implored him to attempt a cure for Lucy, arguing, "But you would
have done so before you moved from the piney woods and came to the city.
Moving to a city sets a man up wonderfully. You are putting on airs. When
you were my family doctor, and used to see my family or my niggers, you
never objected to an investigation of their cases, and you didn't say what you
would do and what not."[85] Then, Sims added, Zimmerman sent Lucy to him
by train, even though Sims had declined the commitment. Zimmerman saw
Lucy as his property and only when she was in good health would he "profit"
from her.

In his re-created dialogue with Zimmerman, Sims hinted that the slave
owners willingly gave him a free hand to practice on their slaves so that he
might effect a remedy for vesico-vaginal fistula. Sims went so far as to im-
ply that the women's masters, out of desperation, *forced* the cases on him.
Sims, however, also wrote to Dr. Samuel Gross that he had promised the masters of the slave women that he would not do "anything that would endanger
their lives or render their condition worse."[86] Sims was the sole judge of his
own ethical limits.

What did Lucy think? This was not a question Sims asked. Perhaps she
did not see a choice but to comply with Zimmerman and with Sims. "Slave
mentality does not appear in a vacuum," writes one modern day scholar. "Its
characteristics—a lack of self-confidence, personal autonomy, and independent thought, a sense of one's own insignificance in comparison to the importance of others, a desire to please the powerful at any cost" are apt words
to clarify what passivity and submission Lucy and her peers presented.[87]

Perhaps, too, Zimmerman regretted Sims's growing specialization as
an urban surgeon and resented his refusal to treat this condition that involved
filth and excrement and female genitals and slaves. Sims, in moving into
Montgomery, left a rural way of life based on reciprocities and mutuality; in

the urban area much of what Sims did resembled a Northern life. His practice was competitive and entrepreneurial, and he sought national recognition for his innovations.

There were obstacles to personal comfort and happiness. Much to the sorrow of Marion and Theresa Sims, their three-year-old son, Christmas Sims, died in 1848 from the same kind of chronic diarrhea which dogged Marion Sims and similar to that which killed so many soldiers during the Mexican-American War. Just when Sims felt he had solved the puzzle of vesico-vaginal fistula with a surgical remedy in 1849, he too became desperately ill once again. In search of an environment more conducive to his own health, Sims migrated from one place to the next in the early fifties and so was especially sensitive to regional conflict over slavery. He described his patients awkwardly as "the cases that occurred to me early and which were given to me for the sake of experiment."[88] By taking such a passive position as the receiver of the cases, Sims avoided a public avowal of the moral responsibility for experimenting over several years on female subjects in bondage.

Sims found that his health, which brought him near death over and over again between 1849 and 1852, depended on good water and, he declared, he preferred the widely heralded Croton water of Manhattan. Representing the city's commitment to sanitary reform, by the mid-1840s a system of reservoirs, tunnels, pipes, and an aqueduct delivered the water from the Hudson River throughout the city.[89] Since Sims had no friends in New York City, his ability to find a new residence and a viable medical practice hinged on the success of his nationally published article on vesico-vaginal fistulas. He had to convince powerful New York City medical practitioners, who were an elite in the medical world, of his skill as a woman's surgeon and of the viability of his politics.

Marion Sims avoided writing about his reliance on slave subjects. In the *American Journal of the Medical Sciences* in 1852, he described the slave women in typically ambiguous and indirect language. This was understandable to some degree since these were the tumultuous years immediately preceding the Civil War. The journal editor may also have made some changes in the presentation. The difference in direct description of the status of the patients is striking between Sims's articles published on the jaw surgery practiced on slaves and the vesico-vaginal fistula surgeries. The former was published in the same journal in 1848 where the latter appeared four years later.

In the early 1850s political and social changes plus changes in Sims's personal life led him to moderate his tone and forgo any public embrace of the use of slaves for innovative and untried surgeries. In the vesico-vaginal fistula article, Sims never referred specifically to the cases of Betsey, Lucy, and Anarcha by name or in terms of their race and bondage. Sims chose rather to describe the surgery in terms of its mechanics and technique. Other physicians' medical articles often followed the specifics of individual cases, one by one.

The tone of Sims's article hid the intensity of his own active interest in the experimental surgery and his commitment to its pursuit. In fact, Sims himself bought one of the slave women so he could continue his operations, and he paid taxes for the others for several years. "In one curious instance the great gynecologist," a scholar reported, "Marion Sims could not secure such permission [for surgical procedure] and actually purchased a patient to operate on her." Nathan Bozeman, Sims's partner in Montgomery after he had left the city, described the case of a young servant who was both Sims's slave and his patient.[90]

Sims certainly was sensitive to the politics of his audience. These were the years just following the Compromise of 1850 and the Fugitive Slave Act, which finally brought the issue of slavery to the forefront. Consequently, in his article of 1852, Sims's personal needs, combined with his own loyalty to the system of slavery, led him to mute the role of slavery in his early surgical experiments. Even in his extensive use of woodcuts for illustration, Sims evaded the issues of slavery and race by portraying his patients as white even when they were African American. Once again in contrast, his woodcuts from an earlier article on jaw surgeries clearly portrayed the patient by race. Perhaps medical practitioners reading the article assumed that the patients were enslaved, given the fact that the operations were experimental and performed in Montgomery; also possible was that the readers ignored the issue when it was not explicit.

After achieving a large measure of success in New York City, Sims did thank his experimental subjects for their perserverance.[91] However, he neglected to mention their bondage:

> To the indomitable courage of these long-suffering women, more than
> to any other single circumstance is the world indebted for the re-
> sults of these persevering efforts. Had they faltered, then would
> women have continued to suffer from the dreadful injuries produced
> by protracted parturition, and then should the broad domain of sur-
> gery not have known one of the most useful improvements that shall
> hereafter grace its annals.[92]

Sims deflected the issue of slavery and medical experimentation partly by singing the praises of his newly emerging expertise in the general treatment of specific female disorders. Slave women, however, knew no privileges because of their gender. Their womanhood offered no protection from the vicissitudes of picking cotton and from the other myriad hardships that attended the life of all slaves. The question, "Aren't I a woman?" asked by Sojourner Truth as she spoke out for a place for black women in the antebellum American women's suffrage movement, expressed the very inability of black women, especially as slaves, to gain recognition of their status as human beings and as women.[93]

In spite of this disparity, Sims's medical career led him to connect the lives of Anarcha, Betsey, Lucy, and others with the lives of all women. What more suitable means of acceptance into Northern life than through exaltation of "the sex." Sims in fact insinuated himself within the boundaries of the Northern and Victorian gender system as he isolated himself from issues of slavery and race. In describing his surgery on the slave women in the 1840s, Sims proclaimed, "I thought only of relieving the loveliest of all God's creation."[94] Indeed, in retrospect, Sims attributed his four-year preoccupation with perfecting a treatment for vesico-vaginal fistula as a reflection of his concern to find relief for women. He had forgotten his original distaste for treating female disorders and now chose to practice only among the white women of the upper and middle classes.

He expressed his admiration of his African American women patients in terms less of beauty and male protectiveness than for their ability to endure pain. They "implored me to repeat operations so tedious and at that time often so painful that none but a woman could have born them."[95]

In the Montgomery of the 1840s, Sims operated openly and publicly on nude African American women, when to do so with white middle- and upper-class women patients would have caused severe repercussions.[96] Sims learned gynecological technique by practicing on live bodies, much preferable and more advantageous in an experiential sense to using corpses. He had already been satisfied with the jaw and mouth surgery he had developed on slave men.[97] Having patients who were his property or were given over completely to his authority and care gave him a carte blanche that did not apply to patients who owned their own bodies.[98]

In treating vesico-vaginal fistulas, other physicians engaged in a similar kind of experimentation in which the potential outcome was unknown and in which the social status of the individual figured heavily in the procedure.[99] When Sims wrote his first article for the *American Journal of the Medical Sciences* about vesico-vaginal fistula, he identified the work of several of these practitioners but maintained his own innovation as the primary source of the technique. The work of the French pathologist and surgeon Velpeau was the most similar, he argued, to his own. In particular, Velpeau used a similar position to Sims's. Velpeau's work, however, was not translated until Sims began his vesico-vaginal fistula surgeries. Mettauer preceded Sims by some accounts, because he performed successful vesico-vaginal fistula surgery at an earlier date, publishing it in the 1840s. Mettauer too performed numerous surgeries, using at least one but probably several slave women on Prince Edward Island, Virginia, as subjects of experimental surgery.[100] Although he experimented with metallic sutures, the larger medical community did not adopt his surgical techniques nor acclaim his methods. Of Mettauer's first three vesico-vaginal fistula patients, a twenty-year-old slave woman was the only failed case.

After a short medical apprenticeship with Sims in Montgomery, Nathan Bozeman continued Sims's practice by using slave women as subjects in experimental surgery for vesico-vaginal fistulas. Bozeman also experimented with technique. Although he adopted the use of silver sutures from Sims, Bozeman did not like the clamp suture Sims employed. Hence he conducted experiments with what he called "button sutures." In these experiments, performed during the early 1850s, he had three patients, all of whom were black.[101]

The use of experimental gynecological surgery on slave women in the antebellum period is further evidence that slave women experienced difficult childbirth. A glimpse at statistics from two Southern practitioners illustrates the prevalence of African American women patients with the tears of childbirth. In 1884, Nathan Bozeman described sixteen cases, of which ten were African American (62.5 percent). Since the cases had accumulated since his early practice in Montgomery, several were undoubtedly slaves.[102]

When Sims hired Bozeman, he was a freshly graduated medical student and had recently studied under Samuel Gross, which made him a good risk, even though Bozeman was previously unknown to Sims. The two worked side by side for a time. While Bozeman assisted Sims with the vesico-vaginal fistula surgeries, Sims instructed his assistant in the new techniques. When Sims's health collapsed in 1849, Bozeman assumed the Montgomery practice. In Sims's absence, he continued to practice and experiment surgically on fistulas, having inherited Sims's practice and his patients. He eventually devised a button clamp to replace the lead shot favored by Sims. Bozeman then published extensively, advertising his own technique while acknowledging Sims as his predecessor in devising the surgery itself.[103]

Less a competitor with Sims and more a follower, Moritz Schuppert practiced surgery in New Orleans. He published an article in 1866, describing several cases and the use of Sims's technique. He described seventeen cases, including many immigrants and several ethnically unidentified patients. Among these were five slave women (29.4 percent). Even in Southern urban areas such as New Orleans, where the ratio of slaves to whites diminished greatly, there were slave women who needed surgical treatment for vesicovaginal fistula. Dr. C. S. Fenner, of Memphis, Tennessee, described four cases he operated on for vesico-vaginal fistula in 1859. Of these, two were African American and one, possibly both, were slaves.[104]

Although these numbers are incomplete, far from disclosing the total number of patients or their racial composition, they are indicative of the presence of childbirth fistulas among the slave population. Sims's own experience in Montgomery adds further testimony.

Sims's surgery was part and parcel of a fairly wide range in a medical practice that concerned slave women and parturition. Slave women had a double handicap which originated in their status as medical subjects—first because they were women, and second because they were slaves. Their bondage created both a vulnerability to objectification by medical men and a sometimes desperate need for improvement in health.

As a corollary to experimentation on slave women but involving all women, a key question was the actual success of Sims's operation. With the subjects of the experimental surgery coming from a less privileged population, there was less follow-up with the initial group to determine if patients indeed enjoyed long-term relief from vesico-vaginal fistulas. Some of the physicians who provided information on the ethnicity of patients published case histories that explored the rate of success of Sims's operation in treating the fistulas. Nathan Bozeman, M. Schuppert, and David Hayes Agnew (1818–1892), a surgeon and the founder of the Philadelphia Agnew Clinic, all reported cases where a woman was mended by surgery but still had incomplete control of urination.[105] Some suggested that time would heal the incontinence. Others argued that gravity helped. Lying down gave the woman relief. The surgery then gave the woman healthier internal tissues and a means to avoid the constant saturation of urine; yet necessity kept her in bed or at least in a horizontal position. Woman patients were often instructed in the self-application of a urinary catheter. Agnew developed a specialty in surgery and wrote a pamphlet on vesico-vaginal fistula in 1867. He stated:

> There sometimes follows a successful closure of the fistula a certain degree of incontinence of urine. . . . To remedy these defects,

tonics, cantharides, and strychnia have been prescribed; yet, after all, time is the great restorer as the parts tend gradually to assume their original condition. Should the incontinence be so great as to produce much discomfort an elastic ring pessary may be passed within the orifice of the vagina.[106]

Thomas Addis Emmet, assistant physician and a partner with Sims in New York City in the 1850s and 1860s, was inclined to call a case cured if there was immediate and complete improvement following surgery. In other words, he injected fluid into the bladder and examined the vaginal tissues (or the tissues damaged by fistula) for leakage. Although this procedure allowed for a measure of success, the ability of the patient to control urination completely was a different matter.

Nathan Bozeman was especially strident in broadcasting what he considered to be Sims's failures in surgery for vesico-vaginal fistula. He maintained that "*not one half* [Bozeman's emphasis] of [Sims's] individual operations before his removal to New York, were successful."[107]

Bozeman described early a case of a young slave who had been Sims's patient, and had then come to him. Sims had operated on this woman, called variously by Bozeman, "a mullatto [*sic*] girl, Louisa, sent to me by Mr. John Bondurant, and Lavinia Bondurant when she was very young."[108] Originally, Bozeman had reported that her first operation occurred at the age of nine; later he reported she was thirteen. Probably her status as chattel made her date of birth uncertain. In any case, in 1850 Sims operated for stones in her bladder. He removed the stones through the septum that separates the vagina from the bladder and hence created a vesico-vaginal fistula. He never completely closed these tears and the woman subsequently came to Bozeman seeking surgical remedy—or rather, her master brought her to the doctor. Bozeman successfully closed the tears using his button clamp, which he promoted as he described the case.

After Sims's death in 1883, Bozeman described other slave women who came to him for further treatment. Again, Sims's surgery had not completely mended the tears. One of the women, Delia, was one of Sims's own servants. According to Bozeman's account, Sims began surgery on her fistulas in 1850 when he and Bozeman worked together to close the wounds. After ten operations, Sims performed his last operation on her, leaving Bozeman to complete the aftertreatment. Bozeman reported that the surgery was a complete failure. Once again, he called upon his alternative technique, using a button suture to hold the sutures, in place of Sims's longer clamp suture fashioned out of shot. Both of the clamps were fashioned as temporary implements to hold the sutures over the critical first two weeks. Bozeman reported positive results.[109]

An accurate rendering of the success of mid- and late-nineteenth century vesico-vaginal fistula surgery is speculative, at best. Doctors Bozeman and Sims were particularly competitive. On the surface, they vied over the technical method of closing the fistula. Bozeman readily granted Sims priority in successful surgery for vesico-vaginal fistula and acknowledged use of his techniques. Nonetheless, he aggressively sought a name for himself by advertising his button suture in medical journals and abroad. In fact, while Sims was busy establishing and running the Woman's Hospital in New York City, Bozeman went to Scotland, England, and France demonstrating Sims's surgical technique for the first time, with the added flourish of his own button suture. Throughout Sims's career, medical practitioners cited the achievements of Sims and Bozeman together, most commonly giving Sims the benefit of the larger contribution.

Sims did not take kindly to Bozeman's intrusions on his success. Following Sims's "Silver Sutures" address before the New York Academy of Medicine in 1857, one reviewer condemned Sims and the New York Academy for going against the protocol of the medical world and seizing the opportunity to elaborate at great length the profundity of his medical achievements in curing the fistula through surgery.[110] In the speech, Sims also attacked Bozeman as a blackguard, one who stole his technique and claimed it for his own.

In his address, Sims proclaimed, "THERE ARE NO ACCIDENTS IN THE PROVIDENCE OF GOD."[111] Sims's allusion to the hand of God in his success with the vesico-vaginal fistula surgery is significant here, because in this same address he attempted to prove empirically that his surgical technique of clamp sutures was more effective than Bozeman's button clamp. During his early career, Sims rarely called upon scientific method, beyond the mechanical techniques of surgery, to further his medical remedies. He had what Steven Jay Gould has called a "Eureka" view of science.[112] He repeatedly reported being struck by a seeming bolt of tremendous insight into medical therapeutics. Most often Sims attributed these to divine inspiration.

In the case of Bozeman, however, Sims felt behooved to prove his adversary wrong. He experimented in several operations using Bozeman's technique. Obviously, Sims's objectivity was tainted with a desire to prove Bozeman wrong and to reaffirm the success of his own clamp suture. This Sims did. He was unable to operate successfully on any fistula patient using

Bozeman's method. He argued fervently that his adversary's technique was a failure. Some around Sims, however, continued to feel that Bozeman was correct, at least in tempering the terms of success for vesico-vaginal fistula. Surgical textbooks routinely included Bozeman's button clamp along with Sims's surgical strategies. Not long after his "Silver Sutures" address before the New York Academy of Medicine, Sims followed Bozeman to Europe, demonstrating his surgery and claiming it as his own. What the struggle between the two demonstrated particularly well was that individual dexterity and ability were key elements in the practice of surgery at this time. Interpersonal jealousies were strong because the medical profession disallowed patents of technical innovations. At the same time, men made careers out of the invention of these very tools.[113]

In his series of operations testing methods to hold sutures in place as they healed, Sims manifested that he was willing to experiment with female bodies in the name of aggrandizing his medical career. Before conducting these surgeries, he had already determined his preferred surgical technique. Sims nonetheless inflicted unsuccessful surgery on women for the sake of his disagreement with Bozeman, and went on to publicize the experiments before the New York Academy of Medicine.

J. Marion Sims never expressed an interest in the origins of vesico-vaginal fistula or in the health of the women themselves. Nor did he concern himself with the extent of recovery made by the patient. He and Bozeman both treated women who were dependent on others for their physical well-being, who were slaves without the right to self-ownership. Sims went on to treat Irish women, and again he felt little obligation to follow through with his surgeries. Certainly neither Sims nor Bozeman saw slavery as a cause of the condition, even though their first patients were slaves. Sims and Bozeman were loyal to the plantation system and to the South. As a defense of slavery, Bozeman argued that women in bondage recovered more quickly than impoverished British victims of vesico-vaginal fistula.[114] For both Sims and Bozeman, loyalty to region and to way of life obviated the necessity of blaming slavery for the large number of vesico-vaginal fistula patients.

Language among physicians dodged the reality of the lives of slave and Irish women with vesico-vaginal fistulas, to celebrate motherhood and femininity. Sims and many other medical professionals operated on the tears without interest in the causes of the condition. They assumed that the surgical remedies were an end in and of themselves. In 1856, Valentine Mott praised Sims this way: "Dr. Sims is entitled to all the honor and all the credit of originality. . . . Go on, Doctor Sims, in your work of charity and benevolence;

although no marble urn or inanimate bust may tell of your honor and renown, you will yet have, in all coming time a more enduring monument; and that monument will be, the gratitude of women."[115] According to Dr. Mott, Sims's surgery created an eternal gratitude among women who suffered from the afflictions—what Columbat called "the disgusting infirmity" resulting from "laborious labor," as translated by Charles Meigs.[116] There was no need then to look further for an understanding of vesico-vaginal fistula. David Hayes Agnew of the famous Philadelphia Agnew Clinic stated: "The successful management of these, in any degree, constitutes one of the most important triumphs of modern Surgery; and if there is any class in this world, more than another, placed unbounded obligations to cherish and respect our art, it is the mothers of the land."[117]

Thomas Addis Emmet, Sims's assistant in New York City, also embraced the work of Sims and taught the surgical techniques to others. He often declared cases cured in the record books. With or without perfection, Sims and Emmet's practice and reputation grew at the Woman's Hospital of the State of New York. Very soon after the opening of the institution, within months, they experimented with new and different surgeries for various female disorders.

In retrospect, the success of J. Marion Sims as the creator of gynecology in the United States depended upon the slave class of African American women who were residents of his hospital in Montgomery from 1845 to 1849. Without access to their bodies he could not have devised the surgical technique that was to bring him international recognition. Among physicians practicing gynecological surgery, Sims had a singular, extenuated access to slave women. And he capitalized on the women's kept presence in the hospital by repeating surgeries on them—surgeries that many others carried out on pigs, dogs, and other animals.

J. Y. Simpson, a renowned obstetrician from Edinburgh, was a medical peer who relied on the vivisection of animals for improving surgical gynecological technique. In 1859 he described Sims's experiments as follows: "Dr. Marion Sims . . . operated twenty-nine different times on one unfortunate patient, using always threads of hemp or silk, and always without success; but that on using metallic sutures in the thirtieth operation a cure was at once effected."[118] Simpson was Sims's rival who sometimes relied on Sims's contributions to medicine and the beginnings of gynecology in his own surgeries. Nonetheless, he reserved a critical sarcasm for Sims's early practice in Montgomery. Simpson wrote in 1863: "Last summer I took occasion to make an extensive series of experiments upon the relative merits of metallic inorganic sutures and ligatures, and upon the relative qualities of different metallic threads. . . . The subjects of the experiments were a number of unfortunate pigs, which were always, of course, first indulged with a good dose of chloroform."[119] Simpson chided Sims for his failure to find more suitable subjects or to use anesthesia.

Simpson's criticisms were to no avail as Sims's focus on gynecological operations led to his eventual medical prominence. He turned to the treatment of female disorders during a time when many medical professionals shared a concern for the health of women. Sims's technique was revolutionary, in a sense, because his operation for vesico-vaginal fistula offered a tangible remedy during a time when medicine had few viable therapies.

The beneficial side of Sims's experiments—his development of a surgical treatment for the fistulas—illuminates the conditions of women's health in the nineteenth century. Slave women in childbirth confronted numerous biological obstacles. Sims's surgery yielded a way to surmount one of them. The origins of the disorder, however, were entangled in the system of slavery itself. Sims's surgery offered no prevention of vesico-vaginal fistula and could provide no assurance for the patient that the tears would not reappear. Sims's migration north freed him of the effects of slavery to some degree, but he continued to treat similar female disorders, which originated, as with the slave women, in the midst of poverty and poor living conditions.

CHAPTER 3

Missions and Medicine

*I*n the winter of 1856, a group of
prominent New York City citizens ventured to Albany to present the New York
State Senate and House of Assembly with a bill called a "memorial," requesting state support for a new institution. Working together, as the Woman's Hospital Association, to facilitate J. Marion Sims's continued surgeries for
vesico-vaginal fistulas, they had already established the Woman's Hospital
in New York City in 1855.[1] The memorialists, as they were called, declared
that after the hospital had existed for a year as a privately funded institution,
demand and need from patients now justified their request for an appropriation of ten thousand dollars. Subsequently the hospital became the Woman's
Hospital of the State of New York. This was but the first of several trips from
the Woman's Hospital in Manhattan, which then comprised New York City,
to Albany, the capital of New York, to report on the institution's growth and
to request state funding.

Those who traveled to Albany included women reformers, highly respected physicians, and elite members of the political community who declared the hospital as a cause of the first order. After Sims had given a lecture
at Stuyvesant Hall in May 1854, urged on by his newly acquired agent,
Henri L. Stuart, some individuals, particularly those inclined to support sanitary reform, saw the merits in his proposal to establish a hospital solely for
the "treatment of diseases peculiar to women."[2] For a more precise meaning,
Thomas Addis Emmet, a New York physician and assistant to Sims at the
Woman's Hospital, later declared that the category of women suffering accidents that originated in labor and delivery was the largest among all patients;
at the hospital there was flexibility in defining admittable patients.[3]

At first there was considerable reluctance among some of the local
medical practitioners to support the institution, particularly among highly

69

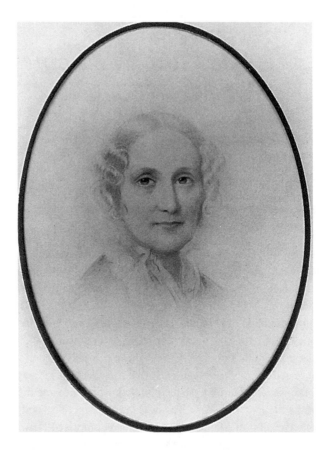

FIGURE 3. Sarah Doremus. *(Courtesy Bolling Medical Library, St. Luke's–Roosevelt Hospital Center, New York.)*

respected doctors such as Valentine Mott and Alexander Stevens.[4] They were members of an elite that sustained its authority in part out of familiarity and through family-name recognition.[5] Not only was J. Marion Sims a stranger to New York City and to the physicians there, but he declared boldly his ability to operate successfully where all others had met with failure. Even after Sims demonstrated his surgical facility before Mott and Stevens, they would not support his initial call for the founding of a hospital to treat women only. However, even Mott and Stevens eventually changed their minds. James Beekman recalled that when the plan for the hospital finally went forth, it was

> signed by every Professor in the College of Physicians and Surgeons, by every Professor in the University Medical College, by every Pro-

fessor in the New York Medical College, by all the leading practitioners of this city to whom it was presented, by every physician to each of our dispensaries, by the surgeons and physicians to all our other hospitals; and when it was sent to Albany, it received the unanimous endorsement of the State Medical Society.[6]

Tremendously important for the original thrust to establish the Woman's Hospital was the energy and enthusiasm of a group of philanthropic women. Led by Sarah Doremus, they founded the institution in January 1855, creating the Woman's Hospital Association. A member of Old New York's elite class and a city merchant's wife, Doremus had been highly active as a women's reformer for decades and was among the hospital's earliest supporters. Fordyce Barker, head of the New York County Medical Society and an accomplished obstetrician, helped to capture Doremus's interest in the cause. With her extensive knowledge of the social reform network, Doremus helped Sims to make critical contacts with key individuals.

Early in the effort to establish a hospital, Sims lectured in Stuyvesant Hall on the need for such an institution before a large and prestigious crowd that included the New York City health inspector and a key leader of the sanitary reform movement, John Griscom.[7] In defense of Sims's brainchild, a newspaper reported that Griscom declared that "a large percentage of the cases of insanity in our insane asylums is due to the neglected diseases of females."[8] Griscom believed such a hospital offered hope and rescue from permanent institutionalization for many women. Laborers and members of immigrant groups often found themselves consigned to insane asylums for illnesses that bore little resemblance to insanity by today's standards.[9]

Furthermore, Griscom captured, in a phrase, a major thread in mid- and late nineteenth-century attitudes toward women. The physical and mental well-being of a woman was diagnosed as almost completely bound up in her womb and its associated organs.[10] In nearly every case, to treat a female's reproductive organs would presumably stop the reflex action by which healthy parts of the body reported sympathetic discomfort or disorder. Therapies to treat reproductive organs went to the essence of a woman's poor health and would ultimately restore her to perfect health.[11] A specifically designated "woman's hospital" spoke directly to the current thinking in medicine and Victorian culture.

At the same time, many women complained of sickness, including reproductive disorders, and sought the care of a physician. Some argued that the reported highly frequent use of blistering and leeches to treat female problems was the result of insistent demand from the women patients themselves. In 1855, Catherine Beecher, a single woman and member of the well-known Beecher family from New England, published the results of a survey of women's health she had collected on her travels. In her statistics of female health she reported a high incidence of a "delicate or diseased" state and of "invalidism."[12]

The ideas of John Griscom, a central force in establishing a public health program for New York City, embodied the marriage of science and religion held by many reformers, men and women alike. Similar to the theology articulated by James Thornwell, Griscom believed that science was a vehicle toward knowing God. His work for sanitary reform involved the use of missionaries from Tract societies who worked closely in neighborhoods spreading Christianity. Their knowledge of the moral makeup of those living in different areas was key to his work in public health.[13] The cause of the Woman's Hospital was another example of a way to use science, in this case the science of medicine, to address human suffering.[14] For both Doremus and Griscom, the overriding direction of change was Protestant and morally based. As a result of the reformers' work to achieve moral perfection of the individual and to address problems of sanitation, community and harmony would replace overcrowded tenements, and other results of poverty.

Issues of morality and religious conversion arose due to diversity and ethnic differences. Unfortunately, all too often reformers identified non-Protestant immigrants as the source of social imbalance and focused on them as the source of problems rather than blaming the political and economic system. John Griscom and Sarah Doremus, at least in part, acted out of a belief that in going into neighborhoods and tenement houses, they would be face to face with the victims of poverty. Victimization was the primary light in which they saw these people. The solution was in their moral regeneration.

From its beginnings, the Woman's Hospital of the State of New York was a unique and pathbreaking hospital. Its establishment, however, was part of a wider movement to create institutions to treat those "less fortunate." There were other much larger hospitals, one of the most important being Bellevue, whose history reached back to the seventeenth century. By the nineteenth century Bellevue was located on the site where it stands today, at the East River on 26th Street. Administration for the hospital derived in part from the state, and during the antebellum period the attending physician and several others were political appointees. The hospital was reorganized and separated from the New York Almshouse in the late 1840s with a new emphasis on treating the impoverished. Bellevue Hospital was not far from the Woman's Hospi-

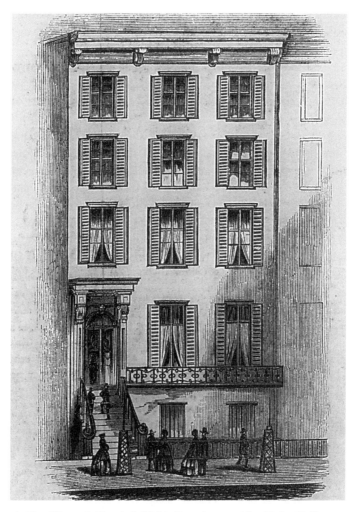

FIGURE 4. First Woman's Hospital, 83 Madison Avenue, New York. *(Collection of the New-York Historical Society.)*

tal; the two institutions were closely connected, sharing a nearly duplicated medical board—for instance, Valentine Mott and John W. Francis—and a number of patients as well. Bellevue Medical College was founded in association with the hospital in 1860. The medical school was successful and drew many student doctors to the area.[15] New York Hospital, another large hospital though not as large as Bellevue, was founded in 1769 as a private hospital. The patients there were less likely to be poor and were more often chosen by their ability to fit admissions criteria.[16] Medical staff from New York Hospital were also often associated with the Woman's Hospital; Fordyce Barker was an excellent case in point.

In the 1850s, 1860s, and 1870s, many neighborhood dispensaries were also founded. One such dispensary bore some resemblance to the Woman's Hospital, and yet it was quite different: Elizabeth Blackwell's New York Infirmary for Women and Children, which was founded in New York City in 1854.[17] Its long-term goal was to provide medical education for women, but, while women were identified as patients, the category of patients treated there was not as narrowly defined as at the Woman's Hospital. The dispensary became a hospital by 1857, and the Women's Medical College associated with it was founded in 1868.[18] A few other medical colleges for women began to appear in this period, though not in New York City.[19]

The first Woman's Hospital in the Western world was in England, established in 1843 by Protheroe Smith, first called the Hospital for Diseases of Woman, then the Samaritan in 1848, and in 1852 the Samaritan Free Hospital for Women.[20] The ovariotomist and father of British gynecology, Spencer Wells (1818–1897), began his ovarian surgeries in the 1840s at the Samaritan and was appointed to the staff in 1854. Lawson Tait (1845–1899), a fellow British ovariotomist and renowned for his skills, practiced at a small hospital, the Crescent in Birmingham, founded in 1871. While the therapies used and the conditions treated varied somewhat, the basic idea became quite popular. None of the English hospitals designated vesico-vaginal fistulas as their singular mission as did the Woman's Hospital, nor did they experience the immediate initial success of the American institution. In America, no other hospital had been established solely "for the treatment and cure of diseases peculiar to females" until this New York City hospital,[21] though lying-in asylums and wards in hospitals had served women in childbirth. (Dr. John W. Francis and James Beekman both hoped to have beds for childbirth at the Woman's Hospital, but these plans never materialized.) In the wake of the success of the first Woman's Hospital, other women's hospitals were established in Philadelphia (1862), Chicago (1865), Brooklyn, and other locations.[22]

As the petitioners went to Albany, they presented a picture of vesico-vaginal fistula victims that contrasted with the experiences of Anarcha, Betsey, and Lucy. They sought support for medical treatment of those "most delicate and difficult diseases of women . . . suffering mothers."[23] Instead of plantation masters imploring the physician to find a remedy for their young slave mothers, women themselves argued for the need to create an institution to treat *all* women sufferers "without regard to place of nativity or residence."[24]

At midcentury, men and women of the Northeast talked about their gender-specific roles at great length. Looking back, it is apparent that American culture designated very specific boundaries based on gender. As the economy changed and industrialism emerged, women found themselves either excluded from the workplace or were given low positions. Women's experience varied by class and ethnicity, but across class lines many people held to a vision of domestic womanhood. Following eighteenth-century ideas of sexual complementarity, motherhood increasingly defined women's difference from men, inferring women's moral purity, submission, and a Protestant piety. The striking contradiction was that women, particularly as active churchgoers and volunteers, helped to articulate and implement a bourgeois notion of womanhood that confined them to the domestic and private realm.[25] At the same time, other women began to speak out for the right of women to vote, to divorce, to keep wages of their labor as their own, and for the right to own property. During the 1840s one such individual, Margaret Fuller, a literary critic, was the first American woman writer to publish a treatise on women's rights. As a transcendentalist she spoke of the existence of a soul in women and of a woman's right to participate fully in education and society.[26] Female reformers presenting a bill to the New York State Senate typified the ambiguity in gender role for many midcentury reformers. On the one hand, the memorialists were proponents of a confining definition of womanhood; and on the other hand, they acted publicly and politically when this was not expected of women. Marion Sims recalled in his autobiography that he asked Sarah Doremus if she was a Warwick, the fifteenth-century man who, though not a nobleman himself, was responsible for crowning kings behind the scenes during the Wars of the Roses and fought among English royalty.[27]

There were no women physicians in the Woman's Hospital delegation to Albany because none had been appointed to the institution nor were any directly mentioned in the hospital records. Just as medicine was garnering a new social authority, meaning, and practice, women in the United States and in European countries found the doors shut to train in medical colleges. Elizabeth Blackwell, believed to be the first American woman doctor, gained admission to the medical college in Geneva, New York, only by accident. Administrators, faculty, and students alike found Blackwell's application ridiculous. The administration, not knowing this, bowed to a student vote. Students wished to defer to what they perceived to be faculty and administration wishes and voted for her admission. The only woman in her class, she received her medical degree in 1849, after which Geneva Medical College refused women admission.[28] In spite of exclusion from most medical colleges and cultural values that defined women as unable to practice medicine, it is important to remember that some women did become doctors and practiced medicine during this period.

Support for the Woman's Hospital included separatist but not necessarily feminist ideas. Women of the Woman's Hospital Association acted out of a belief that women could better serve women patients as administrators and matrons or nurses, and out of a belief that women in sickness constituted a unique medical category that demanded special therapies. Unlike the New York Dispensary for Women and Children, the management of the Woman's Hospital did not pursue appointments of women as medical staff members.[29] Both men and women associated with the hospital linked the institution with a strictly defined and domestically oriented femininity, emphasizing the qualities of self-sacrifice, benevolence, and frailty. Femininity in this definition led to the exclusion of women as medical practitioners on the staff at the hospital.

In the mid-nineteenth century, women who sought entrance into medical school had to abandon the idea of frailty as being essential to their gender. In 1873, E. H. Clarke, supported by many laypersons and colleagues, including physicians at the Woman's Hospital, argued that female reproductive physiology made mental pursuits and intense educational experience incompatible with motherhood and were detrimental to the health of a woman's reproductive organs.[30] Only by denying that medical education could harm their bodies or affect their fertility and menstruation could women defend their interest in becoming doctors.[31] Yet others wanted women as medical practitioners, especially in the treatment of women.

In 1856, physicians and reformers who petitioned the state legislature for support of the Woman's Hospital were focused on a different cause—creating and sustaining an institution to house individuals encumbered by specific female disorders, particularly those associated with motherhood. While the case of vesico-vaginal fistulas was never publicly broached, the concept of a woman's hospital caught on quickly. In 1857, only one year later, Sims was joined by four of the most powerful physicians in the city—John W. Francis, Valentine Mott, Horace Green, and Alexander Stevens—in presenting a further request to the state government for funds to build a new hospital in Central Park.[32] Sims's delegation was successful. Slowly, state funds began to buoy the hospital's annual budgets and the city eventually granted it a block of land. The request for funds now multiplied as the goal became a grand, new, and palatial hospital in uptown Manhattan.[33] Merchants, philanthropists, and politicians joined the campaign, including John Jacob Astor,

William Astor, Peter Cooper, Horace Greeley, E. C. Benedict, and James Beekman.

The year 1857 was also the year that Central Park came into being— and a statue of J. Marion Sims stands in the Park today. Frederick Law Olmsted, the architect of the park, had as his vision an open, safe, and pastoral place where people could move about freely without fear of the perceived dangers of the city. Women, for example, could walk there safely; the park originally even included an ice-skating pond for women only. Creation of this public space was one of many efforts to order geography and social relations in the midst of an enormously dynamic environment. Part of this phenomenon was the movement uptown of many middle- and upper-class people during the mid-1800s. North of Central Park it was still fairly open and unsettled. Downtown, among other places, were areas of extreme poverty: the Bowery, the Five Points district, the Tombs (a large fortresslike prison), and Castle Garden, where the immigrant Irish deboarded. Tenements, saloons, dance halls, and brothels abounded.[34]

Although Olmsted and many others sought to protect women, especially those of the upper class, from the dangers of public spaces, women and men met there often. No matter what one's social status, it was impossible in central New York City to avoid contact with a wide range of people from all backgrounds and classes. In this cultural vanguard of nineteenth-century America, mobility, migration, and diversity contributed to its dynamism. Even in enclaves of socially or ethnically defined populations, there were still other neighborhoods nearby with different demographic makeups. The women who founded the Woman's Hospital Association were but one part of the population.[35]

New York City's position as a national urban center of commerce and industry imbued it with typical Malthusian characteristics. The Erie Canal and growth of railroads contributed to bolstering the city's economic activity and importance. The increasing urban working class was plagued with the attendant poverty and sickness as had occurred in late eighteenth-century England, and the citizens of New York were prone to a high incidence of disease and death. With intermittent epidemics of yellow fever, cholera, and typhoid fever, many people were exposed to death on the streets. Rank smells and drainage, or effluvia, from polluted areas appear frequently in writings describing the city. One such place, the Collect Pond (formerly Freshwater Pond), was typical of the pollution city-dwellers had to deal with earlier in the century. Located at the Five Points neighborhood on the tip of Manhattan, the site was the dumping ground for all kinds of refuse, from the dirt dug for foundations to excrements of all sorts, many of which were toxic. The city finally reclaimed the area and dumped the waste into the Hudson River, then built a large prison, named the Tombs, in the 1830s. Sarah Doremus worked with women prisoners there, who were dealt with harshly.[36]

In addition to polluting their environments, New Yorkers faced the problems due to rapid population growth, especially from European immigrants. They supplied factories and merchants with workers who worked for little pay, but not all were poor. The destitute, however, suffered especially from chronic, financially based panics and often lived in crowded and unhealthy surroundings. Most moved to the southern end of the city, where the Five Points neighborhood became known for its immigrant, largely Irish, residents. Their way of life stood in sharp contrast to Olmsted's vision of life around Central Park.

Reformers responded to poverty and sickness by building myriad asylums and institutions. One writer aptly described the decades between Andrew Jackson's presidency and the Civil War as the years of "the discovery of the asylum."[37] The mortality rate was higher than that of other cities, including London and Liverpool. In New York City, in 1863, one in every thirty-six people died.[38] Even more appalling was the rate of infant mortality. Social reformers saw the creation of asylums as a way to provide care for the so-called worthy poor, often leaving the unqualified to die. Like Malthus, these reformers feared that giving charity to all in need would only perpetuate and multiply the problems associated with poverty. In the controlled atmosphere of the asylum, individuals, or inmates as they were known, could learn regulation and self-government as well as receive assistance in times of need. Sometimes such institutions were supported by the state. One somewhat notorious example in the early nineteenth century was the New York Almshouse, which became a refuge for people suffering from various conditions, including typhus and destitution.

While there are numerous examples of reform activity, and specifically of female reform activity, a celebration in the Five Points area is an illuminating case in point. In 1850, on Thanksgiving Day—which was a newly celebrated holiday—women gathered in the downtown neighborhood to celebrate converting the Old Brewery, a tenement house with an extraordinarily dense population that once housed twelve hundred people, into a Ladies Home Missionary Society. Such an activity represented the impulse to bring Protestant values into neighborhoods settled by those in need—in need, that is, of religious education as well as food and shelter.[39]

Politics were part of the establishment of institutions and of their public legitimation. The Association for Improving the Condition of the Poor, founded by Robert Hartley in 1842, and the Sanitary Association of New York City (1859) were organizations created to effect reform and to gain political standing. Their historical presence symbolized the importance of sanitary reform in the realm of New York politics.[40] The Woman's Hospital Association became part of a movement for health reform.

The Woman's Hospital in Its First Years

Thirty women constituted the original Board of Managers for the Woman's Hospital. For the first eleven years, these managers had virtually complete authority in the administration of the hospital, outside of the power held by the Medical Board and the decisions made by the associated medical staff. Subsequently, a lay board of prominent male citizens became the Board of Governors for the new hospital completed in 1868. The first pavilion for the hospital, funded in part by the state and in part by the city of New York, was completed in 1868 and the second pavilion in 1876. The move to a larger building paralleled changes in the administration of the hospital as well as important changes in the therapies practiced there. In their administrative positions, the men who were lay governors of the hospital acquired authority over the Medical Board and the Women Managers, and simultaneously spelled the end of the Woman's Hospital Association per se. During the second decade, the Board of Lady Supervisors, as they called themselves after 1867, continued, however, to make substantial contributions financially and also to play a considerable role in policymaking.

For the first decade of the hospital's existence, it was housed in a four-story building close to Sims's home. This hospital had only forty beds. From its inception, the female administration intended to treat a variety of women, and they found ways to achieve that end. They instituted a sliding scale for payment in their constitution of 1856, so women from a variety of economic backgrounds could seek medical treatment. Serving women of the middle classes as well as poor women was a given at the institution.

As with other institutions at this time, the Woman's Hospital, throughout its first twenty years, separated the destitute and impoverished in the free ward from the patients who had the ability to pay. The Woman's Hospital administrators were required to supply twenty-five free beds for patients who needed care in order to qualify for state and city grants, including the charter to the land. (The hospital's capacity was forty-four patients in 1855, and seventy-five in 1868.) Surviving notes from the Board of Lady Supervisors indicate that between 1874 and 1875 one-third to one-half of the patients occupied free beds. Between 1855 and the 1890s, patients stayed on four floors, where a graduated fee for boarding defined the class of patient. During the first decade, the boarding fee ranged from three to ten dollars per week. The first floor held the wealthiest patients in single rooms. The next two floors had less expensive accommodations in double and triple rooms. All out-of-state patients had to pay for boarding in the first years, and in the late 1860s they were required to pay a fee just to gain entrance to the hospital. By 1868 they paid a surcharge of twenty-six dollars. Some were able to avoid the cost of boarding if the new Board of Lady Supervisors agreed. That year, residence in the new Wetmore Pavilion ranged from fifteen dollars a week for a single room on the first floor to six dollars and fifty cents for a triple on the third floor.

Not only were the patients spatially situated according to wealth or lack thereof, but a large outdoor department was designed to serve the lowest echelon of patients. Typically outdoor departments of hospitals involved staff physicians who visited patients in their homes. The outdoor department of the Woman's Hospital was unusual in that it included surgery done in the hospital on what is known today as an outpatient basis. The patient went home to recover. In 1849, Dr. John Van Buren instituted the first outdoor surgical clinic of this kind at the New York Almshouse.[41] Dr. Gunning Bedford also had an outdoor department connected to the Lying-In Asylum. He and his associates used this clinic to assist in the home deliveries of babies. Many dispensaries and outdoor departments existed, but rarely did they treat patients surgically. The Woman's Hospital outdoor department was also unique in its location on the fourth floor of the hospital, where it constituted a central part of the activities in the hospital. This exemplifies the relatively modern qualities within this small hospital, even during the pre-Civil War decade.

The patients served by the Outdoor Department were poor and often unable to get a bed in the hospital.[42] The annual reports were slow to document the precise number of patients in this department. Sims's first book of case records, however, shows outdoor patients as early as March 1856. According to the hospital annual reports, there were "many" such patients in 1856, 305 in 1858, and by 1864 there were 683. The number of visits was even greater since these patients often returned for further treatment. In 1870, there were, for instance, 1,701 consultations. That same year, only 173 were patients admitted into the hospital.[43]

Some have argued that hospitals and asylums at midcentury were often designed to accommodate the "worthy poor." Lay stewardship guided these institutions and medical science did not prevail in the administration of hospitals until the early twentieth century.[44] Moral guidance, these historians feel, was as significant as medical therapeutics and hence gave extensive authority to the lay administrators.

The Woman's Hospital was indeed such an expression of private benevolence and lay stewardship, as the managers envisioned their efforts as moral and charitable. Yet it was also very modern, due partly to the emphasis on specialization of its medical staff, which was more advanced than others in the medical profession and similar to that of modern times.

Successful surgical techniques for female disorders apparently appealed to women in many walks of life. One of the benefits of subscribing to the hospital, as was done by all managers as part of their membership on the Board, was to win the privilege of recommending a patient for admission. According to the bylaws of the original constitution, for annual contributions of under three dollars a subscriber could recommend one patient, for five dollars two patients, and for fifty dollars one more patient. These contributions made the donor a member of the Woman's Hospital Association and further augmented the women's power to define the institution. The material implications of this constitutional bylaw are unknown. Whom did these women recommend as patients? Were the patients from tenement houses found through churches or other volunteer groups? Or were they simply friends who were financially sound but ill? The constitution and notes of the managers suggest that some women who sought shelter and treatment in the Woman's Hospital were not destitute. The rends of childbirth may have been more common among the lower classes but certainly were not restricted to them.[45]

The history of the Woman's Hospital of the State of New York thus belies some generalizations that have been made in recent histories of hospitals. Historians have argued that only after the Civil War did hospitals begin to resemble the hospitals we know today. Not until the early twentieth century did treatment in a hospital appeal to anyone except the very poor. Nineteenth-century hospitals have often been depicted as centers of death, putrid matter, horrific odors, and devastating poverty that drove away all but the poorest.

Much of American medical history rests on the premise that modern medicine accompanied modern hospitals and relied on laboratory science. In this framework, scientific technique that was in place by the turn of the nineteenth century focused on the treatment of disease rather than on individual patients. Historians argue that the importance of an individual's makeup, character, and even environment, which were so important in nineteenth-century medicine, spurred the use of germ theory, antisepsis, and aspepsis as well as the more familiar medical therapies we know today. This implementation enhanced the authority of medicine and its practitioners.[46]

Some have asserted that medicine had gained a stronger authority even before scientific practice—that is, laboratory science—was integral to the practice of medicine.[47] The Woman's Hospital is one such example. It used relatively modern medical practices, including clinical treatment and specialization, even before the implementation of scientific medicine. Neither anesthesia nor antisepsis were yet in use when the Woman's Hospital opened. In fact, anesthesia was not employed by the staff until after the Civil War, and the use of antiseptic procedure such as application of carbolic acid did not begin until the 1870s. Still, the hospital in its early years used many surgical therapies and admitted a high percentage of patients from the middle classes.

The Social Geography of the Hospital

As was common in nineteenth-century hospitals, a female board of administrators was active and philanthropically oriented at the Woman's Hospital. One way to understand the network and identity of the women participants in the Woman's Hospital Association is to think of them as part of a city neighborhood. Throughout the nineteenth century, before railroads became part of urban life, particularly during the middle decades, transportation was often by foot. New York City also had a high rate of mobility, with people moving from one neighborhood to another. In the social geography of mid-nineteenth-century New York, even though mobility gave rise to a high turnover in population, certain institutions, especially churches, maintained a stable membership. One of the strongest examples of an enduring community was membership in the Presbyterian churches.[48] Sarah Doremus came from a Presbyterian background, and Marion Sims also had early contacts at the Madison Square Presbyterian Church near his home and the hospital. No doubt this brought him into a circle of individuals, including the women Managers, who came to support him. Not five blocks away was Bellevue Hospital.

The early years of the Woman's Hospital demonstrate the persistence of community and geographic identity of neighborhoods in New York City during the mid-nineteenth century, particularly in institution building.[49] The women who first volunteered there lived near one another and within a mile of the hospital. Many of the first decade's managers lived between Washington Park and Union Square, in a fashionable residential area. Many of the displaced upper class resided there after having left the southern wards of Manhattan that were now inundated by poverty and immigrants. Often the women lived close to one another. Even in this area, one of the "best" places to live in the city, garbage sometimes piled up and the streets became filthy. Interspersed with "some of the finest [residences] in the city . . . were 'tenant houses' with multiple family residences, dram shops, saloons, brothels, slaughter houses, and stables."[50] Though these neighborhoods were strongly defined by class, they were still socially and ethnically mixed. The poor, immigrants, and blacks lived in and among upper- and middle-class families.[51] Women's work at the Woman's Hospital was one way to make order out of the chaos, high energy, and uncertainty of the dynamic that was New York City in the mid-nineteenth century.

Several other asylums stood in the area, including the Nursery for Children of Poor Women, which became the Nursery and Child Hospital. The Woman's Hospital was more than a mile away, on the edge of the city. Sarah Doremus and her associates may have walked to and from the hospital, or they may have used carriages or street cars.

Although many people remembered the first Woman's Hospital as an impermanent institution, the years there were formative. The effort of the women was extraordinary and essential, contributing to its success on Madison Avenue between 28th and 29th Streets for twelve and one-half years. The early hospital itself was much more a neighborhood phenomenon than it would be later, since many of the early Irish patients came from the nearby homes or institutions.

The women had rented the house originally, in 1855, so that Sims could demonstrate his surgery for other physicians in the city in a location just a few houses away from his private residence. He was still frail and somewhat incapacitated by his own past ravages of sickness. Thomas Doremus put up the collateral to make the use of the house possible. The success of Sims and of the Woman's Hospital depended on finding a place for Sims to demonstrate his talents before prominent New York physicians such as Gordon Buck, Alexander Stephens, and Valentine Mott. The women deferred to Sims and his central role in gynecology by situating the hospital near his residence.

Thomas Emmet captured the environment of the hospital well: "The neighborhood was in that desolate transition-state between country and town, in which the picturesque domicile of the recent immigrant and the sportive goat are the most prominent features of the landscape."[52] During the 1850s the Irish, and some Germans, predominated in the immediate vicinity. The residences closer to the East River, at 1st and 2nd Avenues, were homes to a higher percentage of the poor than the central region. There were many old tenement houses, the worst of which were "in bad state of repair, very filthy within, and usually with filthy pestilential surroundings."[53] By 1865, streets to the east side of the Woman's Hospital were a home to laborers, the Irish, and some freed blacks who had been chased out by draft rioters in 1863, while the west side was dominated by a higher class of residence with more space in their homes and a higher level of "sanitary condition." The patients came from all neighborhoods, while the women volunteers lived more comfortably in their neighborhoods to the south and west.

As the city grew, the neighborhood continued to change and in many ways it lost its cohesion. The residences of the women volunteers reflected this process. After the Civil War, they no longer lived in clusters near one another. Typical of upper-class New Yorkers, they lived for the most part along Fifth Avenue above Washington Square. Some clusters of women continued to live near one in 1870, but by 1875 residential dispersal had dissipated this previously shared neighborhood of the first Women Managers.

Besides a geographic and class affinity, many of the first managers were patients of physician Fordyce Barker (1817–1891) of Manhattan. Barker was a European-trained physician who practiced medicine and taught obstetrics at the Medical College of Bellevue Hospital (later he would also teach "Diseases of Women").[54] A native of Maine, Barker was already quite well established in New York by 1855 and was of great help to Sims in organizing the hospital.

In addition to his familiarity with the elite medical community, Barker supplied a list of several women who might prove willing to create an institution such as the one Sims wanted. This first group of women did in fact provide the momentum that made the hospital possible. Thomas Addis Emmet recalled that "at the first meeting held to form an organization Dr. Barker suggested, with a single exception, the names of all the ladies who constituted the first board of managers of the Woman's Hospital Association. He was at the time the family physician to all, with the single exception, and it was through his personal influence that these ladies were induced to assume the responsibility."[55] Barker himself recalled that prominent physicians had advertised Sims's technique "to such of the benevolent, influential and wealthy of the sex who alone are victims of this affliction."[56]

The suggestion is apparent that several of the original women founders shared a bond of suffering and female disorders, as well as class and race. The benevolent women were not simply ministering to the poor and afflicted women out of charity; they too had experienced afflictions either from childbirth or pertaining to female physiology. Sarah Doremus, who gave birth to nine children, might very well have sustained perineal tears, a vesico-vaginal fistula, or a uterine prolapse.[57] Evidence from the wealth and success of Sims's and Thomas Emmet's private practices underscores the recollections of Fordyce Barker that not only poor women suffered from vesico-vaginal fistulas.

As the Victorian period matured and even as society grew more secular, motherhood gained further respect and honor as the central and superior female activity. Women who suffered vaginal, perineal, and/or anal tears were considered not culpable for their poor health. After all, they were bearing children. Benevolence, succor, and medical attention were rightfully theirs, as long as they maintained individual "worthiness" through marriage.

Women's suffering and weakness during childbirth were the very expressions of their femininity. Although their ability to bear children peopled the earth and reflected strength, women deferred to men within the context of the prevailing social order. Their weakness and suffering during delivery expressed subordination of their gender. Many argued that the charity and self-sacrifice of the women managers, together with the suffering of the patients, made the hospital a monument, even a "temple," to womanhood.

The words of Caroline Thompson, an ex-patient, spoke clearly for the Woman's Hospital Association as she delineated the understood relations of man and woman that informed the organization of the Woman's Hospital. In 1857 she joined others in a trip to Albany to argue for support of the hospital: "Gentlemen—to your noble hearts, your generous nature, your chivalry and your gallantry I appeal. To your strength of mind and firmness of purpose, I bring my weakness and dependence. At the feet of your manly nature, I lay the self-devotion—the womanly hearts of my sex. In woman's weakness lies her truest strength."[58]

Despite dwelling on their gender's fragility, the female hospital affiliates did find strength in their womanhood. The women joined one another to minister to those who suffered the unfortunate consequences of their physiology and reproductivity. In the very establishment of the hospital, these women belied female weakness and succeeded in the face of many obstacles.

Women volunteers at the Woman's Hospital encountered no resistance to their activities. "Is it not worthy of them [women], that the first WOMAN'S HOSPITAL that was ever established," declared Mrs. E. C. Benedict in 1859, "has its Board of Directors and all its managers—except the medical managers— ladies!"[59] Dr. John Francis extolled, "We sent [Marion Sims] to the wives and mothers in our city; he laid the sorrows of woman before them; they heard; they sympathized; they spoke; and, lo! the Woman's Hospital springs into existence."[60] Later in the same address he declared, "The Woman's Hospital, my friends, is the work of woman, for the benefit of woman."[61]

Separation by gender, the creation of a woman's hospital, grew out of a sense of propriety and discretion. The women managers saw the hospital as a special place, a "peculiar institution unfit for other than the skill of the Surgeon and the direction of Women laboring to ameliorate the miseries of their own sex."[62] Their supervision of the hospital was a "mission of Work, and love as *moral agents*."[63]

Prominent physicians such as John W. Francis and Valentine Mott saw the hospital's work as a gift to "wives and mothers." "No Christian doubts the sphere of woman's duties," declared Francis, who presided over the Woman's Hospital Association anniversary meetings until his death in 1861.[64] "Wives and mothers" described women who had been stricken by illness while meeting obligations and duties within the "woman's sphere."

Women members of the Woman's Hospital Association were loath to undertake issues of health reform or to advocate education. One former patient revealed the socially dominant female modesty and reticence as she wrote in gratitude for the surgery and care she had received at the hospital in its first years. In doing so she turned to questions of privacy and health reform: "The work which you have generously undertaken is of such a nature that it cannot be proclaimed from the housetops, and thus secure to you the plaudits of the world. It is a work which must necessarily, to a great extent, be done in secret."[65]

People rarely publicly discussed female disorders relative to reproductive organs, and the hospital volunteers were no exception. But the more daring female and male health reformers, on the other hand, challenged this standard of privacy. They envisioned a scientific and balanced public exploration of human health.

The founders of the hospital referred only obliquely to vesico-vaginal fistula, and never mentioned personal physical afflictions. Their voluntarism did not contribute to an ideology or culture of "no more secrets," in which science was a tool reformers used to educate women in female physiology.[66] The Woman's Hospital affiliates intended rather to shelter and give privacy to those who suffered from these ailments. Nonetheless, they shared a belief with the more outspoken health reformers that the physiological well-being of the individual was central to society, a linchpin of social order and stability.

Simply by identifying themselves with vesico-vaginal fistula and accidents of childbirth, Sarah Doremus and her colleagues associated themselves

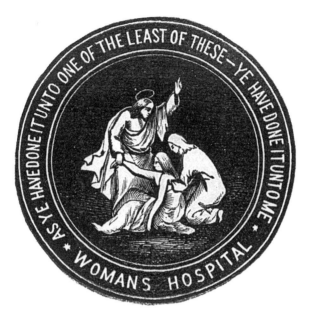

FIGURE 5. The logo for the Woman's Hospital Association, "As ye have done it unto the least of these—ye have done it unto me." *(Courtesy of the Bolling Medical Library, St. Luke's–Roosevelt Hospital Center, New York.)*

in a cause for physical conditions that were publicly unmentionable.[67] Their work was particularly important because they as women associated themselves with the new surgical technique. Undoubtedly women, especially those of the middle classes, may have been reluctant out of modesty to seek medical treatment for these female disorders. The work of Doremus and the others made way for female care and shelter in the hospital and thereby encouraged women to seek treatment. Furthermore, they helped to break down sanctions of privacy by fostering an institution concerned solely with female disorders.

Victorian propriety, however, did impose limitations on the women's activities. Once the hospital was established, there were no efforts by the women to investigate the origins of the so-called accidents of parturition or to educate women in personal hygiene or preventative medicine. Nor did the women managers actively engage in public controversy surrounding midwifery or other women's reproductive issues. The women managers deferred to the medical practitioners for medical therapy and placed the treatments under a veil of silence, to be ethically and medically judged by peers in the profession only.

Sarah Doremus and Her Associates

Looking at individuals among the Woman's Hospital managers and associates clarifies the nature of the institution and illuminates the qualities of the women's voluntarism. For most of the women, the evidence is sparse. There is, however, abundant biographical information on one singularly active member, Sarah Doremus, and some scattered materials for others. The annual reports provided the names of spouses and family connections for some of the women.

Mrs. David Codwise was the first president of the Board of Managers. Her primary concern was money-raising. She was sixty-five at the time of the founding of the hospital, very sick from its inception, and died within the first decade of its establishment. Other members included Mrs. William Astor, Mrs. John Jacob Astor, Mrs. Peter Cooper, and Mrs. Russell Sage—all but the last the wives of men who were also active in supporting the institution. Clearly many of the women managers represented great wealth. Upon their deaths, Charlotte Gibbs Astor, in the 1870s, and Margaret Slocum Sage, in 1918, generously endowed the hospital. Other women also made endowments, but not of the same magnitude.

Husbands were often very prominent citizens. The Coopers and the Astors are obvious examples; John Jacob Astor was the largest property owner in the city. The Astor family built a library in central Manhattan and right across the street was Cooper Hall, built and donated by Peter Cooper. Mrs. E. C. Benedict's husband was known as a member of the New York City School Board, and as a lawyer as well. E. C. Benedict also participated in the governing of the Woman's Hospital, serving on the Board of Governors for many years. R. B. Minturn's wife was among the Woman's Hospital Association's officers during the first years of the institution. Robert Minturn came from a patrician family and was a prominent businessman. His interests, similar to others of his status, included working for public health through the Association for Improving the Condition of the Poor, which had a strong religious component.[68] After the Civil War, Mrs. George T. M. Davis was very active on the Board of Managers. Her husband also served on the Board of Governors. Davis accrued his riches from railroad investments, reflecting the surge of new wealth that accompanied the post-Civil War era.

During the first year of the Woman's Hospital Association, eight of thirty-four women managers were wives of doctors, including the wife of Fordyce Barker. These husbands were also involved with the hospital, often as consulting physicians. This changed quickly, however, so that by 1857 there were only four wives of physicians. Rarely were the wives of consulting or staff physicians members of the hierarchy of the hospital management; besides Sarah Doremus, these were usually wives of businessmen. Fordyce Barker's wife was an exception, maintaining an active role on the Board of Managers for many years. Wives of staff physicians were also active in other institutions, particularly the Nursery and Child Hospital. Theresa Sims never engaged in reform activities for the institution, except to give donations.

Among the women managers in the first decades of the hospital, Sarah Platt Haines Doremus stood out as the most important volunteer, serving from 1856 until her death in 1877. She exhibited tremendous energy as a reformer and at the same time exemplified the religious and benevolent impulse that brought Sims's surgical technique and the Woman's Hospital Association together. Physicians at the Woman's Hospital remembered her because she worked on a daily basis to keep the hospital afloat in its early years. This is how Thomas Addis Emmet, assistant and partner to Sims as well as a prodigious writer and keeper of records, recalled her activities:

> Mrs. Doremus is the one most clearly associated in my mind with all the early struggles made from day to day. . . . I well recollect on more than one occasion, when we met in the morning, Mrs. Doremus had said: "Doctor, we have not a dollar in the house and it will soon be time for me to go out to get something for dinner. The Lord will provide in time."[69]

> She had a large acquaintance, and would not go far before she would meet some one who would give her what she needed and he would fill her basket to be sent back by the butcher boy.[70]

The first years of the hospital's existence were slim indeed. Money came, but for a new and bigger hospital. The Civil War also came and diverted energy in other directions. Doremus continued to work on a day-to-day and individual basis to keep the hospital afloat.

Doremus was born Sarah Haines in 1802. Although a woman of phenomenal accomplishment, her achievements were largely unsung in her day. She simply gave herself over to myriad causes throughout her adult life. Certainly her wealth and social status made this possible, but her commitment was the key ingredient. At the age of nineteen she married Thomas Doremus, who became a wealthy New York merchant. Together they had nine children, one son and eight daughters. All eight girls were born between 1822 and 1838, a birthrate of roughly one child every two years. Her son, also named Thomas Doremus, became a physician and a chemistry professor at the Medical

College of New York Hospital. Social status alone could not shelter Sarah Doremus totally from the difficult emotional lessons and the physical stress of bearing such a large family. Two daughters died in childhood and three others predeceased her.

The demands of motherhood were insufficient for Sarah Doremus's enormous energy and impulse to "do good." She was involved in several organizations, associated with philanthropy, evangelicalism, and Presbyterianism. In the 1840s she participated in missionary organizations, working to send women on missions to China; she was also a prominent member of a New York City Tract and Mission society.[71] From this activity she began visiting women prisoners, and eventually participated in the Women's Prison Association. In 1846 she, with Abigail Gibbons and Catherine Sedgewick, established an asylum for women who were recently released from the Tombs prison downtown. This halfway house was located at 121 Tenth Avenue, and later was renamed the Isaac T. Hopper Home. The mission of the asylum was to prevent recidivism among the clients by offering the women ex-prisoners moral guidance and shelter after leaving prison. Doremus followed Catherine Sedgewick as the second director of the home.[72]

In 1850, Sarah Doremus was a founder of the New York House and School of Industry, an institution concerned with the lives of the poor children of New York. There were many street urchins in New York at midcentury, who lived much more independent lives than middle-class children of the time. Reformers, including Sarah Doremus, thought of street kids as the number one urban concern and responded to their large numbers with a variety of reform programs.[73] The goal was to provide work and education for children too poorly clothed to attend public school. In 1867, Doremus became president of this institution.

In addition to this association, Doremus contributed to the founding of the Nursery and Child's Hospital. Originally called the Nursery for the Children of Poor Women, under the leadership of Mary Delafield Dubois and Thomas Addis Emmet's aunt, Charlotte LeRoy, Sarah Doremus and others devised the institution to address the high rate of infant mortality among foundlings. Mostly the deaths fell among children of women serving as wetnurses, which led the reformers to create an asylum to care for infants of wetnurses.[74]

Dubois, LeRoy, and Doremus, along with others involved in the institution, recognized that after wetnurses gave birth, then sought employment suckling other people's babies, their own children often failed to thrive, since they were deprived of the nutrition they needed. The reformers strove to assist these women, yet many infants still died. Alternative nutrition was rarely satisfactory and living in the asylum was not necessarily healthy. The great rate of sickness among the young children sheltered in the house forced the women directors in 1857 to expand the nursery into a hospital attached to New York Hospital.[75]

There was a different asylum, the Marion Street Lying-In Hospital, where "worthy" married (but impoverished) women found refuge during parturition. At Marion Street, volunteers urged women to hire themselves out as wetnurses after childbirth in order to gain respectability. The unfortunate consequence was a pattern of mothers driven by employment to ignore the well-being of their own newborns.[76]

The Nursery and Child's asylum encouraged wetnurses to better themselves by leaving their infants in the asylum and earning money through their profession. As the hospital served as an intermediary for the hiring of wetnurses, the policies worked to screen the women's health to avoid spreading disease through contaminated milk. The Nursery and Child's Hospital had an admissions policy based on ability to prove membership among the worthy poor, including medical certification to insure the quality of the woman's milk. Significantly, the structure and practice of Nursery and Child's led to an increasing involvement of medicine in the practice of wetnursing. The hand of charity was balanced by the hand of judgment.[77]

Through her vast experience with asylums and reform institutions, Doremus brought administrative knowledge and fostered connections in a network of individuals involved in benevolence. Many noted the importance of her contributions to the Woman's Hospital as they reminisced about the early years. She helped to maintain provisions for the hospital and meanwhile worked public channels to strengthen the fledgling institution. Because she was in her fifties and a well-seasoned reformer by the time she began to work for the Woman's Hospital, she was indispensable for her community ties. The director of Nursery and Child's Hospital, Mary Dubois, for instance, through Doremus's influence became one of the first members of the Board of Managers of the Woman's Hospital.

The height of Sarah Doremus's career as a religiously motivated reformer came with her creation of the Woman's Union Missionary Society in 1860. As with much of her voluntarism, she established this group across denominational lines. Doremus headed the society for fifteen years, working out of her home and publishing *Missionary Crumbs*, a journal of missionary activity. Here Doremus demonstrated her ability to challenge boundaries for women's roles—engaging women in foreign missions—building a kind of public role as Christian mother to the community.[78]

For several years, Sarah Doremus served as treasurer of the Woman's Hospital Association. Her contacts were on a one-to-one level, seeking out individuals who had the wherewithal to provide food and rent for the hospital. Several times she went to James Beekman (1815–1877), a wealthy New York citizen. During the war, Doremus sought loans through him from hospital building funds in order to meet the rent of the "little temporary hospital," as Marion Sims called it.[79]

City politician James Beekman joined forces with the Woman's Hospital Association, and he headed the financial and political efforts to find a new and bigger location for the new hospital. He was not involved directly with the women managers as they ran the hospital at 83 Madison Avenue. Beekman became increasingly dedicated to the hospital during the last twenty years of his life, presiding over the Board of Governors after 1868.

Beekman's political acumen aided the Woman's Hospital in its quest for state financial support. With wealth inherited in 1833 from his father and uncle, and without a doubt part of the patrician elite of Old New York, Beekman pursued an education and traveled in Europe. He was especially interested in government. In 1850 he was elected state senator in New York, and again in 1862. Along with Minturn, he was a member of the Union League in New York City. These connections, of course, helped the needs of the Woman's Hospital.

Analogous to Sarah Doremus's extensive female reform activity, James Beekman had a strong and powerful interest in hospital administration. Besides presiding over the Woman's Hospital Board of Governors, he was vice-president at the New York Hospital and director of the New York Dispensary. In this capacity, Beekman became engaged in the then-current discourse over hospital construction and proper ventilation. He had gained experience during the Civil War caring for large numbers of injured soldiers through New York Hospital.[80]

Sarah Doremus's ability to communicate and work well with James Beekman enhanced her contributions to the well-being of the Woman's Hospital. In the context of her personal goals, however, Doremus must have held her supervision of the hospital's religious services as most important. She urged all patients to attend services on Sunday. The rules allowed no visitors in the hospital during that time unless the visitors also wished to attend. Doremus invited various ministers to preside over the weekly gathering. Each meeting of the Board of Managers also began with a tract reading. The annual reports document that she kept the institution very well stocked with

Bibles. After all, Doremus started her voluntary activities as a missionary for the New York Tract Society.[81] She became president of the Board of Managers in 1867 and remained so until her death in 1877, but resigned from her religious duties in the hospital in 1873, due to ill health.

Comparing Doremus with Margaret Slocum Sage demonstrates some similarities and differences among the early managers. Sage (1828–1918) was twenty-six years younger than Doremus, and she was childless. One might say Sage experienced some loosening, or at the very least shifting, of the gender system as she grew up. While Doremus had studied only at home, Margaret Slocum was educated at the Troy Seminary, which provided a rigorous and pioneering program in the education of women. She taught for a few years before marrying Russell Sage, becoming his second wife in 1869. Margaret Sage's reform activity included the Women's Christian Temperance Union and women's suffrage. Unlike Doremus, Sage articulated issues of women's rights within the context of Victorian culture.[82]

In Margaret Sage's generation, Caroline Lane (Mrs. David Lane) was a volunteer who was younger than Doremus—by thirty-nine years. She became active in the organization after the Civil War and served second only to Doremus in the Board of Lady Supervisors (as the managers were removed). Lane's generational perspective derived from her experience with the Women's Central Association of Relief (an auxiliary of the Sanitary Aid Commission) during the Civil War. Her role was to work in the transport of soldiers to hospitals from the front, and provided her experience in giving medical care and learning nursing and hospital organization. The expertise of Caroline Lane suggests the shifts in female voluntarism at the Woman's Hospital from the sixties to the seventies, a move away from moral reform toward the scientific philanthropy of the post-Civil War era. Her choices in a public life were different from those of Doremus.[83] Other women from the original Board of Women Managers were among the group of New York women who founded the Women's Central Association of Relief, including Peter Cooper's wife and the Astors.[84]

Though each was a member of the Woman's Hospital administration, these women's lives suggest generational changes and changes in the history of the institution itself. Sarah Doremus exemplified the antebellum moral reformer and participated in an unbelievable number of reform activities. Her religious impulse shaped the original institution. The motivation of the other two women included religion but incorporated a changing idea of how to effect change and how to manage institutions.

The Evangelical Mission

The original group of women in the Woman's Hospital Association conceived of the new institution as an asylum governed by religious philanthropy. They chose a chapter from Matthew as their creed: "As ye have done it unto one of the least of these, ye have done it unto me."[85] On the hospital seal, these words circled an image of Christ with two women. One is prostrate, held up by another. Christ is holding the ailing woman's hand with his own left hand uplifted, as if to minister to her condition.

Such a Christian motto meant that these women saw the founding of the hospital as a refuge for women who were injured by childbirth. Their womanhood bound them together. Those who offered supplication identified with those who suffered vesico-vaginal fistulas, tears of the perineum, or other "accidents of parturition." Matthew's message was explicit. Those who extended food and shelter to the suffering would reap the reward of salvation; those who failed to do so would be eternally damned. At the same time, the creed of the hospital implied that those women who suffered tears of childbirth (or similar female disorders) were poor women. They were "the least of these."

Although the public and explicit rationale for the hospital persisted in emphasizing service to the poor, the category delineated by gender transcended class. The women managers meant by "the least of these" all women who suffered from wounds and disorders of childbirth, or the female reproductive organs.

Religion and voluntarism provided alternative avenues of expression for women. Volunteers clearly sought to "do good" through their weekly meetings with one another, their visits to the hospital, and other related works. In the name of benevolent reform they strove for amelioration of poverty and suffering, expecting personal religious rewards on judgment day. They were in no way committed to such radical social change as abolition that challenged the fundamental institutions of their society.[86] The mission of the Woman's Hospital Association was conservative, seeking to restore a sense of community many in the patrician class associated with the Old New York of the early nineteenth century—before the rise of the new merchant class and the new working class.[87]

Nonetheless, the group of women who oversaw the hospital in its early years were not entirely homogeneous, nor were the women utterly submissive to the more powerful male figures involved in the hospital—from politicians through surgeons. There was a strain of religious enthusiasm that affected the tenor of activity and eventually led to conflict within the institution. The nature of the religious revivalism led some of the women to see themselves as equal to men in the common quest for spiritual righteousness.

The symbol of the Great Physician on the Woman's Hospital Association logo is important because of what it reveals about the mission of the hospital and Sims's role in it. The Great Physician or God the Physician was part of Calvinist thought and essentially portrayed God as a healer. In this symbology, healing brought the mind and the body together. Such was a concept of deep tradition in the Presbyterian Church. Sims and Doremus were both Presbyterians; likely many others involved in the institution were as well. Among women reformers, Presbyterianism was prevalent and frequently represented a fair degree of wealth.[88] Many Protestants, including Presbyterians, were ecumenically oriented and often participated in reform activity across denominational lines. Many associated Christianity with nationalism, and religious revivals in New York City during this time led in the same direction.[89] Belief in the symbol of a divine healer also connected the strength of Sims's religious convictions with his role as a physician, and in particular with his role as a physician to suffering women. Even though slavery was a burning political topic and North and South were more and more divided, the union of these two qualities in one man helped to obscure his recent practice in Montgomery. The symbol itself was somewhat problematic, however, since the implication was that Sims was Christ.

Sims himself conceived of his treatment of vesico-vaginal fistula and the creation of a woman's hospital as a kind of religious mission. In 1854 he wrote from New York City to his wife in Montgomery, "The *cause* . . . is at the top of my throat, it fills my brain. It is the grand moral object of my professional life" (Sims's emphasis).[90] Before the New York Academy of Medicine he elucidated his sense of commitment as he pursued surgical experiments in Montgomery. "I now stood alone—alone! did I say? no, I was not alone, for I felt that I had a mission, if not of a Divine character, at least but little short of it, of Divine origin. I felt that the God who had called me to this good work . . . was with me, and would not desert me."[91] Since women in slavery were never treated as "the loveliest of all God's creations," Sims must have had other women in mind—women resembling more closely the women of the Woman's Hospital Association.[92]

Through the establishment of a hospital specializing in women's diseases, the Woman's Hospital Association hoped to implement the assurances Sims expressed for the wide philanthropic implications of his surgical innovations. Sims, the women who supported him, and others of their time perceived Christianity and science as complementary, not conflicting. During

the first eleven years of the hospital's existence, they banded together to create the administration of the Woman's Hospital, to unite science (in medical
practice) and Christianity (in reform activity).

The collective intention of the women volunteers was to provide a charitable institution where women, predominantly poor women, might gain relief from disorders associated with female physiology. Their interest grew out
of knowledge of Sims's vesico-vaginal fistula surgery. They conceived of
themselves as "angels of mercy," regarding their own moral and religious contributions to the rhythm of the house and hospital at 83 Madison Avenue to
be equally important to the medical therapies. Moreover, they knew that their
contributions of money, their fund-raising, and the daily acquisition of gifts,
ranging from turnips to kindling, were vital to the survival of the Woman's
Hospital. The medical renown of the early surgical gynecologists (who considered themselves most often simply physicians) snowballed, while attention paid to the demands of these women diminished.

In the first years, Sims's surgery provided the impetus and the mission
for the establishment of the Woman's Hospital. His strongly religious perspective combined with his medical skills to win the support of the women
volunteers. Marion Sims's decision to move to New York City in the early
1850s had been risky. After several years of frequent moving and traveling,
Sims found a home on the edge of New York, on the east side of Madison
Avenue between 28th and 29th Streets. Although New York City was growing at a rapid rate, there were few houses in Sims's neighborhood. From his
parlor window he had a clear view of the East River.[93] Some immigrants lived
on the outskirts of the city near him; he could hear the farm animals of Irish
families. Sims was also on the outskirts of the practicing medical profession
in New York, where he had trouble winning the support of the powerful professional elite. His own vulnerability and struggle at this time aligned him
to a degree with the Blackwell sisters and other women practicing medicine.

By the early 1850s, the economic stress of Sims's prolonged sickness
had begun to wear down his family. Their income from various property, including the sale of their slaves and the inherited wealth of the Bartlett Jones
estate, pulled them through lean times. They were able to keep boarders in
their house at 89 Madison Avenue in New York. Boarding payments provided
crucial income before Sims's practice was to start again. Even in the early
1850s when Sims was a migrant practitioner, so to speak, patients from Montgomery, who sought Sims's skills, followed him north for treatment.[94] As destitute as Sims remembered himself and his family to be in their first years in
New York City, they never failed to have a housekeeper, and a wetnurse when

needed. Eventually Theresa Sims sold their property in the South, including the slaves, and they made New York their permanent home.

When Sims felt reasonably assured of a successful medical practice and professional recognition, he declared: "I don't doubt for a moment the success of the great object of my life. I only fear the failure of my health; but I am now well, and I pray God to continue his blessing on my efforts. Give me health, and even without money I shall accomplish wonders with the aids now at my command."[95] Indeed, Sims's restoration to good health took on qualities of the miraculous. Sims evinced powerful religious ideals at this juncture in his life. He later described each breakthrough he achieved in the Montgomery experiments as a moral rebirth that kindled and explained his medical success. About the surgical cure for vesico-vaginal fistula he said "that it was the result of a Providential train of circumstances over which I had no control, and that it pleased God to lead me in this direction in spite of my predilections."[96] Sims argued that it was the hand of God that propelled him to success. Hence, he came to see his work in gynecological surgery as having a divine origin.

In letters written in the 1850s both to his father and to his wife, Theresa, in Montgomery, Sims urged both to self-denigrating humility before God. Much to his relief as an outsider and as a Southerner, he found a Presbyterian church on Madison Square in New York City that won his praise and membership.[97] The more abolitionist cast of Henry Ward Beecher's sermons in Brooklyn did not inspire Sims for obvious reasons. In his letters, his joy and enthusiasm at being alive translated into an experience of religious rebirth.

In his ministrations to his close family, Sims's letters took on a tone of self-righteousness. In late December 1854 he wrote to Theresa, urging her to undertake a public statement of religious rebirth.

> Have we done our duty to our children, to ourselves, to our God? We have not. . . . Why wait a moment? A public profession of the religion that I know glows in your heart is all that is needed. The power of your example will do more for the moral elevation and religious culture of the rest of us than whole volumes of sermons. Your whole life is a sermon, Why not, then, preach it? Your heart is full of religion. Why not, then, openly declare it? If you do not take first step forward, then we shall remain in darkness and doubt.[98]

Doubtless, Sims was confident of the success of his personal repentance. He took it upon himself also to call upon his wife to cleanse herself of moral and religious backsliding. Religious messages and accounts of sermons are frequent in his letters to Theresa throughout the 1850s and 1860s. Whether she too underwent a religious rebirth is undocumented, as is most of her life. That she remained loyal to J. Marion Sims is clear.

Any remorse or internal conflict Marion Sims might have felt in his previous experimental surgeries or from the sale of his loyal slaves found release in his turning to religious fervor.[99] His revival impulse followed the pattern of much religious activity in the antebellum period, exhorting the individual to bring about individual perfection through internal moral control or self-government. In 1855, Sims also wrote a forceful letter to his father. He once again reported great confidence in his own mission in life—that of saving women from miserable afflictions through his surgery. As he had done with Theresa, Sims joined his own moral failings with those of his father. "You and I, my dear father, have both been very bad men, considering we were almost faultless in all the duties and relations of life. We have been mere *moralists*. We thought ourselves as good as anybody, and far better than most people. We never dreamed of our own sinfulness and utter unworthiness" (emphasis Sims's).[100]

Enthusiasm and piety colored Marion Sims's letter to his father as he sought to instruct him in winning spiritual cleansing and redemption. "How are we to acknowledge that we are rebels, that we have taken up arms against our Father? He has said nothing but an *unconditional surrender* will suit Him, and He has pointed out the only way that he will receive our approach. The Saviour is the way." (emphasis Sims's).[101] Throughout his life, then, Sims had held to an overriding religious faith. But religion grew in importance in the early fifties, when he left his home behind. In 1854 he wrote Theresa, "This expatriation . . . almost made me mad."[102]

At the same time, medical practice was an art for Sims, and he thought of himself as laying his accomplishments upon "the altar of science," a metaphor brilliantly capturing the tension in his thought. Some contemporary scientific thought, "Huxley, Tyndall and Darwin," he claimed, flew in the face of the values he cherished.[103] As a physician, Sims's religion was particularly important. This was not unusual in this era and reflected to a degree a very different concept of the origins of disease and sickness held by both physicians and laypersons. Physicians, such as Sims was, coming out of a rural context, were central figures in their communities. They were called upon to interpret death and to demonstrate science. Medicine was truly a practice, more grounded in everyday life than theology. Physicians and ministers, in fact, sometimes quibbled over who should prevail in the sickroom. Practicing medicine for Sims was the quintessential expression of doing good works.[104]

Thomas Addis Emmet and His Irish Loyalty

Religious benevolence bound the early institution together. Points of tension were never too far beneath the surface. One early issue was the suggestion of female medical practice at the hospital. Initially, the Women Managers had suggested that Sims hire a woman assistant surgeon. In fact, they had demanded it as part of the hospital constitution: "Article XVI. The Surgeon's Assistant must be a woman."[105] Sims began his residence in New York City on good terms with Elizabeth Blackwell. Although Elizabeth Blackwell was partially blind and hence was not a surgeon herself, her sister Emily, who was a co-physician with her and Marie Zakrzewska at the New York Infirmary for Women and Children, had excellent credentials. Marie Zakrzewska, who was a Prussian immigrant with extensive experience as a midwife and who received her M.D. degree from Cleveland Medical College in 1856, remembered that Sims lost his enthusiasm for working with the Blackwells as his hospital began to take shape.[106] "He later learned from his professional brethren, as well as from a wider public, that women physicians were by no means popular and could in no way forward his plans."[107] Vitally serious about her career, Zakrzewska fought a long hard battle to win her degree and in 1862 established the New England Hospital for Women and Children.[108]

Though she was only thirteen years old at the time of the incident but would eventually become a neurologist and a pediatrician, Mary Putnam Jacobi recorded the incident with anger in her history of women in medicine: "Emily Blackwell was the woman who should have been chosen. She had an education far superior to that of the average American doctor of the day, a special training under the most distinguished gynaecologists of the time—Simpson and Huginer [sic]—and had received abundant testimonials to capacities."[109]

When the Woman's Hospital was being established, Emily Blackwell had served as an assistant to James Y. Simpson and had worked with William Jenner. She was probably the most qualified woman surgeon in the world.[110] Her experience included obstetrics and early gynecological surgery. The Women Managers, whatever their original motivation, submitted to Sims's maneuvers to appoint T. A. Emmet as his assistant instead. The by-law became, "The Surgeon's Assistant shall be such a person as the exigencies of the case require."[111] Adding insult to injury, the Women Managers appointed the widowed sister of Henri Stuart (Sims's agent and not a physician), supposedly in Blackwell's stead, filling a supervisory rather than a medical role; she later became matron of the hospital.

With little concern for women's rights or debates over the role of women, Thomas Addis Emmet had a mission of his own that was at variance with that of the Managers and concerned the politics and cause of the Irish. Although he was born in Virginia, Thomas Addis Emmet (1828–1919) held strong and direct ties with Ireland. His grandfather, Thomas Addis Emmet (1764–1827), was a Protestant fighting for Irish liberation from Great Britain. Subsequently he was banished from Ireland but not before he and his wife spent time in jail for their role in the United Irish uprising of 1798. As a result of his participation in the same rebellion, Emmet's great-uncle, Robert Emmet, who was renowned as an orator, was martyred, hanged in France.[112] The United Irishmen, both Protestant and Catholic, sought independence from the colonial rule of Great Britain and carried out the uprising, inspired in part by the recent occurrence of the French Revolution.[113] After emigration, his grandfather "[Thomas Addis Emmet] was considered the foremost advocate in New York and was ranked along with Daniel Webster and Charles Pinckney as perhaps the three finest in the nation."[114] The grandfather died the year before the younger Emmet's birth. His death was followed by one of the largest funerals ever held in the city. A prominent attorney in New York and a leader in the Society of United Irishmen, he was "the most honored" of the group among Irish exiles in America.[115]

The year after the death of Emmet's well-known grandfather, a controversy stirred among the city's Irish over funds for a memorial to the senior Emmet. Following Catholic Emancipation in 1829, an act of Parliament that gave Irish Catholics in Ireland limited rights as citizens, the unity of the 1798 uprising had begun to splinter. The conflict between Irish Protestants and Catholics arose again in the use of funds gathered for the Emmet Memorial.[116] For those connected with the United Irishmen, freedom of religion remained very important, and that included the younger Thomas Addis Emmet. The context of Irish politics, the struggle for freedom, ethnic loyalty, and the American Revolution became highly symbolic for the ideology of the younger Emmet.

Emmet's background included wealth, prestige, a wide family network in New York City, and a strong sense of political identity and moral responsibility. His great-grandfather, Robert Emmet, had been a physician who published a medical text in Latin in 1742 on diseases of women.[117] Emmet's grandfather had a medical degree but later became a lawyer. His son John Patten Emmet was the father of Thomas Addis Emmet.[118] After studying medicine, John Patten Emmet married the daughter of a Presbyterian minister and became a professor of chemistry at the University of Virginia, Thomas

Jefferson's only appointee. Thus Thomas Addis Emmet was a Southerner and grew up in Virginia. As a child, after his father's early death, Emmet spent virtually every summer in New York City with his uncle, Bache McEvers, who was also a physician.[119]

To no one's surprise, the younger Thomas Addis Emmet also became a physician. He studied at Jefferson Medical College in Philadelphia, just as Sims had done earlier. In 1850, soon after completing his education, through a connection with an Irish Patriot—who, he claimed was his only friend besides his family in New York City—Emmet won an appointment as a resident physician at the Emigrant Refuge Hospital on Ward's Island in the East River near Manhattan. This hospital, established largely for immigrants from Ireland during the peak of the Famine Migration, had just opened. Those fleeing Ireland in the years of the famine, in the words of scholar Hasia Diner, "more than those before or those afterward, represented the landless and the poor; who just could not remain at home."[120] Besides often being in poor health and destitute as they embarked, Irish immigrants traveled across the Atlantic Ocean under miserable conditions, including overcrowding and a general lack of supplies. Many who died on the trip were simply thrown overboard. Typhus was rampant, and the establishment of the Emigrant Refuge Hospital was an effort to isolate victims of the disease and to offer them medical treatment. Within a few weeks of beginning his practice at the hospital, Emmet caught the disease himself. But he recovered and returned to the institution to continue his practice.

Emmet's experience among the desperately ill immigrants intensified his already strong pro-Irish sentiment. Later he wrote at length about British mistreatment of the Irish, and about the horrendous conditions immigrants endured in their migration.[121]

After three years of resident appointment at the Refuge Hospital, Emmet gained a city appointment as Visiting Physician in 1854. At that time, Emigrant's Refuge Hospital became the state-run New York Emigrant Hospital on Ward's Island.[122] The State Commissioners of Emigration took charge of the institution, and Emmet felt honored to have won the appointment ahead of others who were many years his senior. While acquiring knowledge of anatomy and practice in pathology during his years on the island, Emmet completed thousands of autopsies and kept extensive records. Several years on Ward's Island also brought extensive experience in childbirth. Emmet worked there until he and the State Commissioners were replaced—the positions were subject to political patronage.

Politics in New York City were machine run and often corrupt, reflecting the complexity of the urban population. While the numbers of Irish immigrants grew and helped to form a new urban proletariat and maintained a city political machine, national political controversy was heating up. In the 1850s, African Americans and Irish competed for jobs and the political crumbs of favor. There were abolitionists, for example Horace Greeley and Lydia Maria Child, who focused their reform efforts on ending slavery. Harriet Jacobs, in her slave narrative, recounted her move to New York City as an escaped slave, her intense fear of recapture, and revealed the common sentiment of racial denigration of African Americans. The Fugitive Slave Law of 1850 angered abolitionists, but others in New York City wantonly captured anyone they identified as a potential runaway and sought bounty rewards for shipping them back to the South. This activity was countered by the formation of the underground railroad set up by African American abolitionists to usher off the captured victims.[123]

As African Americans, freed and enslaved, suffered from segregation and widespread prejudice and were faced with the difficulty in finding work that would provide a decent wage, the Irish were also struggling at the bottom rungs of the ladder. Many Irish worked in the needle trades, in textile factories, and as prostitutes. Others worked on the waterfront and in heavy labor, such as those who built the Erie Canal in the 1810s and 1820s. Irish women often worked as domestic servants in New York City. As one author has written, in the early nineteenth century the Irish were not white; in their home country of Ireland, they had a racial identity and were considered less by the English. In an American society structured by racial categories, they often shared a kind of complementary status with African Americans, and the situation easily became competitive. Cultural caricatures of both ran rampant.[124] Prejudice against the Irish interfered with their ability to make a living. In America many targeted them as the source of disease and filth in cities. In New York City, tension over slavery and impending war set the Irish and the African Americans at odds with each other. The Draft Riots in New York City in 1863 erupted out of the conflict felt throughout the city on all class levels over ethnic loyalties and the onset of the Civil War. On a very fundamental level, Irish Americans balked at being drafted to fight against slavery when the African Americans themselves were not allowed to fight, and upper- and upper-middle class whites could buy their way out of the draft.

Looking back, it is easy to assume New York City was a stronghold for Northern sentiment, a pro-Union Army, and a hotbed for antislavery efforts in the antebellum era. However, reconstructing the story of social diversity and relationships during this period forces our interpretations of political loyalty and commitment to change. Before the Civil War, social divisions drawn in part along lines of religion and prejudice were in no way confined to slave-owning regions. Catholicism was the object of widespread xenophobia. Although definitions of race changed, segregation by race permeated much of American society. With some exclusion based on the nature of the woman's problems and a set of rules governing behavior, the Woman's Hospital proudly admitted everyone. In contrast, Bellevue had a segregated wing for its African American patients. The Protestant women administrators were willing to tolerate Catholicism and the Irish—but only within a context of their own design. Often the Irish Catholic patients became a mission for the reformers. Among medical staff there was tension as well. During and after the war, the reform efforts of the women administrators turned more to their loyalty to the North, but Sims and Emmet were both loyal Southerners, as was T. Gaillard Thomas, another key physician at the institution from 1861 through the first decades. In this way and in other subtle ways, race and ethnicity came to play in the history of early gynecological surgery.

Though Thomas Emmet's ancestors were not Catholic, his loyalties were clearly to the Irish cause; so much so in fact that he converted to Catholicism not long after he began working at the Woman's Hospital. His wife's involvement in the Church was the reason he gave for his conversion; no doubt loyalty to the Irish cause influenced him as well.[125] Catherine Duncan, whom he married in 1854, was from near Montgomery and was known to Sims since her childhood. As were many Victorian women, Emmet's wife was sickly. He met her at a water cure and retired after marriage with her to a cottage to help her recoup her strength. This was following the birth of their first child.

In finding a position at the Woman's Hospital, Sims's long-standing friendship with Emmet's wife helped to break the ice for him. Emmet recalled that Sims also shared some of his sentiment for the Irish since his heritage was Scotch-Irish. Sims's preference for a young surgeon whose wife was a childhood friend over Emily Blackwell with her impressive credentials is more testimony to the original embrace of gender roles at the hospital—excluding women from medical practice—than it is to Sims's embrace of the Irish people. For a few months, then, Emmet worked at the Woman's Hospital temporarily as Sims's assistant. After the conflict over hiring a woman assistant had passed, Emmet won the official appointment as Sims's assistant and quickly became the Assistant Surgeon, often operating on his own.

Excluding Emily Blackwell from practicing medicine at the hospital clarified the hierarchy at work in the Woman's Hospital, which mirrored the society at large. The influence and significance of the authority of the women was clearly demarcated. Within these boundaries, the Board of Managers contributed handily to the first decades of the institution.

Even though the two sexes worked separately in the administration of the hospital, they shared a cultural belief in the proper roles of men and women. This language was shared by all involved in the hospital throughout the first decades, including physicians. Establishing administrative divisions and articulating a gender code in the constitution for the Woman's Hospital helped, to borrow a phrase from woman's historian Linda Kerber, "maintaining boundaries" of delineated gender activity, without necessarily describing exactly how people acted.[126]

Noteworthy in the hospital administration was a framework for authority that derived from ideological separations of the public and private spheres by gender. Literally adhering to sexual segregation of labor, the women supervised internal affairs, inside the hospital—from checking linen supplies and groceries to managing the nursing staff—while the men governed external affairs, from maintaining the grounds to raising funds from state government. There was only limited overlap in delineated tasks. While the rules were very specific and both women and men relied upon this sexual division as constitutional structure for the institution, in fact the managers were as active publicly as the governors, simply cloaking their work in a cloth of domestic benevolence.

Originally the emphasis in public discourse of the institution lay in the realm of a sex-based notion of motherhood and women and developed only after the Civil War into a language with a class base. In their creed, "As ye have done it unto the least of these, ye have done it unto me," the managers expressed their motive of benevolence and charity while they demonstrated their allegiance to their sex. While they held to the confining code of womanhood in the nineteenth-century Victorian era, they ignored, or failed entirely to see, the economics of its applicability. The language of domesticity assigned women the keeping of the hearth and the maintenance of the home. By the use of female servants at home, the wearing of clothing sewn in sweatshops by women, and the employment of matrons and servants in the hospital, the status of the hospital administrators depended on the broader activities of lower-class women.

Crucial to the dynamic and growth of the Woman's Hospital and the medical practitioners there was the availability of human subjects for exploration of the so-called science of woman. In New York City, these subjects were predominantly Irish. At the hospital there was a steady majority of Irish patients in the first years. Their experiences are described in the next chapter.

CHAPTER 4

Patients and Practice

————⟫⊛⟪————

*I*n the first casebook of clinical records for the Woman's Hospital, the number one entry is Mary Smith. She became a legend at the hospital, somewhat larger than life, representing the hundreds of Irish vesico-vaginal patients who came to the hospital in the first decade of its existence.[1] As an Irish woman, she was certainly not alone, for New York City at midcentury was a city of the Irish. In 1851, at the height of Irish migration to the city, 175,735 Irish-born people were living there, comprising 27.9 percent of the city's population.[2]

As was common among the Irish women patients at the Woman's Hospital, Mary Smith had also immigrated during Ireland's Great Famine. Between 1848 and 1850, the famine had peaked in its devastation, killing more than one million people through starvation and malnutrition. The migration to escape these conditions lasted from 1845 through 1855.[3]

As if a prototype for Malthus's *Essay on Population,* the Irish had reproduced at a very high rate from the late 1700s through the 1820s, only to experience several small famines, including one between 1800 and 1801 and another between 1816 and 1819.[4] A cholera epidemic and typhoid also raged in the early 1830s. While these may have been the "positive checks" Malthus predicted as a "natural" way of maintaining a population balance, in fact the population rebounded from the early famines and was beginning to experience a lesser rate of growth. The age of marriage went up, and women had their first children at an older age. In 1801, Ireland and England became one country, but in reality Ireland was a British colony, with natives, in particular Catholics, having little or no voice in their government. There were some pockets of manufacturing and industrialization in Ireland, but the economic relationship with Great Britain dictated that Ireland serve as a market for English goods and maintain an agricultural economy at home.[5] Potatoes

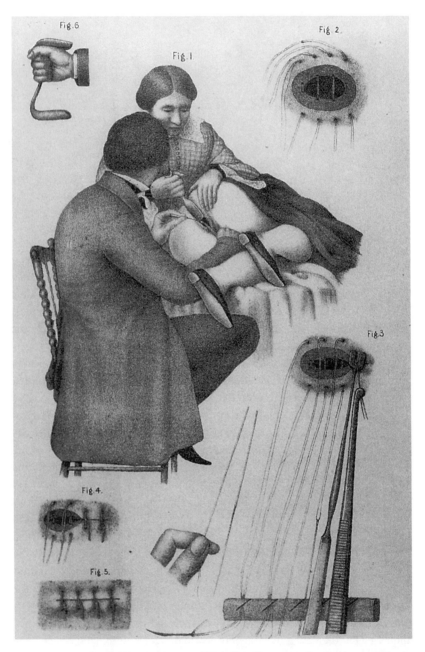

FIGURE 6. Sims and Margaret Brennan, illustrating the steps of vesico-vaginal fistula surgery and the Sims's Position. Dr. Henry Savage, the illustrator, practiced medicine at the Samaritan Hospital with Sir Spencer Wells. In Henry Savage, *The Surgery, Surgical Pathology and Anatomy of the Female Pelvic Organs*, 3d ed. (New York: William Wood, 1880), 117, Plate 24. *(From the Special Collections, Southern Illinois University School of Medicine.)*

gained in popularity because the soil could produce so much more of them per acre than any other crop.

For the most part, until the Great Famine, Irish farmers succeeded in growing enough to feed the British, which was their primary task, and themselves. *Phytophtera infestans*, the potato blight responsible for the famine, was first noticed in the Irish potato harvest of 1845. The crop failure appeared suddenly in a dry rot that destroyed the harvest at the end of the season. During the years of the famine, England was very slow to respond to the needs of the Irish people. At first, the government assumed the famine would last for only one season and calculated that the Irish would be able to endure what seemed to be a minor setback. Unhappily, the famine continued for several years, with the greatest period of starvation in the years 1846 and 1847. Slow to react in the beginning, the British multiplied their error by declaring the famine over prematurely, bringing work projects and what little welfare assistance they offered to an end too soon. The famine killed one of every nine people in Ireland. Although this number was less than that of other major catastrophes in history, the percentage affected was still extraordinarily high, with fatalities more than one million. Yet outside of Ireland, the history of the Great Famine has until recently been largely ignored and seldom told.[6] Many people were not only unable to feed themselves, but also lost their land.

Many of the patients of the hospital were thus Irish. The hospital on Madison Avenue was in a ward where Irish and native-born lived together. There were tenements, but not many boardinghouses. Many of the immigrants were single women, and often they were young. Although families split up in the process of emigrating, individuals, even single youth, managed to sustain their familial ties, often staying with a relative.[7] Irish women frequently found work as servants, wetnurses, or doing piece work in the needle trades and on the streets.[8] Physical problems, most often a result of childbirth, brought them to the Woman's Hospital.

With the help of Thomas Addis Emmet's clinical records, we know some of the details that brought Mary Smith, and others, to the institution. In 1855, at the age of thirty-five, having recently arrived from western Ireland, Mary Smith sought admission to the Woman's Hospital.[9] Her labor for the birth of her first child began in Ireland on a Sunday, fourteen years before her admission in the Woman's Hospital. During her first days of labor, Emmet recorded that the only intervention the midwife offered was a footbath. Likely the midwife also helped her to change positions or perhaps to walk around. However, there is no way to uncover the details of this birth beyond the record left by the physician and the injuries to Mary Smith's body. After four days of labor, birth attendants, using some form of diagnostic measure, listening perhaps for fetal heart tone with an ear to Mary Smith's abdomen, discovered that the infant was dead. As was the practice for many midwives in time of crisis, they sent for the physician. The physician came but did nothing to speed the labor or to facilitate delivery, as far as Mary Smith could remember many years after the birth. In looking back to reconstruct the event, her memory was influenced by her relationship with Sims and Emmet.[10] What she told them was likely different from what she might have recounted for a female relative, for instance. After a week of labor with the dead child likely far advanced in the birth, the corpse was finally delivered. Mary Smith sustained tremendous tears following the birth but miraculously went on to bear two more children. Of the three children she bore, only the middle child was still alive. Where her family was, or if her husband lived, is not noted in the record. She seemed quite alone.

Forty-two years after his first encounter with Mary Smith, Emmet remembered in 1899 the circumstance of the occasion with great detail. The moment symbolized for him his medical practice and charity among the Irish immigrants. Marion Sims was there, as was Margaret Brennan, in her capacity as Sims's nurse. In Emmet's eyes, Margaret Brennan was an Irish woman beyond comparison (whether she was an immigrant or not is not recorded). Although she had no educational background and was unable to read and write, she stayed at the hospital for thirty-seven years as a nurse and was integral to the success of the surgeries. Focusing on Mary Smith, with Emmet serving as the audience, Sims demonstrated the position for pelvic examination and the use of the speculum. Details were vague but Emmet remembered Smith was "a most offensive and loathsome object."[11] Although Emmet, unfamiliar with vesico-vaginal fistulas, could not comprehend the nature of the woman's trouble, he saw a large gray mass in her vagina. Sims, however, discovered a vesico-vaginal fistula among the scar tissue. Scar tissue often masked the fistulas, and part of Sims's skill in the surgery was to be able to identify fistulas behind the scars and to repair them. Working with his characteristic speed and dexterity, he retrieved the mass, which in fact included a wooden ball from a fishing net, from her vagina. Emmet reconstructed that earlier, in Ireland, a physician had embedded the ball in Mary Smith's bladder to forestall a herniated prolapsed bladder. Now, after all these years, tissue adhered to it. Her surrounding and external tissues were profoundly excoriated from the continual seepage of urine. So many years later, Emmet still remembered her anguish and screams of pain as Sims extracted the ball.

This was just the beginning of her medical experiences with Sims, for she eventually underwent at least twenty-four operations. In 1861, just before Marion Sims's unexpected departure for Europe, he repaired Mary Smith's tissues so that her bladder was held in place and no longer prolapsed into her vagina. Although this was something of an improvement in her condition, the traumatic birth had destroyed her urethra and she remained unable to retain urine in her bladder. In retrospect, Emmet was somewhat critical of Sims's abandonment of the case at this point.

With Sims's departure, Emmet, at the age of thirty-three, became the Surgeon-in-Chief for the hospital. Emmet recalled that because the managers of the institution were not happy with Emmet's conversion to Catholicism, they appointed him only with great reluctance. With time they came to admire his contributions to the institution, but only grudgingly. Ignoring their complaints and acting with a fair degree of autonomy, he returned to Mary Smith and used what we know today as plastic surgery techniques to rebuild her urethra. With this surgery, Mary Smith regained the ability to control her urine for several years, during which time she worked as a nurse at the hospital. Later, to Emmet's regret, she turned to Sims for further surgery, to remove stones in her bladder. Emmet lamented the fact that Sims destroyed the delicate tissues of her urethra in the extraction of the stones. She then became, in Emmet's words, "incurable."[12] After a horrible and fruitless struggle to overcome her fistulas and damage from childbirth, Mary Smith became a "common street beggar" and eventually died after a street cart ran her down.[13]

Many questions come to mind when considering the story of Mary Smith's childbirth and subsequent injury, known among physicians in the mid-nineteenth century as an accident of parturition. Emmet's meticulous records give us a rare window on childbirth of the past. Many of the births were horrific, with for instance, cases where the fetal head was delivered but not the infant's body, for hours, even days.

Why was vesico-vaginal fistula so prevalent, even to merit the founding of the Woman's Hospital of the State of New York? How has childbirth changed? What were the experiences for diverse women during this period of economic change? How did the historical experience of birth mirror cultural and social changes? Unfortunately, for the most part the documented births were unpleasant. Their outline and clinical detail, nonetheless, help to elucidate the lives and choices of women who otherwise had no voice or historical presence. The best way to tease apart this narrative of Mary Smith is to begin with the question of the origin of the condition that led to such prolonged labor. Then, following the chronology of birth, we will explore the conditions of labor and finally its outcome.

Where did the vesico-vaginal fistulas originate? The earlier cases of Anarcha, Betsey, and Lucy, as also many of the later cases treated at the Woman's Hospital, began with a prolonged labor. Notes of physicians and a diagnosis of a contracted pelvis suggest that rickets may have created a mis-shaped pelvis, which subsequently meant difficult childbirth. Thomas Addis Emmet analyzed many statistics that he gathered in his medical practice, and he used them in part to find the critical factors at the onset of vesico-vaginal fistulas. Although he was careful to keep clinical records and designate key variables, he does not include rickets or a contracted pelvis in his explora-tion of the etiology of the disease. Hence Mary Smith is not described as having a contracted pelvis. During this time, other physicians sometimes de-scribed women with vesico-vaginal fistulas as also having contracted pelves, or rachitic pelves. It was not until 1881 that *The Science and Art of Midwifery*, written by prominent New York obstetrician William Thompson Lusk, linked vesico-vaginal fistulas and the effects of rickets: "Yet, it is impossible to study the cases of vesico-vaginal fistula reported by Emmet without arriving at the conclusion that the existence of contracted pelves is frequently overlooked."[14] Lusk did not include recognition, if indeed he understood the disease in these terms, of nutrition and poverty as part of the context for the condition of rick-ets. While the standard Irish diet of potatoes and buttermilk was remarkably adequate until the famine, nutritionally the food lacked vitamins A and D, which are necessary for the absorption of calcium and for the prevention of rickets.[15] How well the diet sustained a pregnancy is another issue. The con-ditions preceding and during the Great Famine made the presence of rickets in the Irish population likely.

In this era when the new science of obstetrics was so rudimentary, how did physicians recognize rickets or a contracted pelvis? As with much of nineteenth-century medicine, a key element was the identification of what was normal in childbirth. Building on previous knowledge of the pelvis as inflexible and the potential source of dystocia or difficult childbirth, Jean-Louis Baudelocque, an eighteenth-century French obstetrician, developed techniques of external pelvic measurement known as the "external conjugate of the pelvis." Published in 1781, his method of pelvic mensuration was used for one hundred and fifty years before roentgenography or X rays replaced it.[16] The instrument used to measure the pelvis was the "pelvimeter." Baudeloque's techniques became more understood in 1851 through the work of a German obstetrician, Gustav Adolphus Michaelis.[17] Helping to disseminate the concept of pelvimetry as put forth by William Smellie, Baudeloque used his measurements as a guide to determine whether a woman's pelvis was adequate for birth and whether it was normally formed. While Baudelocque was cautious in his advocacy of the accuracy of external measurement, he was far ahead of his time in understanding the connection between rickets and pelvic measurement. Michaelis's work further demonstrated the inadequacy of external pelvimetry, but his work was not heralded until the twentieth century.[18] In twentieth-century diagnostic practice, however, the availability of X-rays made the technique of external measurement wholly inadequate and misrepresentative in diagnosis.

In 1839, Carl Naegele, another German obstetrician, published *The Obliquely Contracted Pelvis* in German. This work described with words and drawings the qualities of a rarely known misshapen pelvis, a condition not associated with rickets, and its influence on childbirth. One chapter explored rachitic pelvic deformities, which were distinct from the obliquely contracted pelvis.[19] In America, Charles Meigs also mentioned rickets as causing pelvic deformities and difficulty in labor.[20]

One further layer of ambiguity in scientific use of the technique came from a very different discipline in the late eighteenth and early nineteenth centuries. Pelvimetry was also a tool of early physical anthropology and was used alongside the measurement of skulls. Different modes of measurement appeared as a basis of comparing women's bodies, in particular across cultural lines and ranking them, as was the case with skull measurements, in a linear fashion from highest to lowest. Similar to the scholarship that led to the formation of the American School, the use of pelvimetry was profoundly embedded in perceptions of racial differences and went on to emphasize sexual differences and variation in the experiences of giving birth.[21] "Normal" then eventually was reckoned to belong to the representative pelvis of the top-ranked category—the European, but not likely the Irish woman. While there was overall a tendency to rank the female European's ample or capacious pelvis as the highest classification, scholars never used or compared pelves to the extent they had relied upon craniometry in the nineteenth century. The two measurements connected with each other because for obstetrical purposes the measurement was intended to compare the size of the fetal skull with pelvic size to predict the ease or difficulty of birth. The highest rank of pelvis—as distinguished by its ethnic origin—did not necessarily relate to the greatest ease in giving birth. Linked to cultural gender roles, the pelvis became the measure of comparison of women while the skull was the measure of men. Women had a superior size of pelvis, and hence were suited to giving birth; men had the superior-sized skull, and the implication is obvious.[22]

Throughout the population, rickets occurred among the nutritionally deprived and resulted in identifiable bone malformations among children and young adults. Even if pelvimetry was of little use in assessing a woman's likely childbirth experience, through the technique some physicians discovered the importance and presence of rickets in gestating women. Although Lusk did not have access to our twentieth-century knowledge of vitamins and nutrition, unlike Naegele he was aware of vesico-vaginal fistula by name and by incidence among his patients. As with Naegele, Lusk did see that rickets resulted in a misshaped pelvis that was both flat and shallow and, in Naegele's words, most conspicuously the pelvis was marked by a *"contraction of the inlet* anteroposteriorly and *enlargement of the outlet"* (Naegele's emphasis).[23] This condition obviously contributed to difficulty in birth, especially prolonged labor. Lusk also noted that in his practice in New York City, more foreign-born patients suffered from rachitic pelves than the native-born. Lusk, more clearly than Naegele or Meigs and at a time after Sims and other practitioners at the Woman's Hospital had already treated many hundreds of cases of vesico-vaginal fistula, noticed the connections between rickets, childbirth, and vesico-vaginal fistulas.

Today, nutrition experts and medical professionals have access to knowledge about the vitamin and mineral deficiencies that led to the condition of rickets. Nineteenth-century physicians described symptoms, but did not treat the origins of the disease. Even though today we have knowledge about the effects of malnutrition, there are still millions suffering from it and dying. In Ethiopia and Khartoum there are hospitals, one a twenty-one-year-old Fistula Hospital, that treat women with vesico-vaginal fistulas who incurred them during prolonged labor, much as nineteenth-century women had done. The World Health Organization identifies malnutrition and poor living conditions as primary causes of vesico-vaginal fistula.[24]

In addition to rickets, possible causes of fistulas included tissue damage from the use of pessaries (presumably used to keep their uteri in place), and also the presence of syphilitic ulcers, cancer, or what we would recognize today as cervical and vaginal infections.[25]

Ethnicity was a factor which also influenced the incidence of vesico-vaginal fistulas. As a component of social structure today and in the nineteenth century, it reflects the economic and social status of certain groups. Ethnicity also may determine the quality of health care, rather than be a reason for certain medical conditions.

In his 1868 text on vesico-vaginal fistula, Emmet described in detail seventy-three cases from the Woman's Hospital.[26] Although he was inconsistent in reporting the ethnic origins of the women, he did write down that many of them were Irish. In 1899, Emmet recalled that "out of 200 cases, 58% had been immigrants" (from Great Britain, Scotland and western Ireland).[27] Several other physicians, contemporaries of Emmet and Sims, reported on victims of vesico-vaginal fistulas from various ethnic origins. Dr. M. Schuppert described several women on whom he operated in New Orleans. Some were German immigrants, others were Irish. In addition, Schuppert treated slave women. Dr. Nathan Bozeman also reported on several afflicted slave patients.[28]

There is no way to determine precisely the extent of those injured by vesico-vaginal fistula. Because the condition was not fatal, records of its occurrence are very limited. While most of the patients were immigrants and members of ethnic groups considered as "other," vesico-vaginal fistula's prevalence seemed fairly high throughout the total population. Fleetwood Churchill, a physician in an Irish lying-in hospital and author of a well-used text in midwifery, somewhat reluctantly suggested before the establishment of the Woman's Hospital that "perforations of the coats of the vagina, anteriorly or posteriorly, with the subjacent organs, the bladder or rectum, is [*sic*] not very rare."[29] In the 1856 memorial for the Woman's Hospital, presented in Albany, advocates described patients as coming "not only from New York and the adjoining states, but also from Louisiana, Mississippi, Tennessee, Canada, and even from Central America."[30]

In the nineteenth century, women from northern Europe spent long winters indoors; upper-class women, particularly those of European origins, found paleness fashionable and sheltered themselves from the sunlight, thus depriving themselves of a crucial source of vitamins necessary for the absorption of calcium. Ethnicity was a social category, to a degree artificially separating those who suffered from vesico-vaginal fistula. Just as not all the Irish were poor or malnourished, not all the vesico-vaginal fistula patients were Irish, African American, or poor working-class women.

Even though the Great Famine had a substantial effect on the lives of immigrants, and on the experience of childbirth, the culture and politics of Ireland also played a part. Ireland shared the controversy of midwives versus other medical care but also had a fairly long history of male midwifery and medical attendance.[31]

In his book *Vesico-Vaginal Fistula* (1868), which described patients from the Woman's Hospital, Thomas Addis Emmet reported that many of the Irish

A COMPARISON BETWEEN DIFFERENT MODES OF DELIVERY. — AVERAGE TIME IN LABOR. — AND MEAT. — WHERE VESICO-VAGINAL FISTULA RESULTED.

MODE OF DELIVERY		CURED			IMPROVED			NOT IMPROVED			DIED			RESULT NOT GIVEN	
		No. of Cases	Hours in Labor	Weeks under Treatment	No. of Cases	Hours in Labor	Weeks under Treatment	No. of Cases	Hours in Labor	Weeks under Treatment	No. of Cases	Hours in Labor	Weeks under Treatment	No. of Cases	Hours in Labor	Weeks under Treatment
Forceps.		67	60.29	16.82	5	35.30	25.40	1	48.00	8.00	–	–	–	1	36.00	4.00
Ergot and Forceps.		8	46.00	12.42	–	–	–	–	–	–	–	–	–	–	–	–
Craniotomy.		11	47.77	14.45	2	57.00	16.00	–	–	–	1	103.00	6.00	–	–	–
Version and Craniotomy.		2	22.50	9.00	–	–	–	–	–	–	–	–	–	–	–	–
Version.		3	9.00	7.53	–	–	–	–	–	–	–	–	–	–	–	–
Version and Forceps.		2	46.00	36.00	–	–	–	–	–	–	–	–	–	–	–	–
Traction made to deliver the body, pains having ceased after birth of head.		9	77.22	8.33	–	–	–	–	–	–	–	–	–	–	–	–
TOTAL OF CASES OF ARTIFICIAL DELIVERY.	Number of Cases.	100	–	–	7	–	–	1	–	–	1	–	–	1	–	–
	Av. Time in Labor.	–	71.67	–	–	76.00	–	–	48.00	–	–	103.00	–	–	36.00	–
	Av. Time under Treatment.	–	–	15.24	–	–	22.85	–	–	8.00	–	–	6.00	–	–	4.00
TOTAL OF CASES DELIVERED BY THE UNAIDED EFFORTS OF NATURE.	Number of Cases.	27	–	–	2	–	–	2	–	–	–	–	–	1	–	–
	Av. Time in Labor.	–	50.81	–	–	39.00	–	–	26.00	–	–	–	–	–	48.00	–
	Av. Time under Treatment.	–	–	19.68	–	–	34.00	–	–	4.00	–	–	–	–	–	73.00
TOTAL OF CASES DELIVERED BY USE OF ERGOT.	Number of Cases.	6	–	–	–	–	–	–	–	–	–	–	–	–	–	–
	Av. Time in Labor.	–	61.66	–	–	–	–	–	–	–	–	–	–	–	–	–
	Av. Time under Treatment.	–	–	34.83	–	–	–	–	–	–	–	–	–	–	–	–
TOTAL OF CASES WHERE MODE OF DELIVERY WAS NOT STATED.	Number of Cases.	13	–	–	–	–	–	–	–	–	–	–	–	–	–	–
	Av. Time in Labor.	–	55.00	–	–	–	–	–	–	–	–	–	–	–	–	–
	Av. Time under Treatment.	–	–	14.92	–	–	–	–	–	–	–	–	–	–	–	–
TOTAL OF ALL CASES.	Number of Cases.	146	–	–	9	–	–	3	–	–	1	–	–	2	–	–
	Av. Time in Labor.	–	64.38	–	–	61.91	–	–	33.33	–	–	103.00	–	–	42.00	–
	Av. Time under Treatment.	–	–	16.82	–	–	25.44	–	–	5.33	–	–	6.00	–	–	41.00

FIGURE 7. Chart on the origins of vesico-vaginal fistula by Thomas Addis Emmet from his essay, "The Necessity for Early Delivery, as Demonstrated by the Analysis of One Hundred and Sixty-One Cases of Vesico-Vaginal Fistula." (*Transactions of the American Gynecological Society* 3 [1878]: 116.)

	TIME UNDER TREAT-			THE SAME COMPARISON MADE WHERE THE CHILDREN WERE STILLBORN. — WITH THE CONDITION OF THE BLADDER DURING LABOR — AND ESCAPE OF URINE AFTERWARDS.											
TOTAL.				STILLBORN.				CONDITION OF BLADDER DURING THE TIME OF LABOR.				ESCAPE OF URINE AFTER LABOR.			
No. of Cases.	Av. Time.		Percentage on the Mode of Delivery.	No. of Cases.	Average Time in Labor.	Average Time in Treatment.	No. of very Large Children.	Emptied, Number of Cases.	Not Emptied, Number of Cases.	Average Time of Retention, in Hours.	No Mention made in History of Case.	No. of Cases from Delivery.	No. of Cases after Delivery.	Average Number of Days after.	No Mention made in History of Case.
	Hours in Labor.	Weeks under Treatment.													
74	68.55	17.13	45.90	34	76.64	15.58	12	8	6	67.50	20	13	16	8.57	5
6	46.00	12.42	3.78	6	46.00	13.50	2	2	-	-	4	8	2	11.50	1
14	61.25	14.07	8.70	13	53.33	15.00	4	2	4	57.25	7	6	4	10.16	1
2	22.50	9.00	1.24	1	28.00	9.00	-	-	-	-	1	-	-	-	1
3	9.00	7.33	1.80	2	13.00	7.50	-	1	-	-	1	2	-	-	-
2	48.00	36.00	1.24	2	46.00	36.00	-	-	-	-	1	-	-	-	2
9	77.22	8.33	5.59	8	78.00	8.75	1	1	3	71.33	4	3	5	11.00	-
110	-	-	68.32	66	-	-	19	14	13	63.27	38	27	23	9.06	10
-	62.82	-	-	-	66.07	-	-	-	-	-	-	-	-	-	-
-	-	15.48	-	-	-	13.70	-	-	-	-	-	-	-	-	-
32	-	-	19.88	16	-	-	7	3	4	50.25	8	-	13	10.34	3
-	44.44	-	-	-	46.73	-	-	-	-	-	-	-	-	-	-
-	-	21.37	-	-	-	12.31	-	-	-	-	-	-	-	-	-
6	-	-	3.73	5	-	-	4	-	4	86.25	1	3	1	2.00	1
-	61.66	-	-	-	64.00	-	-	-	-	-	-	-	-	-	-
-	-	34.83	-	-	-	41.00	-	-	-	-	-	-	-	-	-
13	-	-	8.07	-	-	-	-	-	-	-	-	-	-	-	-
-	55.00	-	-	-	-	-	-	-	-	-	-	-	-	-	-
-	-	14.92	-	-	-	-	-	-	-	-	-	-	-	-	-
161	-	-	-	86	-	-	30	17	21	66.83	47	30	43	9.67	14
-	58.61	-	-	-	62.39	-	-	-	-	-	-	-	-	-	-
-	-	17.32	-	-	-	15.45	-	-	-	-	-	-	-	-	-

patients who came to the hospital had only recently arrived in New York City—perhaps a month earlier. A European colleague had questioned him about the large number of vesico-vaginal fistula patients, implying, Emmet seemed to think, malpractice among American obstetricians. Emmet's response was to compile records and document the origins of the cases. He discovered that many of the vesico-vaginal fistula patients came to the United States already suffering with the tears of childbirth. They "often averaged a little less than one month between the date of their arrival in the country and their admission to the Woman's Hospital. . . . Great Britain, and the poorhouses in the west of Ireland and northern portions of Scotland had sent this country the accumulation of years."[32] Once an institutional locus became known to the European medical world—especially England and Ireland—where women with the condition could be treated, governments and welfare organizations sent them to New York City. Mary Smith, too, came to the hospital soon after her arrival.

The origin of vesico-vaginal fistula may have had to do with the nature of the practices governing childbirth. Did the childbirth itself cause the fistula, or was it somehow due to the medical or lay supervision and/or intervention in the birth? Although Ireland's population was predominantly rural, hospitalized and medically governed childbirth was much more common there than in the United States.[33] Immigrants who had come from small farms, however, still often adhered to folk remedies and used local healers.[34] Emmet, in identifying with the Irish as his people, impressed upon the Irish patients to pursue a more middle-class way of life. Irish American professionals witnessed the stereotyping of the Irish as filthy and disease-ridden and sought to help change that characterization. As Emmet collected his clinical data, he identified nativity as a key factor in the etiology of vesico-vaginal fistula. His view of the significance of race or ethnicity was paramount in describing the incidence of the condition and in identifying the obstetrical treatment of the patient, thereby vindicating American physicians.

Another way to look through the narrative of one birth as exemplifying a larger experience is to ask what Mary Smith expected as she prepared to give birth to her first child before she left Ireland. Apparently she went to a midwife as the primary expert and support for her expected delivery. How much preliminary prenatal care there was cannot be known. Probably not much, except through an informal web of social relations and the spiritual and religious communality among her female friends and family.

As we look back to discover the history and origins of vesico-vaginal fistula, we lose sight of the overriding fear of death that accompanied pregnancy, labor, and delivery.[35] A laboring woman could easily die during labor—often because of prolonged labor with no skillful intervention or assistance. Puerperal fever was a major killer of women following birth, especially those under medical supervision. This disease was common in hospital wards when unwitting doctors did not know to wash their hands and carried a killer streptococcus bacteria to their patients.[36] By reading between the lines of a clinical record we cannot easily unearth the fears and feelings of those made objects in the medical arena.

The practice of midwifery was much stronger spiritually than obstetrics, and it was associated with a cosmology that united the physical and spirit worlds. It was also less hierarchical and hence more "democratic" than the physician/patient relationship.[37] Midwives, who were severely affected by the colonization of Ireland by England, implicated in the persecution of Catholicism, and became lost in the devastation of the Great Famine and immigration, were undoubtedly absent when they were needed most. Perhaps the twenty-one-year-old Mary Smith and women like her were familiar with the consequence of vaginal tears and urinary incontinence, but likely this was not their greatest fear in childbirth.

Mary Smith's case was emblematic of Irish vesico-vaginal fistula victims. How did her labor go? For one, it was extremely prolonged. There was a full week between the onset of labor and the delivery of her first child. In these cases, lengthy labor typically caused the impaction of the fetal head on the mother's *symphysis pubis*, her bony pubic floor. In the seventy-three cases described in Emmet's text on vesico-vaginal fistula, the average length of labor was sixty-four hours, nearly three days and nights. Emmet defined labor as the period beginning with the rupture of the bag of waters. Hence, the average three days and nights varied according to the intensity of contractions and did not always include the unremitting contractions known today as hard labor. On the other hand, depending on the individual and the circumstances, this measurement could describe an unfathomably long labor. Part of the difficulty determining the measure of a normal nineteenth-century birth is that there was no absolute standard of a birth, as is true even today. In the nineteenth century, when medical science was just beginning to establish the parameters of a "normal" birth, physicians collected and published lengthy statistical reports of their obstetric experiences and recorded the difficulties or extraordinary circumstances that occurred, but variations still persisted. In his tabulations of clinical records for vesico-vaginal fistulas, Emmet included length of labor as a key factor.

Notwithstanding the lack of a standard, Emmet's clinical descriptions of births preceding incursion of vesico-vaginal fistulas leave no doubt about their extreme difficulty and the suffering involved. Alternatives for the parturient besides lying in bed seemed few. The most striking fact throughout these descriptions is the prevalence of births that were close to completion, up to the last stages with the head out or nearly out, yet full birth did not occur for excruciatingly long periods of time. Several times Emmet described the infant's head as crowning, having reached the perineum (the perineum being the skin stretching between the vaginal and anal opening), when the final strong uterine push simply dissipated and the birth stopped prematurely. Sometimes the head of the infant was born hours, or even days, before the rest of the body came. Emmet noted the ineptitude of those managing the births in these cases. The result would certainly involve the woman's extensive loss of tissue.

With births such as these, medical practitioners who described the situations had differing versions of how far the fetal head advanced before the birth was blocked. Besides the Emmet examples, Marion Sims also described instances of fistula occurring after a birth in which the head could not get past the cervix; in other words, the dilation of the cervix was insufficient to admit the passage of the fetal cranium. Others described a birth in which the infant was nearly born, but was held back by the rigidity of the perineum. Today, in hospitals in industrialized countries, such instances of an inflexible perineum obstructing birth do not occur. Present-day routine episiotomies obviate the possibility of such an occurrence. They were, however, controversial in Sims's time and were performed only infrequently.[38]

Closely tied to the damage caused by the impacted head of the infant was the frequent retention of urine by the woman in labor. In the cases described by Emmet, several women endured lengthy labors, sometimes for days—without urinating. Mary Smith's labor lasted one week, and she did not urinate for the duration. A bladder distended with urine represented a serious obstacle to the speedy and smooth progression of labor. Others were unable to urinate for several days after giving birth. As Emmet himself said, "Beyond question, in the majority of cases, a neglect to empty the bladder has, by retarding the progress of labor, proved an indirect cause of vesico-vaginal fistula."[39]

Texts on midwifery written by early nineteenth-century physicians noted that full bladders often resulted in fistulas and cautioned doctors to determine their presence during labor.[40] If the woman in labor could not relieve herself, catheters were sometimes suggested. Emmet, however, did not publicly urge medical professionals to encourage urination during labor until the

publication of his gynecology text in 1869. Even then, he described urine retention as an indirect cause. In a paper presented before the American Gynecological Association, he urged his audience to understand the blockage a
distended bladder presented in the birth canal as the fetus pushed toward delivery.[41] A full bladder was a physical impediment to birth and undoubtedly
contributed directly to a prolonged labor.

   Why did some women fail to urinate during labor? This happened so
commonly as to suggest that women either assumed a passive role in labor
or were overcome with fear and anxiety. They certainly distanced themselves
from their own biological functioning. It is also appropriate to question the
direction and guidance, if any, they received during labor. Later, after the
1860s, some physicians were more eager to apply a catheter than to assist
the woman in urinating on her own. Churchill, in his text on midwifery, urged
physicians to encourage women to change position in order to facilitate labor and to prevent a full bladder.[42] Unfortunately, the largely oral—as opposed to written—history of female midwifery prevents knowing their
practices during labor. Although there were variations among cultures and
individuals in midwifery, it is virtually certain that these women did not often use catheters to drain urine from the bladders of women in labor; probably they did not use them at all. Many physicians recognized that before
using instrumental intervention, physicians had to find a way to empty the
woman's bladder, if not voluntarily then with the use of a catheter. These historical clinical records help us to see that, in this time of extensive conflict
in several countries between medicine and midwifery, many women received
little or no assistance and experienced a high level of fear and discomfort in
childbirth, especially when the labor did not progress. They may then have
been unable to move from bed, and even unable to relax the pelvic muscles
enough to urinate. Nor did they know to get up out of bed, change position,
or walk during labor to help speed delivery.[43]

   Unlike the centuries-old female-dominated practice of midwifery, male
medical dominance in childbirth was very new. While medical education was
increasingly denied to women and efforts were made to stop the practice of
female midwifery, no recognition or reciprocal acknowledgment of the experiential knowledge of female midwives occurred.[44] This was a great loss,
particularly for women giving birth. An excellent example lies in the history
of the use of ergot. Ergot, an oxytocic found in a rye grain fungus, was one
of the tools midwives had used for centuries to speed labor through the in-
tensification of contractions. Learning of the drug potential but lacking par-
ticulars of dosage, physicians began to use ergot early in the nineteenth

century. Its utility as the expediter of labor and birth was quickly embraced. Unfortunately, when misused, especially when overdosed, ergot caused violent contractions and fetal death.[45] When ergot failed to speed the contractions and bring labor to its conclusion, physicians had the option of using instruments. Sometimes these medical instruments themselves played a role in the incidence of vesico-vaginal fistula. Physicians disagreed about the use of forceps and changed their patterns and position on the matter over time. Many listed the misuse and clumsy handling of the forceps, even a catheter, and occasionally the tools of craniotomy during delivery as a possible cause of vaginal damage.[46] Others argued the need to resort to instrumental intervention more readily. The difficulty lay in the fact of the prolonged labor itself. Without instruments the woman might persist in a fruitless labor until both she and the infant were dead. David Hayes Agnew, a well-known Philadelphia practitioner, reflected the opinion of many medical educators of his time in his text:

> Wounds of the vesico-vaginal septum terminating in fistula follow both the legitimate and the criminal use of instruments. The maladroit use of the vectid in attempts to rectify a vicious position of the foetal head, or of the perforator in performing craniotomy, may cause this accident, as these instruments are liable to slip and open the bladder. Even the forceps have been charged with playing an important part, I know of no means so well calculated to prevent the accident as the timely employment of this instrument in skillful hands.[47]

Forceps were beneficial, but only when managed by "skillful hands." Both Sims and Emmet joined Agnew to strongly argue for the use of forceps as a *preventative* measure. In 1858, Sims wrote in a published letter to Fordyce Barker: "These fistulas are sometimes produced by laceration, but most commonly by a slough which is generally in proportion to the duration and degree of impaction, whether instruments are used or not. Instruments are often blamed for injuries which are produced, not by their use, but by the want of timely application; in other words, by the prolonged pressure of the foetal head, before they are resorted to."[48] Emmet reiterated the same argument several times: "I do not hesitate to make the statement that I have never met with a case of vesico-vaginal fistula, which, without doubt, could be shown to have resulted from instrumental delivery. On the contrary, the entire weight of evidence is conclusive in proving that the injury is a consequence of delay in delivery."[49]

In a publication of 1878, Emmet put forth what he considered to be his ideas concerning "the cause of the injury [vesico-vaginal fistula] . . . and . . . the means and mode of preventing it."[50] In this paper Emmet urged "the necessity for an early delivery," with obvious emphasis on the intervention in labor with forceps. Emmet added that the use of forceps presented a viable option in a prolonged labor only if the bladder of the parturient woman was empty. He then advocated the use of a catheter preceding the use of forceps.

There was an animated discussion following Emmet's paper among the physicians present, including Dr. Fordyce Barker, Dr. John Atlee of Lancaster, Pennsylvania (an acclaimed ovariotomist), and Dr. White of Buffalo, New York (the obstetrician involved in the renowned Loomis Trial of 1850).[51] These men were unable to agree on the proper moment of intervention in labor with forceps. During much of the nineteenth century, there was reluctance among medical men to intrude in labor and an accompanying uncertainty about the proper time at which to do so. Emmet argued that the forceps should be used when the fetal head receded from the cervix. Others disagreed. Whenever the forceps might be applied, Emmet never maintained that the use of forceps would eliminate fistula altogether, only that forceps would help to prevent tears.[52] Discourse focusing on Emmet's research into the origins of vesico-vaginal fistula became a debate over the use of instruments and medical procedure. In a similar vein in 1880, Mary Jordan Finley, a medical student at the Woman's Medical College of Pennsylvania, presented a doctoral thesis on vesico-vaginal fistula. The thrust of her argument was to advocate the use of forceps. Like Emmet, she argued that, more often than not, physicians waited too long to apply the forceps: "It is true that improperly applied and rudely handled forceps may cause a laceration of the vaginal wall. Yet it is scarcely conceivable that even they could do more damage than the long continued pressure."[53] She added that "the distention of the bladder undoubtedly assists in bringing about this unfortunate result."[54] Also in accord with Emmet, Finley saw the failure to urinate during labor to be of some consequence. Yet she and Emmet both focused their arguments on the great advantage in expediting labor through the intervention with forceps.

Emmet's line of reasoning was not above question. We might interpret his statistics either as a defense of the use of forceps in childbirth, or as a critique thereof. More than 50 percent of the cases examined in either of Emmet's texts originated in childbirth where forceps were employed. At the same time, such prolonged labor argues indeed for the necessity of instrumental intervention. However, the fact that a substantial number of women experienced such intervention and still sustained the tears of vesico-vaginal fistula suggests that the use of forceps was not absolute assurance for good health following childbirth.

Here we have clear evidence of physicians in the 1870s urging one another on in the use of forceps. This clarifies the history of childbirth and its relationship to the use of forceps. While physicians gained access to forceps in the late 1700s, many years passed before they used them with ease or regularity.[55]

Even in relation to the use of technology, a substantial part of the history of childbirth is a rite of passage. Physicians came into cultural authority as representing science and the social structure of the larger political and economic system when they began to supervise childbirth.[56] With eighteenth-century changes in the Western world, including various degrees of embracing industrialization and capitalism, women came to symbolize "nature's body." They were the link between men and nature; nature and women's bodies were now objects for the study of science. Following the work of the eighteenth-century scientist Carolus Linnaeus, female breasts became the basis of the natural history classification of "mammals."[57] Childbirth and women's medicine were the proving ground for shifts in cosmology in the eighteenth and nineteenth centuries. Physicians with forceps in hand, even though they would not use them for decades, became a symbol of power—instruments they could retrieve for problematic births.[58]

Women were both active participants and victims in the creation of this rite of passage. In part, social class provided a set of guidelines or a combination of what their mothers had done during birth and what their friends and culture put forth as a pattern. For some women, tangible problems arose from various sources such as rickets and nutritional deprivation and/or a whole gambit of family-inherited potential weaknesses in birthing, and perhaps also some social context, such as famine or slavery. These women's births and lives were woven into the textured pattern emerging for childbirth, and for women's health as well.

A present-day French physician, Michel Odent, puts forth a radical notion for arranging or situating childbirth today—devised for the individual parturient woman. He argues that laboring women alone and left to themselves (with help nearby if necessary) can best and most easily give birth. While contention arises from his ideas, the underlying concept is that women know how to give birth without medical intervention because they have the same knowledge and capabilities as other animals. What happened in the eighteenth and nineteenth centuries was further manipulation and distancing of all humans from the most natural act of birth—civilization, if you will. Odent's view of birth shifts our perspective enough to help to explain how women and men created and supported a birth ritual in which women lay flat on their backs in feather beds covered with sheets and clothing. A male physician supervised, with his eyes averted and only his hands allowed to feel his way through birth under the sheets. Each and every birth did not happen this way, but that prototype emerged as a childbirth ritual of the dominant culture.[59]

None of these issues were clear or felt by physicians in the mid-nineteenth century. In fact, many complex and confounding aspects of their surrounding culture—especially those emanating from social and economic relations—prevented them from seeing the limitations to their arguments. Just as Emmet was quick to defend the medical practitioner and to urge the practitioner on in the use of forceps, so he easily condemned the midwife for the misuse of ergot. By the 1870s Emmet, like others, including Fordyce Barker, sought to eliminate the use of ergot to speed a labor that had stultified—a prolonged labor in which dilation had ceased and the fetus no longer made headway into the birth canal—the characteristic labor of the vesico-vaginal fistula patient. Emmet claimed that the case histories of women to whom ergot was administered showed that many were attended by "irresponsible women," reaffirming his belief that the medical profession was blameless and the use of forceps a necessity.[60] He included the use (or rather the misuse) of ergot during delivery as a central factor in understanding the origin of vesico-vaginal fistulas. The reality was that male medical practitioners frequently joined female midwives in the use of ergot and they, not the midwives, were most likely to misuse it.[61]

Doctors also resorted to the use of craniotomies, and traction when the labor failed to progress. Many physicians were reluctant to use these tools, since the outcome of such interferences was often fatal for the infant or possibly damaging for the woman in labor.[62] In the instance of a craniotomy or the use of traction, the infant had no chance of survival. During a craniotomy the skull of the fetus was perforated and emptied so that the fetal head could collapse and pass through the birth canal. Traction involved manually pulling on various parts of the infant in order to complete delivery.

Resulting from unknown factors but doubtless including overdosage of ergot, a penetrating and dark side of nineteenth-century childbirth, accompanying cases of vesico-vaginal fistula, was the high percentage of stillbirths. In the cases described by Emmet in his text on vesico-vaginal fistulas, at least fifty-nine of the seventy-three births were stillbirths. In his article of 1878 he quantified the number of stillbirths at 50 percent among the cases he

TABLE 1. *Childbirth Statistics from Vesico-Vaginal Fistula Cases, 1861–1867*

Ethnicity	% Still-births	Average Length of Labor (hours)	% Forcep Deliveries	Average Age at V.V.F. Birth (years)	N
U.S.	78	66	51	30	39
All Non-U.S.	100	59	52	27	29
Irish:	(100)	(60)	(62)	(30)	(21)
Not Indicated	100	75	60	29	5
Total (average)	89	64	52	29	73

Source: Thomas A. Emmet, *Vestico-Vaginal Fistula from Parturition and Other Causes with Cases of Recto-Vaginal Fistula* (New York: William Wood & Co., 1868).

compiled. Table 1 shows that among immigrant patients at the Woman's Hospital before 1868, the rate of stillbirth was 100 percent. While there was a common ground among all the women represented in the table, such an absolute certainty of stillbirth among the group ethnically defined as "other" gives us pause. Although the rate of infant mortality was tremendously high in this period (in 1850 New York City overall, death consumed 52 percent of children under five), the immigrant infant and child mortality was even higher.[63]

A first reading of Emmet's book *Vesico-Vaginal Fistula* is shocking. It parades case after case of stillbirth and horrendous labor all in a clinical and flat tone. The book is organized by the nature of the wound or fistula, and cases were selected by their exemplariness for medical procedure. Emmet's policy and that of other physicians was to use the lowest social category—the poor Irish state patient, for instance—as public clinical evidence to discuss in a journal or book. For the most part, physicians spent their energy trying to save mothers and became inured to the death of unborn or newly born children.

Emmet presented his information somewhat haphazardly. Occasionally he failed to describe the outcome of a birth—whether the child survived or not. David Agnew reported that twelve of eighteen births were stillbirths among his vesico-vaginal fistula patients. Stillbirths were not unknown among the population as a whole.[64] Such a high rate of death, a fairly late age for many women giving birth to their first child, and often a very large child at birth suggest that further unexplored gestational metabolic problems—perhaps gestational diabetes—influenced such bad birth outcomes. Whatever the case, the prevalence of stillbirths stands in stark relief for the modern reader.

What remains unclear is how the mother rebounded from the loss of a newborn, particularly when the death followed an instrumental delivery. To some degree, at least, scholars ought not to separate the health of mothers from that of their infants. Though Emmet may not have considered the connection between the infant's death and the health of the mother, the connection seems certain. The fact that 59 of 73 of Emmet's case studies originated in the delivery of a stillborn child underscores the tie between the mother and the child.[65] Death of the child, combined with the intervention of instruments during birth, especially those employed to destroy the fetus, almost certainly slowed the mother's ability to recover.

Mary Smith's case exemplified one woman's inability to recover. Repeated surgeries could not render her able to engage in her life fully. Other cases showed some ambiguity in recovery. Indeed, according to some, Sims's surgical triumph at midcentury was not as perfect as it might have seemed. Both Thomas Addis Emmet and Nathan Bozeman reported instances of failure of the surgeries Sims performed. Lax in the keeping of records, Sims lacked rigor in surgical follow-up. Although cases were almost routinely labeled "cured," in fact a "cure" was not defined. Presumably a patient might have recovered from the fistula and ceased to suffer incontinence, only to endure a subsequent pregnancy. The process of childbirth and delivery might reopen the scar tissue or somehow aggravate the vaginal tissues to create new tears. Also, a woman with a contracted pelvis would repeatedly suffer from prolonged labor. William Lusk maintained that such a woman would be more likely to suffer further complications after several pregnancies. Even after the perfection of Sims's technique, repeated operations were common in the treatment of the condition and suggest that completely rectifying the tears was a difficult process, and not one accompanied by guarantees of success.

Mary Smith's clinical record opens a window on childbirth experiences and the incidence of vesico-vaginal fistulas. The graphic and horrific detail of her clinical record and the statistics charting others underscores the difficulty of these women's lives and their need for health care. The following chapter charts the course of medical innovation that accompanied surgeries for vesico-vaginal fistulas at the Woman's Hospital.

CHAPTER 5

A School for Gynecologists

———— >●<————

$\mathcal{T}$reating vesico-vaginal fistulas surgically represented part of what made the Woman's Hospital so significant and well known, and celebrated across generations of physicians. Beyond that there was the medically historical moment in midcentury New York City, involving several innovative surgeons and a network of institutions, philanthropists, women reformers, and patients—all of whom were essential to the dynamic that existed at the Woman's Hospital. Although the ramifications were felt for many decades and the hospital and the surgeons are still recognized today, the surge of attention to medical practice and change had peaked in the 1860s and early 1870s.

Professional publications present important documentation of the unfolding and specialization in gynecology. In 1862, soon after the establishment of the Woman's Hospital, the first volume of the *Bulletin of the New York Academy of Medicine* was published, recording activities from the Academy's meetings in New York City from 1860 through 1862. Its contents reflect the priorities of medical scholarship, the texture of medical exchange in New York City, and the role played by doctors and medical workers at the Woman's Hospital. Included were transcriptions of papers read at meetings, including the discussions that followed, and the names of the individuals who were present and participating. Interspersed throughout is a variety of information deemed important to the Academy but not part of formal presentations. Involved in the journal's publication were all four surgeons who would later, in 1872, serve together as head surgeons and constitute the Medical Board at the Woman's Hospital: T. Gaillard Thomas, Edmund R. Peaslee, Thomas Addis Emmet, and J. Marion Sims. Sims, who was back briefly from Europe, participated in the Academy's meetings. Also prominent was Fordyce Barker. Others included G. T. Elliot, Alexander H. Stevens, and Augustus

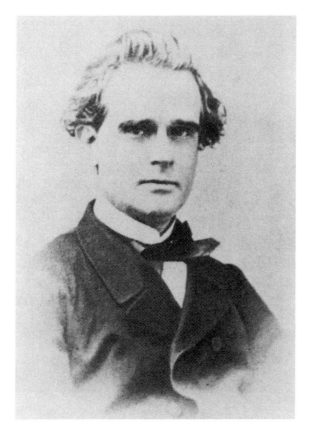

FIGURE 8.   J. Marion Sims. *(Courtesy of the Bolling Medical Library, St. Luke's–Roosevelt Hospital Center, New York.)*

Gardner. Topics reflected an interest in gynecology, such as amputation of the cervix and treatment of uterine diseases. Included in volume 1 was a report of the vaginismus case discussed in chapter 1 of this book.

Theodore Gaillard Thomas (1831–1903), who was almost the same age as Emmet, began his association with the Woman's Hospital in the early 1860s. When Sims prepared to leave the country, he asked Thomas to join Foster Swift in providing clinics for the outdoor department. Like Sims, Thomas was born in South Carolina. Growing up on Edisto Island, the son of an Anglican minister, Thomas experienced a society based on a rice culture and large plantations that typified the Carolina coast. This was a community that fostered the creation of the Gullah language among African Americans

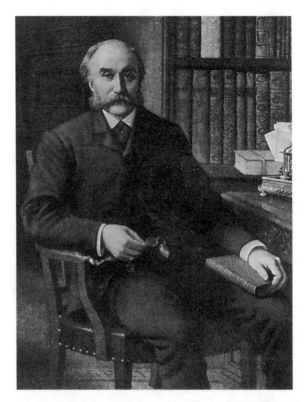

FIGURE 9. Thomas Addis Emmet. *(Courtesy of the Bolling Medical Library, St. Luke's–Roosevelt Hospital Center, New York.)*

and made other noteworthy contributions to agriculture and society.[1] Thomas was not directly tied to the slave economy in his adulthood but he, Emmet, and Sims had a strong bond as a result of their antebellum Southern ties.

As Sims had done approximately thirty years earlier, Thomas attended the Medical College of South Carolina.[2] He graduated in 1852 at the age of twenty-one and went to New York on a steamship, seeking experience and adventure. Although he never wrote about his coming of age, he surely gained clinical experience beyond measure in the two hospitals where he interned: Bellevue Hospital and the Emigrant Hospital on Ward's Island (under the supervision of Emmet). Along with Emmet, Thomas practiced on Ward's Island during peak years of the Irish migration. Following the pattern of the best physicians in his day, Thomas then spent two years abroad, in Dublin and Paris. In Dublin he worked under A. H. McClintock, a renowned obstetrician at the Rotunda Hospital. With his travels and studies abroad, Thomas gained acquaintance with the study of pathology and clinical medicine. His later writings revealed the broad classical background in languages and history he acquired in the course of his education. After he returned to New York, he established a practice with John T. Metcalfe, a prominent New York obstetrician also associated with the Woman's Hospital. Metcalfe invited Thomas to be a partner in Metcalfe's thriving private practice. As he emerged as a key figure in the creation of the specialty of surgical gynecology, Thomas's experiential strength lay with obstetrics. Without a doubt his gynecological innovations emerged out of the practice of medical governance of childbirth, known by some then as male midwifery.

Although both Emmet and Thomas volunteered to serve the Confederacy at the beginning of the Civil War, neither found his way into military service. Thomas thus became a key figure at the hospital during the war years, along with Thomas Addis Emmet. Somewhat earlier than the time of his initial position at the Woman's Hospital, Thomas had won an appointment as visiting obstetrician at Bellevue Hospital, where he practiced for many years. Thomas held a position as professor of obstetrics and also taught clinical diagnosis at the Bellevue Medical School, replacing Gunning S. Bedford as Head of Obstetrics at Bellevue Medical College in 1862. Bedford, a prominent obstetrician in his own right, in 1850 had started the first outdoor clinic in obstetrics in New York City. In 1863 Thomas resigned the Bellevue position to become Professor of Obstetrics at the College of Physicians and Surgeons. After two years he became Professor of Obstetrics and the Diseases of Women and Children at that institution. In addition, Thomas was consulting physician at Nursery and Child's Hospital—where Sarah Doremus volunteered and which was associated with New York Hospital—Elizabeth Blackwell's New York Infirmary for Women and Children, and Roosevelt Hospital, among others.[3]

Thomas's example is important because his various associations, and in particular his several years at Bellevue Hospital and the Bellevue Medical School, illustrate the web of hospital activity that connected the Woman's Hospital throughout Manhattan. The exchange was among physicians, medical faculty, women health reformers, and patients. Medical education and hospital work were becoming closely intertwined, in fact remarkably separated from more traditional academic campuses.[4] Even though the Woman's Hospital was a small institution, its base was very large, involving patients, physicians, and administrators from the biggest hospital in New York City—Bellevue— only a few blocks away. In the years immediately following the Civil War,

Bellevue Medical School gained a competitive edge over other area schools, especially New York Medical College.

With twelve hundred beds and serving the poorest and most destitute of the sick, Bellevue Hospital by the 1860s had become an important source of clinical experience for medical students. In 1861 it opened Bellevue Medical College.[5] In 1860, for example, the hospital had treated over 11,000 patients and handled 474 births, suggesting the breadth of opportunity offered to medical students.[6] Beginning in 1849, Bellevue Hospital had offered clinics taught by either a visiting physician or surgeon. (This was Thomas's original position.) The visiting physician or surgeon, who was obliged to be in attendance as a physician at the hospital during the school term, taught in an amphitheater clinic. He began with the introduction of a patient's case history, then brought the patient before the students and described his diagnosis and method of treatment.[7]

Thomas's extensive background in obstetrics and childbirth served as a foundation for his development of medical techniques and strategies. Working with Emmet at the Emigrant's Hospital in the early 1850s provided him with extensive childbirth experience. In 1852, the hospital had a total of one thousand beds, including three wards containing seventy beds for obstetrics.[8] John Metcalfe was a prominent obstetrician there and enhanced Thomas's reputation and expertise to an even greater extent. When Thomas taught clinical medicine, his lectures mixed obstetrics with surgical gynecology.[9] Medical students' opportunities for clinical instruction were very rare in antebellum America and not a required part of their education. The formal opening and reorganization of Bellevue Medical College contributed to the changes that would move tentatively toward more rigorous standards for medical instruction, especially the inclusion of clinical medicine and the use of hospitals. In New York City, Bellevue Hospital was of central importance in providing subjects for clinical study and lectures in surgical amphitheaters. Even though they were not paid positions, physicians actively sought appointments as attending and visiting physicians at hospitals.[10] More senior members of the medical community held the positions of consulting physicians.

A small group of medical men dominated the clinical scene in most of the hospitals in New York City.[11] Often sons of these men followed them into medical practice. Included among the elite practitioners were Thomas and E. Randolph Peaslee (1814–1878).

In the early 1860s Thomas represented the new generation of practitioners. Emmet was the same age as Thomas and rose rapidly to positions of authority, first at the Emigrant's Hospital and then at the Woman's Hospital.

Although Thomas's presence is quite low-key in the discussions following the papers in the *Bulletin of the New York Academy of Medicine*, by the end of the decade he had gained stature and a visible authority among practitioners around the world. In 1868, he published a major text on gynecology, *A Practical Treatise on the Diseases of Women*, which was quickly translated into several languages, and a new edition was published the next year.[12]

Peaslee was the only Northerner among the four chief-surgeons-to-be. He was a New Englander, born in New Hampshire, and only one year older than Sims. Peaslee studied at Dartmouth and eventually enrolled at Yale Medical School, where he received his degree in medicine in 1840. After finishing at Yale, Peaslee went to Europe and pursued the study of histology (the microscopic study of tissues) and physiology. With a strong background in several languages, Peaslee was particularly intent on gaining knowledge from German medical scholars in these areas. In this regard, Peaslee was among the earliest American scholars to become adept at the use of the microscope and in particular to pursue advanced training in areas that combined the chemistry of physiology and the study of tissues with the use of the microscope. In 1851 Peaslee began to teach at New York Medical College as a Professor of Physiology, Pathology, and Microscopy, but he did not move to New York until 1858, after ending his teaching career at Bowdoin and Dartmouth colleges.[13] His New York Medical College appointment eventually included a lectureship in obstetrics and diseases of women.[14] In 1857 he published a book on histology, serving to introduce American physicians to European scholarship. After he moved to New York City, he also served as attending physician at the Demilt Dispensary, where he offered his expertise in surgery and the diseases of women. Established in 1851, the Demilt Dispensary served the East Side of Manhattan where there were many tenements and many Irish patients.[15] He also held a teaching position as Professor of Gynecology at Bellevue Medical College, after Thomas left there. As with the other surgeons at the Woman's Hospital, Peaslee's private practice was extensive as well and supported him handsomely. A Yankee through and through, Peaslee became attending surgeon at the New England Hospital for soldiers in New York City through an appointment by the U.S. Surgeon General.

Another associate of the Woman's Hospital visible in the Academy proceedings was Fordyce Barker (1817–1891), who, in addition to being foremost in founding the hospital, also served as a consulting physician there. Having studied midwifery at Bowdoin College in Maine after medical studies in Boston, Edinburgh, and Paris, he went on to teach at Bowdoin for several years.

He then moved to New York City and held an appointment as a faculty member for the Bellevue Hospital College. He taught there for thirty years, holding the position of Chair of Clinical Midwifery and Diseases of Women.[16] Throughout the fifties, sixties, and seventies, Barker was also closely involved in the activities and growth of the Woman's Hospital. He published widely, writing on obstetrics and female disorders of the reproductive organs. In the first volume of the *Bulletin of the New York Academy of Medicine*, Barker was strongly in evidence as a senior member of the medical world, thoroughly engaged in discussing disorders, female conditions, and medical practices. He frequently spoke up during discussions, especially during one exchange regarding classifying diseases of the cervix.[17] It is clear from the publication that Barker worked closely with the New York Academy of Medicine and frequently served on various committees.

These practitioners and those who associated with them in various institutional settings were part of a medical world where paradigms of knowledge and concepts of scientific truth were shifting profoundly. The most important historical quality of the Woman's Hospital was that, from its beginnings as a hospital, it provided a medical workshop. First Emmet offered workshops and then the phenomenon grew. Here a core of talented and ambitious surgeons collectively addressed the problems of female disorders and devised therapies for treating them. They taught one another surgeries, they practiced at clinics where they also instructed medical students, and they invited physicians from outlying areas and Europe to visit their hospital. Young doctors sometimes gained appointments as attending physicians in the outdoor department of the Woman's Hospital and learned gynecological procedures. Peaslee and Thomas both mentioned bringing their senior classes to the Woman's Hospital regularly.[18] Peaslee recalled that in 1871 one thousand physicians had visited the hospital.[19] This tradition continued well on into the twentieth century, when the physician who devised the Pap smear was associated with the Woman's Hospital.

Many of the early physicians articulated a self-conscious set of aspirations for the Woman's Hospital. They began communicating among themselves in the mid-1850s, in the temporary quarters of the house on Madison Avenue. As several years went by, the plea for the funding of bigger facilities became more strident. Increasingly, medical proponents of the hospital declared the contributions of hospital-associated physicians to the creation of gynecology as evidence of the hospital's importance. On celebratory occasions of back-patting and fund-raising, the medical staff detailed the way in which the hospital represented a nucleus of very important activity.

John W. Francis, for instance, always presented the main address at the annual meetings. Although a practitioner of heroic therapies, Francis was nonetheless aware of the unique contributions being made at the Woman's Hospital and supported Sims's surgical practice wholeheartedly. In 1859 he praised Sims, saying his operations generated interest and imitation in "that peculiar department of female disease."[20]

In the first years of the Woman's Hospital Association annual anniversary events, the word "gynecology" did not appear in the texts of those giving addresses. Even in the late 1860s, Emmet waxed eloquent and enthusiastic about the dynamics of the Woman's Hospital without mentioning the specialty as gynecology. "I do not think that I am extravagant when I state that this Hospital has been the instrument of opening a field of observation from which a stock of information is to be gained hereafter, for the profit of the human race, greater than the whole store already accumulated since our professional knowledge was reduced to a science."[21]

Emmet expressed a kind of medical positivism, describing a progressive path in the unfurling of a new medical science, specifically in gynecology. In his memoirs he also expressed belief that the early years of the Woman's Hospital were immensely innovative and significant in contributions to medical practice: "I believe no one in the profession ever had the like opportunity afforded them for clinical teaching as I had, nor so great a number of listeners, who put in practice in his teaching intelligently and without delay. A revolution was effected in an incredibly short period and these clinics made the Woman's Hospital known throughout the world."[22]

Emmet was not alone in his belief that instruction and education were critical aspects of the success and power of the hospital. In 1871 Thomas declared, "It is the mission of this institution to spread abroad, to publish to the world, and to force a recognition of what will do more for the advancement of Gynaecology than any other discovery."[23] Thomas here referred to teaching Sims's surgical method for closing vesico-vaginal fistulas. The next year Thomas added, "This hospital [is] proving not merely a local sanitorium but an institution of learning, a school of instruction to other lands. . . . Physicians unfamiliar with the advances made by modern gynaecology come here to learn."[24]

Thomas, Emmet, and Peaslee all articulated a sense of the Woman's Hospital as historically momentous in creating a new branch of medicine:

> Since . . . establishment [of the Woman's Hospital], the progress of this department has been far more rapid than that of any other branch

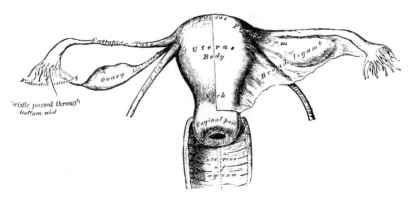

FIGURE 10. Anterior view of female pelvis. In Henry Gray, *Anatomy, Descriptive and Surgical*, 10th Eng. ed. (Philadelphia: Lea Bros., 1883). *(From the Special Collections, Southern Illinois University School of Medicine.)*

of medical science and art; and it must be conceded that this Hospital has contributed more than any other single cause to this result. If gynaecology has also progressed more rapidly in this than in other countries, it is largely because we have had this source of stimulation and of experience in our possession. Its influence has also been very great abroad, since it has served as the model for Hospitals for Women within the last ten years, not only in several of the large cities in this country, but also of England and upon the Continent.[25]

In the first years of the hospital, attention turned to the cervix and problems associated with displaced uteri. Physicians compared the position of a patient's reproductive parts with the standard depicted by *Gray's Anatomy* (see figures 10 and 11). The original therapies bridged the gap between the treatment of female disorders that had predominated and was ongoing, and the radical new approaches in surgery. Therapies in place before surgery included technologically based intervention. Many physicians throughout the Victorian period relied on the use of various appliances. Charles Meigs and Hugh Hodge were central figures in devising these instruments, the former developed a ring for the prolapsed uterus and the latter a pessary for the same purpose. Also available were several different pessaries and a variety of bougies, tent sponges, and individually devised variations of tools.

In his presentation during the spring of 1860 before the New York Academy of Medicine, Edmund Peaslee opened a discussion of the use of pessaries, asking if and when they were valuable in treating female complaints.[26]

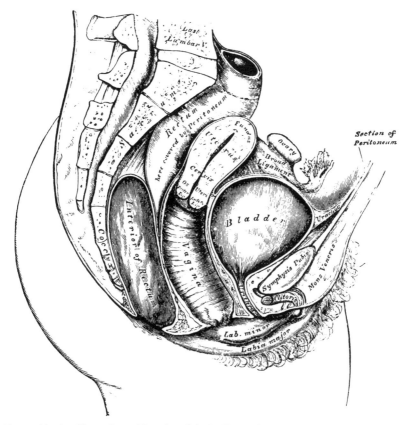

FIGURE 11. Ancillary view of female pelvis. In Henry Gray, *Anatomy, Descriptive and Surgical*, 10th Eng. ed. (Philadelphia: Lea Bros., 1883). *(From the Special Collections, Southern Illinois University School of Medicine.)*

Peaslee strongly advocated the use of pessaries in the treatment of uterine displacement—anterior, posterior, or downward. Augustus Gardner responded to Peaslee's seeming defense of the use of pessaries by stating that he found all forms of pessaries to be completely useless and ineffective and suggested the uterine sound, a stemlike tool that passed through the cervix to probe the uterus, might be a better instrument. While the uterine sound provided a means of examining the uterus internally, it carried dangers with it, particularly in the form of possible puncture of the uterus. Gardner was a New York physician and Professor of Diseases of Females and Clinical Midwifery at New York Medical College. He attended occasional operations at the Woman's Hospital and was closely aligned with J. Marion Sims, but he was never formally connected to the hospital. He spent time in Paris in the 1850s and was influenced by medical practice there. His writings often concerned conception and the maintenance of marital bonds, being very staunchly opposed to abortion and contraception.[27]

While Peaslee and Thomas each took issue with Gardner's descriptive diagnoses of various patients and his remedies, Sims was more sympathetic to Gardner. He appeared to take a middle road, characterizing cases in which pessaries had served patients well. At the same time, Sims described patients who only recovered from uterine displacement by the surgical incision of the cervix. One of the ultimately most controversial surgeries, yet one of the most common during the first decades at the hospital, was the splitting of the cervix, originally performed with a kind of knife, later revised to a technique using scissors.

Throughout the first volume of the *Bulletin*, Sims's emphasis was on facilitating conception and pregnancy. In one case he described a patient who wore a pessary only long enough to conceive, and went on to bear a child and enjoy fairly good health, particularly as represented by the placement of her uterus. For Sims, good health and ability to conceive and bear children were all one in the lives of women. For his part, Gardner, like Sims, discussed early surgeries at the Woman's Hospital—examples from 1855 of cervical incision—and voiced his hearty approval and willingness to duplicate the surgical methods employed by Sims.[28]

In the first volume of the New York Academy of Medicine's *Bulletin* is a paper from the spring of 1862 by Augustus Gardner on the "Amputation of the Cervix" (the same meeting where Sims presented his paper on vaginismus). His paper was but a small part of a great expenditure of energy and attention spent on the cervix during these midcentury years. "Amputation of the Cervix Uteri" addressed treating a variety of symptoms, from a prolapsed uterus to leukorrhoea—cases, Gardner said, both "local and reflected," by removing at least part of the cervix.[29]

At the Woman's Hospital in the first years of its existence, Sims and Emmet frequently resorted to amputation or excision of the entire cervix (that which protruded beyond the vaginal wall). Although case records indicate success with these surgeries—"cured"—problems still ensued during recovery. There was, at the same time, an accumulation of knowledge from experience, a realization, for instance, that the cervix was not entirely expendable. Once, while operating in the presence of Valentine Mott, Sims accidentally perforated the abdomen of a woman and was forced to think quickly, rapidly closing the wound and managing to save her life.

Sims eventually saw that pregnancy could not follow the excision of the cervix, and he became much more tempered in his use of the operation, virtually abandoning it by the 1860s. Emmet wrote in his text that since 1865 "I have not resorted to [amputating the cervix], in consequence of seeing . . . such results follow my own handiwork. It was a favorite mode of treatment both with Dr. Sims and myself in the Woman's Hospital."[30]

When Gardner practiced cervical amputation, one of the symptoms he cited, leukorrhoea, was a vaginal discharge, often called the "whites" among various Woman's Hospital physicians. It probably originated in one of a variety of different bacterial sources or infections not recognized by these practitioners. For Gardner and others in the Academy, surgery now seemed a therapy of great potential.

Important to the proponents of much of the early gynecological surgery—Gardner, Sims, Emmet, Thomas, and most other physicians in their circle—was a different perspective on disease, called reflex theory, which posited that the uterus was the central organ in female physiology, as was also the underpinning for John Griscom's remarks cited earlier. In this framework, various disorders, especially nervous disorders, stemmed from the uterus; in treating the uterus a woman could achieve health and balance throughout her system. Female physiology was read completely through reproduction, puberty, menstruation, and childbirth. Seen within a closed system of energy, nervous depletion in one locus led to stimulation in another. For medical practice, the result was an overriding emphasis on the reproductive organs.[31]

Surprisingly little was known about the human female cycle. Medical writings emphasized the role of semen but showed little understanding of the ovum or the role of the ovaries in reproduction.[32] Fertility was misgauged by nineteenth-century physicians, and menstruation was largely misunderstood. For instance, one other article by Gardner in the 1862 *Bulletin* addressed the case history of a woman he claimed was misdiagnosed with tuberculosis, suffering instead from "vicarious menstruation," in this case bleeding from the lungs.[33] Gardner, influenced by M. Huguier of France, and Sims and Emmet found themselves looking at the cervix, using the speculum, to begin to probe the mechanics of reproduction. Their task in part was to determine the pathological from the normal state of the cervix. This was much more easily done by examining live patients than those in the deadhouse. Medicine still had a great deal to learn about the physiology of human reproduction.

Science and medicine misunderstood the relationship between menstruation and conception. Until the discovery of hormones and their role in reproduction, doctors routinely advised women that their most fertile time was right after or during their periods.[34] Doctors in the nineteenth century often blamed ill health in women on the absence or tardiness of their periods. In the late nineteenth century, one doctor reported there was an "old idea of the noxious influence of retained menstrual blood."[35] A school of German physiologists influenced James Y. Simpson to believe that menstruation was a kind of "vicarious respiration" without which carbon built up in the female body.[36] Doctors used this as a premise for directing the use of emmenagogues, abortifacients, and for the administration of bleeding, even among pregnant women.

Some physicians believed that pregnancy itself was a disorder because the menstrual flow ceased and caused congestion in the woman.[37] Others believed that women who had no periods sometimes bled from other parts of their body—"a vicarious menstruation"—from their lungs or their breasts, for instance.

Among medicines prescribed were emmenagogues, herbs, and various pharmaceuticals given by mouth, to cause menstruation to return. These herbs and medicines were often the same as those used by midwives.[38] Doctors used emmenagogues as abortifacients to produce abortions. These physicians were limited in their ability to determine if a woman was pregnant, especially in the early months. Cessation of menstruation could indicate pregnancy as well as some other disorder. Not until the 1840s did American law and social ethics sanction against abortions. Until that time, ending a pregnancy that happened before quickening had no meaning separate from miscarriage. Miscarriage and abortion were interchangeable concepts. After the 1840s, abortion became illegal and doctors played a part in identifying abortion as criminal. Still, as a recent scholar points out, physicians continued to practice abortions under many guises, yet succeeded in separating women from their pregnancies by denying the validity of quickening as a turning point in pregnancy.[39] Quickening was the moment when fetal movements evoked awareness in the mother, what we often designate as a kick. Involved was the mother's authority in sensing life within through feeling and touching. Physicians began to intervene in this designation of life as they slowly found other ways to recognize pregnancy.[40] With the criminalization of abortion in the 1840s, quickening no longer figured definitively as the identifying point of life during a pregnancy. Despite their participation in the debate over abortion, doctors were under no ethical compunctions to remove themselves from the control of menstruation and felt strongly that regular menstruation was the key to health for women.[41]

Another form of treatment of the cervix was cupping and leeching. Doctors sometimes prescribed the application of leeches to the cervix itself. Charles West provides a case in point. In his 1857 text on diseases of women, he detailed the use of leeches and praised the results in cases of what he called "congestive dysmennorhea." He did caution against the possible escape of a leech and the need to pay close attention to the therapy.[42] In the 1870s and 1880s physicians persisted in the employment of leeches.[43] Leeches were applied to the breast, to the temples, and also sometimes to the anus. Some argued that the use of these bloodsuckers was preferable to surgery.

Anodynes were another common form of treatment. In midcentury and in the Victorian period many women depended upon strong painkillers— opium and morphine occasionally—to avoid great discomfort. As anesthesia became known, some physicians used chloroform or ether to ease painful menstruation (dysmenorrhea).[44]

Caustics, blistering, and cautery were other therapeutics used to treat the cervix. Physicians commonly applied silver nitrate there as well. Charles Meigs and Gunning Bedford both frequently diagnosed leukorrhea (vaginal discharge due to inflammation) and treated it with an application of silver nitrate directly on the cervix.[45] This and other local treatments often created scar tissue and possibly exacerbated the ill health of the patient.

Doctors at the Woman's Hospital, and elsewhere, continued to use these therapies throughout the nineteenth century. Emmet frequently used silver nitrate in his therapies for the cervix, and Thomas occasionally prescribed the use of leeches. At the same time, practitioners, often experimenting with new therapies, showed little fear of admitting they performed a wrong surgery. Many physicians, rather, were confident that they were pioneers in a new medical practice and felt they had some leeway to make errors. In the hospital's first seven years Emmet and Sims experienced great freedom in their ability to devise innovative new surgeries.

For New York surgeons and physicians, the Woman's Hospital provided excellent access to cases. In addition to the autonomy in medical practice that the Medical Board enjoyed vis-à-vis the Lady Supervisors of the hospital, Sims, Emmet, Thomas, Peaslee, and other practitioners benefited from the number of patients. Unfortunately, these patients came from a social class that was vulnerable for use in untried surgeries—either because of gender, ethnicity, or economic status. The Irish predominated as patients at Bellevue Hospital as well as at the Woman's Hospital of the State of New York. The nearby Nursery and Child's Hospital also had mostly Irish patients, including parturient women. The interlocking network of physicians and administrators—

Emmet's relatives, Sarah Doremus's expansive philanthropy, the overlap of visiting physicians at these institutions—all helped to supply patients as objects of surgical practice.

In the first six years at the Woman's Hospital, Sims gathered experience and knowledge for the culmination of his career as a gynecologist. Emmet and Thomas and many others were part of the era's growth in the surgical treatment of women. Emmet wrote later that Sims

> was so fertile in resource when I first knew him that he perfected scarcely a tithe of the brilliant conceptions passing constantly through his mind, and it was impossible to see him perform the most simple operation without learning something new.
>
> He was perfecting and devising new instruments, studying modes of exploration, and planning different surgical procedures, all in a field too new to find any precedent to aid him in the experience of others.[46]

The first volume of the New York Academy of Medicine's *Bulletin* reflects the dynamic of the experimental surgeries at the Woman's Hospital in its first years. As was the pattern for many papers, Augustus Gardner's paper on cervical amputation focused primarily on one case, which concerned a woman's prolapsed uterus following several births, and the removal of her cervix. The woman was married to her cousin, a situation that resulted in several miscarriages and stillbirths; in addition, she suffered from venereal disease and possibly tuberculosis. In an appended paper, the attending physician, who had also been part of the surgical team for the cervical operation, described the patient's last childbirth. Gardner developed his method and his presentation to mirror and honor Sims and Sims's surgery for the amputation of the cervix—copying use of his speculum and the position he chose for the patient.

While Gardner's case was apparently not from the Woman's Hospital, most of the first-time surgeries there were performed on similar cases of childbirth injuries. Many Woman's Hospital patients suffered lacerated perineums or recto-vaginal and vesico-vaginal fistulas. Also common was uterine prolapse, often caused by multiple pregnancies. Almost as soon as the institution opened its doors, the doctors at the hospital treated a variety of complaints. There were cases of menorrhagia, or heavy bleeding during menstruation, and dysmenorrhea. Others were there to recover from previous medical treatment. Cases of amenorrhea (lack of menstruation) and troubled puberty also made their way to the hospital or to the outdoor clinic. Tumor patients came, too, although the treatment of cancer was eventually denied at the hospital. Still other patients suffered the effects of gonorrhea or syphilis. Finally, there were those who complained of sterility.

Cervical amputation was one of the first surgeries developed by Sims and Emmet. Other surgeries performed included clitoridectomies, and narrowing of the vagina (elytrorrhaphy), which were spun off from the numerous strategies used for incision of the cervix. As Gardner suggested, the surgery seemed likely to suit a wide number of female complaints. This surgery and others, such as incision of the cervix, became popular among some physicians but eventually met criticism in the medical community and lost favor. Surgeries such as these were accompanied with changes in the diagnosis of symptoms and the priority given to them. Sims, Emmet, Thomas, Peaslee, and other associated American gynecologists may have devised new techniques and medical instruments, but their greatest innovation was the willingness to operate.

Debate over the cervical surgeries lasted decades. By the time of Sims's death, he, Emmet, Thomas, Peaslee, and others had developed a language of specifically designated and carefully delineated symptoms—although ambiguities persisted even into the 1880s.[47] In an article in the British journal *Lancet*, which Sims wrote when he was living in London, he introduced the topic of cervical surgery in the 1860s as a remedy for "painful menstruation," sometimes called dysmenorrhoea. Physicians did make distinctions at times between painful menstruation and dysmenorrhea, but ambiguities in language and diagnosis persisted. The symptoms were not clear-cut, but the surgery, according to Sims and Emmet, offered relief from pain *and* likely fertility for a childless woman.

In 1826 Scottish physician Jack Mackintosh had used a bougie to open the cervix in a case of dysmenorrhea. While Mackintosh did not operate, he began the practice of dilating the cervix with a variety of tools and made possible the subsequent use of surgery. The bougie was a tool used first to open the male urethra when urination ceased and the urethra tightened up. As it had for the male urethra, the bougie mechanically forced the cervix open. Mackintosh followed the use of the bougie to break the strictures of the canal with graduated sponge tents. As the treatment progressed, larger tents were introduced until the cervix seemed to be of sufficient width to allow the menstrual flow. Mackintosh was not concerned with sterility so much as he was with women incapacitated during menstruation, or the "monthly molimen," to use a nineteenth-century phrase. Doctors used Mackintosh's technique throughout the century, usually for cases of little or no menstrual flow—amenorrhea, or for flow of normal quantity, but not for cases of menorrhagia. Sims and his associates, however, utilized various similar therapies, surgical and otherwise, on cases ranging from amenorrhea through menorrhagia.

In 1844 Sir James Y. Simpson utilized Mackintosh's technique and added his own surgical procedure. In addition to the use of bougies and sponge tents, Simpson employed his tool, a lithotome caché, to incise the cervical canal. He inserted the tool into the cervix, and when reaching the os internum (the opening to the body of the uterus), he sprung open a built-in knife as he pulled the lithotome back through to make an incision the length of the canal. Simpson performed this surgery, without the use of anesthetic, in his office. Patients frequently left immediately to return home. Some physicians reported severe hemorrhaging and complained of the dangers associated with the procedure, but Simpson denied their reports.[48]

Simpson used the procedure in cases of what he called "obstructive dysmenorrhoea." Sims and Emmet shared Simpson's mechanical model for the functioning of female reproduction, and also Simpson's faith in cervical incision. Emmet considered himself a mechanic in his approach to surgery.[49] Sims articulated a simple theory of menstruation in his text, *Clinical Notes on Uterine Surgery*. Although Emmet eventually revised his ideas concerning the complexities of the cervix and uterus, the theoretical underpinning of Sims's and Emmet's surgeries in the first years was a belief that pain in menstruation often emanated from a blocked or obstructed cervix that would not admit the menstrual flow.

In the London *Lancet*, where chapters of *Clinical Notes* were serialized before their publication as a book, Sims defended his use of cervical incision, in response to many highly critical letters from British doctors. Obstruction in the cervical canal alone, he maintained, caused the symptoms of dysmenorrhea. "Its action is mechanical. . . . It [dysmenorrhea] is only a symptom of real disease. It may be inflammation of the cervical mucous membrane; retroflexion; fibroid tumour in one wall of the other . . . all of which are but so many mechanical causes of obstruction, which must be recognized and remedied if we expect to cure the dysmenorrhea."[50]

Other American physicians had already turned to an investigation of the cervix as the seat of female sickness. In 1854 Charles D. Meigs, the eminent Philadelphia obstetrician, published an article for the AMA on "diseases of the neck of the uterus."[51] In his writing, Meigs provided several colored plates depicting the cervix in various states. (Within a little more than two and a half decades, A.J.C. Skene, of the younger generation of gynecologists, supplied photographs of the cervix, demonstrating the rapid changes that occurred within the field.) Although Meigs was not inclined to pursue surgical therapies, he was interested in the use of the ocular, the viewing of internal female reproductive organs. Meigs wanted to determine the pathology of the cervix and to demonstrate its various disorders. He was ambivalent about the use of the speculum and about invading female privacy with visual inspection, yet he pursued an interest in determining the "normal" weight and measurements of the cervix and uterus, which he called the "ideal" or "standard."

Drawing from the French, as Meigs had also done in 1854, Augustus Gardner described the "raspberry" cervix, that is, an inflamed cervix. Once again, like Meigs, he did not describe Sims's or anyone else's surgery for incision of the cervix, since Sims only began using the technique in the mid-1850s. Later, in 1860, Gardner expressed great admiration for Sims's vesico-vaginal fistula surgeries and amputation of the cervix, and he used Sims's operating technique as a model for his own.[52] While Sims and Emmet differed widely from the way Meigs practiced medicine, they did share with him a premise that the uterus (with the cervix as its mouth and neck) was the central organ governing the health of women and girls. Meigs articulated this theory over and over again: "It is, at least, certain that sexual diseases do give rise to severe distress in distant regions of the body . . . the radiating point of the mischief being concealed within the depths of the pelvis, and wholly masked by the constitutional disorders thus set on foot by it."[53] Following this same line of reasoning, premised in reflex theory, in his text Sims described a Southern patient who suffered menorrhagia plus fainting, blindness, nervous attacks, and sterility. Sims diagnosed a retroverted uterus and a closed cervix and applied three days of sponge tent therapy to the cervix. He described her as cured, "and [she] subsequently became a mother."[54] Although the woman suffered a wide variety of complaints, Sims, like Meigs, determined that the cervix and a malposition of the body of the uterus caused all the symptoms. Most often, however, Sims would call upon incision of the cervix rather than "mechanical dilation" through the use of sponge tents.

Like Meigs, Sims privileged definitions of the normal female reproductive organ. He devoted an entire section of his *Clinical Notes* to the "normal position" of the uterus. He argued that there was confusion among doctors over the definition of the "normal" because of a lack of live subjects: "One [author] will tell us the uterus is about two and a half inches deep, while another will say it is less. Both are right; for the uterus, an erectile organ, full of blood, is larger and longer in the living body than in the dead. The knowledge of one is gained in the clinic; of the other in the dissecting room."[55]

Sims and Emmet each defined the uterus as an erectile organ, analogous to the penis, recalling epistemologies prior to the nineteenth century that posited that male and female represented in essence one sex rather than two.[56] They drew from their clinical experiences at the Woman's Hospital to derive an understanding of female physiology.

Sims's and Emmet's First Surgeries on the Cervix

The work of mid-nineteenth-century physicians in the field of gynecology clarifies the manner in which they based their diagnoses and medical practice on what they knew through experience. First, through the use of the speculum, the doctors were able to see the vagina and the vaginal wall. In America, Sims greatly enhanced the visual scope through innovation in tools and position of the patient. One physician-historian, James Pratt Marr, suggests that "Sims and Emmet knew a great deal about vesico-vaginal fistula, but Thomas surpassed all others of his time in his knowledge of the anatomy of the pelvic floor."[57] Further innovations made the cervix more accessible and visible. Symptoms and disease were thought to radiate from the newly glimpsed locus, the cervix uteri. The uterine sound helped to make the body of the uterus somewhat available to medical examination. Expanded surgical technique later made the ovaries and the uterus accessible; the process of diagnosis and therapy then turned to these organs of reproduction and remained extremely dynamic well into the twentieth century.

From their shared experiences at the Woman's Hospital where they worked for some years together and in their private practices, Sims and Emmet developed a theory of uterine pathology which suggested that uterine position, as well as the condition of cervical tissues, was critical to the health of the woman. At midcentury there were many women who suffered from severely malpositioned uteri, including prolapses to the point where the inverted uterus was distended outside the body. Emmet and Sims argued that anteflexion (or the bending forward) of the uterus often caused dysmenorrhea and that cervical incision cured anteflexion. Another key to their use of the cervical surgery was a determination that enlarged, or hypertrophied, cervices caused difficult menstruation. Both of these arguments depended on an ability to describe the healthy or "normal" physiology.

Incisions on the cervix were to Sims a prime example of the absolute utility of surgery over other therapies. He berated "mechanical dilatations" of the cervix for their ineffectiveness and dangers. Sponge tents, he argued, introduced infection and inflammation to the internal abdominal cavity, possibly causing a pelvic abscess. In the worst circumstances this resulted in septicemia or peritonitis, both producing death for the patient—blood poisoning, severe and irreversible systemic infection. Sponge tents were kept in place for days and days. The cervical canal was artificially kept open (as in birth, miscarriage, or abortion), and the possibility of infection was great. The threat was even greater in the mid-nineteenth century when very few American surgeons heeded standards of cleanliness, let alone antiseptic procedures.

Sims prided himself on replacing what he saw as outmoded techniques with what seemed to him to be a cure-all operation. First, he argued, concerning painful menstruation, "I lay it down as an axiom, that there can be no dysmenorrhoea, properly speaking, if the canal of the neck of the womb be straight, and large enough to permit the free passage of the menstrual blood."[58] The cause of menstrual pain was mechanical and lent itself freely to surgery. The task was to "straighten the canal" and to free the canal from any stenosis. "The fact is, that most of the diseases of the uterus are as purely surgical as are those of the eye, and require the same nice discrimination of the true surgeon."[59]

In the first years of the Woman's Hospital, the surgeries on the cervix were more radical, involving incision on both sides of the external os per surgery. Results from the surgery were less than perfect. Sims recalled, "I have frequently been compelled to repeat the operation [cervical incision], and I remember several patients on whom I have operated as often as three times in the course of a few months and even then the result was not wholly satisfactory."[60] The case of a thirty-year-old Irish woman provides an example. In 1858 she had been married several years with no pregnancies. She was diagnosed as having dysmenorrhea and painful intercourse with her husband, as well as being nervous. Eight days after her admission, she had her cervix divided laterally, with its posterior lip removed. The records report that "although the largest sound could be pushed into the fundus without difficulty, yet to facilitate conception the canal was more dilated by a lateral incision on each side and extended well up into the body of the organ [uterus]."[61] The history reported her cured and released in three months' time, although the possibility of such a cure resulting from the surgery is questionable. Clearly, the surgeons found the restoration of her fertility most important, and proceeded in that direction, according to their mechanical theories of conception.

Another Irish woman, twenty-three years of age, came into the hospital in 1859 complaining of painful periods. The diagnosis included "flexure" of the uterus forwards toward the bladder—anteflexure. She was in and out of the hospital over a two-year period. First, a surgeon split the mouth of the uterus. After the use of various therapies, including applications of chromic acid, she had surgery again. Emmet once again split the cervix, this time employing his standard incision backwards to the vaginal juncture. The records report her "cured." The casebooks have many examples such as these of repeated surgeries in which the rationale is not always clear or consistent.

Finally, an example of an extreme case occurred in 1862. This case is extreme because of the violence and mutilation of the surgery, and also because of the rarity of its use at the hospital (at least in the records). It was a case of clitoridectomy. The twenty-four-year-old woman, who was unmarried, complained of painful periods, convulsions, and some bladder irritation. Sims first slit the neck of the uterus laterally, then he amputated the clitoris, "for the releif [sic] of the nervous or hysterical condition as recommended by Baker Brown." Baker Brown's surgery included removal of the labia minor or nymphi. The casebook reported little benefit from these surgeries, so Emmet performed his surgery on the cervix instead, in 1863. Little information was given on the woman's life after surgery.

Isaac Baker Brown was a British surgeon who performed many operations on women in the 1850s and '60s. He gained a wide reputation because he developed a use for clitoridectomy on women with nervous disorders, most often what he described as excessive masturbation. Brown caused a large stir because of his avowed and frequent use of the surgery to remove radically the clitoris in patients. Many felt that he failed to inform his patients about the effects of the procedure. After a lengthy hearing, the London medical community censured him in 1867 by removing him from the British Obstetrical Society.[62]

Sims was aware of Baker Brown's publications and attempted to use Brown's operation of clitoridectomy at the Woman's Hospital. Later he was in London at the time of the Baker Brown controversy and most certainly was aware of it. Sims, however, did not use the surgery with much regularity. Only three clitorectomies were recorded in the 1877 tabulations for the entire history of the hospital. The accuracy of the record is not above question, however, especially in cases involving controversial surgery. In 1862 Sims and Emmet combined the surgery with the repeated use of cervical incision.

Two of the recorded and published cases concerned venereal growths on the clitoris. Thomas, in his teaching clinic, cited one young woman who had been a patient in the outdoor clinic. After three years of marriage, she had contracted syphilis and died in 1869 following surgery to amputate her clitoris. Dr. Harry Sims, Sims's son, performed an autopsy and declared her death caused by peritonitis, an infection of the abdominal cavity.

Operations on the cervix were considered minor and rarely threatened the lives of patients. The number who may have died from the surgery is unknown. There were some who bled heavily from the surgery and died after they had left the physician's headquarters. Others developed what was called pelvic cellulitis—inflammation and infection in the uterus. This too could be fatal. Lack of antiseptic methods combined with repeated invasions of the sensitive and vulnerable uterine regions caused mortal disease. Often surgeons prescribed daily probings with the uterine sound to keep the cervical canal open. In retrospect, Sims and Emmet prided themselves on their cleanliness, but others undoubtedly lacked interest in sanitary measures.

A striking ambiguity in the procedure for cervical incision—both in effect and in the devising of the technique—was its relationship to abortion. Physicians performed abortions in the nineteenth century by dilating the cervix with sponge tents until the uterus voluntarily emptied itself of the fetus and placenta.[63] Certainly the *surgical* dilation of the cervix would also cause an abortion. In 1847 Simpson said of his technique, using a knife and a sponge tent, "it places the parts in somewhat the same condition as that which they present subsequent to miscarriage. . . . Women after aborting usually soon again become pregnant."[64] Sims dodged the issue of abortion, never referring explicitly to a surgical procedure to induce abortion. Meanwhile, doctors were prominent among those who devised sanctions against women ending pregnancies before their terms were up, and created the new category of "criminal abortion."

Comparing case records to published accounts of surgery on the cervix at the Woman's Hospital brings into relief the process by which Emmet and Sims created a consistent and seemingly rational basis for the surgery of cervical incision. In a sample drawn from the case records, there is ambiguity in the symptoms given as a cause for surgical incision of the cervix. As the surgeons determined a pathology of the uterus and the cervix, a language evolved that described what ought to be and what was. Their perceptions changed over time, and so did their diagnoses. As they wrote articles later, they applied newfound symptomology and diagnoses to cases they had earlier acted upon within a somewhat different nosological framework. Dysmenorrhea, for instance, was a catch-all symptom suggesting need for the surgery. Anteflexion later was identified as the key symptom indicating need for the surgery; and finally endometritis, in the 1870s.

By the 1860s physicians recording the cases referred to the incision of the cervix as "Emmet's operation for dysmenorrhoea due to anteflexion."[65] Even though the surgery became routine, its rationale depended upon undetermined standards of normal physiology. Female reproductive organs change during the menstrual cycle, as a result of gestation and birth, and during the transitional times of menarche and menopause.[66]

Over several years, a discourse emerged to describe the need for incision and/or excision of the cervix uteri. Sims argued originally for the surgery in cases of hypertrophy of the cervix. If the cervix were elongated, or conical in shape, protruding into the vagina for more than half an inch, that was indication of need for the incision. Later, doctors would argue that there was no fixed shape or length of the cervix, and that these standards were of no utility in judging its health.[67]

Emmet varied Sims's original surgery to incise only below the cervix. Sims, in the first years of the hospital, practiced a bilateral cut, following Simpson, and moving from the os externum to the front vaginal junction, with a mirror cut to the posterior. Sims also removed tissue within the canal in the bilateral surgery. In the mid-1860s, Emmet articulated a diagnosis of anteflexion of the cervix itself, not the uterine body, as the chief pathology calling for the surgery. There was nonetheless great uncertainty in diagnosing malposition of the uterus. By the late 1860s, doctors defined anteflexion as a condition of long-standing origin, as opposed to sudden trauma, in which the body of the uterus or the cervix tipped forward.

Meigs, on the other hand, had argued earlier that in cases of retroversion (as opposed to retroflexion) the uterus and cervix stayed in a straight line, rather than one part bending or flexing toward the back of the body.[68] Perhaps this confusion helps to explain why in the case records of the Woman's Hospital there is little distinction made between anteflexion of the cervix and that of the uterus. However, by the late 1870s, when the procedure was the subject of criticism by American physicians, Emmet referred specifically to anteflexion of the uterine neck alone as reason for surgery. He developed an elaborate etiology of anteflexion, isolating puberty as the inception of the condition—an imbalance in the growth of the cervix as opposed to the uterus. Peaslee and Sims, on the other hand, referred to stenosis (or closure) of the cervical canal as the rationale. Neither of them saw adolescence as particularly important in creating the condition leading to dysmenorrhea.[69] Perhaps a patient's history of venereal disease could have resulted in stenosis.[70]

Close examination of a sample of fifty-five patients at the hospital demonstrates the degree of confusion surrounding the surgical technique and the way in which the language of diagnosis changed over time. All these women were patients between 1858 and 1871. Complaints in their case histories of dysmenorrhoea and cervical abnormalities determined their inclusion in the sample. According to one tabulation, a total of 236 incisions of the cervix were made at the hospital between 1855 and 1875,[71] though there is no accurate record of the total number of these surgeries. Emmet, the chief keeper and supervisor of the institutional records, shied away from using the casebooks extant in the late 1870s, even though he drew freely from the records of vesico-vaginal fistula patients.[72] At that time, Emmet preferred to draw from statistics of his private practice. The surgery had become very controversial.

Sims made the number of surgeries for cervical incision a point of notoriety. In his *Clinical Notes*, first published in the *Lancet* in 1866, he bragged that he and Emmet had performed the surgery many times. "I cannot now tell how many hundreds of times (certainly more than five hundred) the operation of cutting open the os and cervix has been done by Dr. Emmet and myself at the Woman's Hospital and in private practice."[73] This estimated figure was often repeated in medical journals as medical practitioners reviewed the feasibility of the surgery. The figure was probably accurate, since Emmet too noted that "during the past six or seven years [before 1865] we have performed the operation several hundred times for various purposes, in hospital and private practice."[74]

The surgery developed ahead of a scientific rationale for it. Of the fifty-five case records studied, fifty seemed to require surgery on the cervix, and nine had amputations of the cervix. Before 1865, "anteflexion of the uterus" did not appear on the case record. There were two cases of simple "anteflexion" before 1867. There were no cases of endometritis or metritis. (This diagnosis became common in the late 1860s.) "Dysmenorrhea" was a symptom that appeared very consistently throughout the case records.

Doctors used the description of anteflexion only as experience allowed precision. In the first ten years, there was an occasional reference to "flexure of the cervix" or simply "flexure" without indicating the direction of the bend (ante- versus retro-). Although Emmet in 1869 argued that anteflexion of the cervix alone created a need for the surgery, among the cases only one indicated exactly "anteflexion of cervix." Perhaps, in the later cases, recording physicians assumed that the reader would know that the anteflexion rested in the cervix. There was a diagnosis of "anteflexion and endometritis" that appeared in nearly all cases between 1867 and 1871. Twenty-three case records indicated anteflexion and/or endometritis; seven of these listed endometritis and anteflexion side by side—the standard case calling for incision of the cervix. Of these twenty-three cases, eighteen underwent surgeries for incision of the cervix. As surgeons gained experience and clinical knowledge, their descriptions of symptoms changed; likewise, their medical comprehension of menstrual disorder changed. Eventually, medical therapies themselves changed.

In the antebellum years, Emmet and Sims frequently operated on the cervix, convinced of the appropriateness of their surgeries. In the cases from these years, retroversion (tipping back of the uterus) was given as a reason for surgery, though Emmet explicitly excluded retroversion as a proper cause for surgery in the late 1860s, as did Peaslee later.

Throughout the period, in the case records hypertrophy of the cervix and the "cauliflower" cervix were legitimations for the retroversion surgery. Dysmenorrhea, a broad and poorly defined symptom encompassing cramps and discomfort during menstruation, was also described in many cases, as were nervousness and a tendency toward hysteria. Finally, doctors sometimes diagnosed closure of the cervix and then proceeded to split the cervix laterally, then using the uterine sound daily to prevent the tissue from reclosing.

James Y. Simpson revealed the difficulty in diagnosis when he argued in 1847 that even a normal cervix might require the surgery. The key, he maintained, was "a want of relation between the quantity of fluid secreted, and the quantity allowed" to escape.[75] For Simpson, obstruction of menstruation sometimes accompanied by hypertrophied cervices, inflamed cervices and misplaced uteri caused dysmenorrhea.

Changing the physiological underpinning, Emmet argued that flexion caused obstruction to the circulation of the uterus—what he and Meigs, among others, designated as a faulty nutrition of the organ. If the cervix were bent at a sharper angle than normal, a uterine dysfunction would result. In addition, endometritis was added as a diagnosis to uterine and cervical flexure in the 1860s. Emmet used the term to describe cases of inflammation of the uterus, a way of refining the concept of inflammation.[76] Both endometritis and metritis were diagnoses for visually inaccessible regions of the uterus. By 1889, the diagnoses maintained their utility and gained some precision in their definition. Physicians found ways to pinpoint areas of suspected inflammation by touch and through the use of the speculum.[77]

In his text, Emmet noted that medical practitioners faced many obstacles in their diagnosis of the uterus and inflammation. "We have no means of judging as to the full extent of disease within the uterine canal, or with accuracy, as to its locality, when situated beyond the range of our vision."[78]

T. Gaillard Thomas, in his text published in 1869, set out to clarify the ambiguities of inflammation as a diagnosis of uterine disease. Out of forty-six chapters his book included seven chapters on the identification, pathol-

ogy, and treatment of uterine inflammation, particularly in the form of endometritis and metritis.[79]

Thomas and Emmet shared an interest in theories of inflammation, and
they also shared the use of endometritis as a diagnosis. In the sample of patients analyzed here on previous pages, Emmet's therapies and practice are
evident in the years after Sims left the hospital. As he explored further the
use of inflammation as a diagnosis, and as he became disinclined to use cervical incision, Emmet relied more and more on the use of hot water injections and local applications of chromic acid to treat uterine disorders. In 1869,
just a few years after he had openly defended Sims's words in *Clinical Notes*,
Emmet noted: "Division of the cervix, for the relief of dysmenorrhoea and
sterility, has been a favorite practice for years past with many of the profession. Scarcely any operation in surgery, however, has been proposed, where
so little judgment, as a rule, has been exercised, and where so frequently its
indiscriminate performances has even amounted to malpractice."[80] While
Thomas Addis Emmet did not abandon his use of cervical incision, he did
combine other therapies with it, and as time went by he was less and less
inclined to use it. From several years of practicing the surgery, he was also
able to identify and treat cervical lacerations and devised ways to manipu-
late surrounding tissue in the treatment of postsurgical cervices, which, in
retrospect, represented early plastic surgery.

Criticisms from other practitioners also surfaced. Edward Tilt, a British gynecologist, had harsh words for those who felt that surgery was the most
valuable therapy in the treatment of cervical disorders. He was particularly
skeptical of Emmet's and Sims's surgery on the cervix. Tilt preferred the use
of sponge tents. "INSTANTANEOUS DILATATION—Says America, with accustomed
audacity, this gradual dilating is slow work; take this instrument shaped like
a lithotrite, wriggle it into the cervix, and then open the blades; what matters
if the circular fibres of the cervix do give an audible crack? is not the woman
under chloroform?"[81] One American medical writer, reviewing Thomas's text,
cried out: "We have a sensational literature, a sensational drama, and we are,
we fear, drifting toward a sensational gynecology. Iatro-mechanical ideas have
an irrational and unmerited preeminence; each day brings forth a new machine for stretching, or cutting, or rectifying the womb; and some wonderful
feat of the knife is blazoned to catch the credulous."[82]

Thomas also practiced the cervical incision, but not as much as Sims
and Emmet. He did emulate Sims's technique for vesico-vaginal fistulas, however, and he went on to innovate several gynecological surgeries, from
Caesarian sections for extra-uterine pregnancies to ovariotomies.

When Sims first published his articles in the mid-1860s urging the use of cervical surgery in the treatment of painful menstruation, he met further objections. The more criticism he received, however, the more adamant he became about its successes. For Sims, the response from the British medical community was, more than anything else, a sign of recognition for his accomplishments. "For when so many eminent men step out off the beaten track to discuss their soundness, it is almost a guarantee that there is truth at the bottom, the whole of which they cannot at once accept because it does not tally with old preconceived notions."[83]

In response to the chapters printed in the *Lancet*, Henry Bennet, an English physician and author of a widely read text on obstetrics and the diseases of women, suggested that the symptom of pain during menstruation was not necessarily pathological. He, like others, felt that Sims's surgical cure was overdrawn and might interfere a great deal with the normal functioning of the female body. Bennet argued that the cause of dysmenorrhea might be from inflammation of the uterus rather than from an obstruction of the cervical canal. He also suggested that a "constitutional dysmenorrhea" might provide a more accurate description of painful menstruation in women. In other words, Bennet argued that some women were simply more inclined to have difficult periods and certainly did not require surgery.[84] Sims said "that organic change may be inflammation, or it may be the cause of inflammation, or it may exist independently of it. But whether inflammatory or not, its action is mechanical."[85]

T. Spencer Wells also took issue with Sims's incision of the cervix. Like Bennet, he thought the surgery was dangerous and fruitless. Wells's response to Sims's manuscript is noteworthy because he reacted first and foremost to the use of the speculum during surgery. This, Wells argued, offended the modesty of the patient. "There is not such difficulty encountered in performing any operation on the uterus by the touch alone, and in the dark."[86] Wells was a pioneer in the performance of ovariotomies, which he, unlike others, apparently saw as no threat to the sensibilities of womanhood. In this latter practice, which involved abdominal surgery, he could see all of the organs involved, but from a different angle.

One further letter to the *Lancet* in response to publication of "Painful Menstruation" was from British physician G. T. Gream, who voiced strong distrust for Sims's uterine technique. Gream argued from the bad result of a case he treated for sterility and dysmenorrhea suffered by a woman of noble standing. He performed surgery similar to Sims's division of the cervix and the woman became pregnant immediately. Unfortunately, she soon suffered a miscarriage, barely escaped with her life, and was never able to bear children.[87] While Sims denied the likelihood of miscarriage following his surgery, he himself, in response, discussed a similar case, differing only in that the woman died.[88]

Sims maintained that scar tissue from the surgery would close the canal to some degree and prevent miscarriage; however, from other vantage points, the outcome seemed unpredictable. Ironically, the procedure he advocated for treatment of infertility would not only cause an abortion if pregnancy was underway, but cervical incision would at the very least complicate a subsequent labor and delivery of an infant. He denied such problems, instead mentioning only women who were able repeatedly to become pregnant following the surgery.

Perhaps Sims, in an underhanded fashion, was practicing abortions and taught the procedure to students. No doubt he developed his surgical technique on the more vulnerable, probably impoverished, patients at the Woman's Hospital without fearing possible accidental abortions in the process. Sims was convinced that his medical therapies healed women and thus made it possible for them to become pregnant. "How often do we hear even medical men say, 'If she could only have a child it would cure her.' To this I always feel inclined to reply, 'If we could only cure her, she would have a child.'"[89]

In his years abroad, Sims visited major hospitals and often operated there, in such places as the Charity Hospital and Hôtel Dieu in Paris, demonstrating his surgical technique and spreading the word about the Woman's Hospital in the State of New York. He and Emmet had operated extensively together, but now Sims once again was in many ways on his own. His clientele changed and he began to practice among wealthier patients. He had a newfound interest in sterility (particularly female infertility), which he shared with Augustus Gardner. Before Sims left for Europe, in 1856, Gardner published his text, *The Causes and Curative Treatment of Sterility*, which located the cervix, the external os (entering on the vagina), and the internal os as the "seat of inflammatory diseases, both acute and chronic."[90] He and Sims believed that conditions of the cervix were responsible for sterility. Sims had focused a great deal of attention on the treatment of sterility from the time he began practice at the Woman's Hospital. In 1866 he published *Clinical Notes on Uterine Surgery with Special Reference to the Management of the Sterile Condition*, a well-received textbook among medical students that was translated into several languages. Although Sims conducted these explorations into reproduction and experimental surgery independently, his work affected the reputation and medical practices of the hospital.

Various cervical surgeries were not the only questionable operations outlined in *Clinical Notes*. Sims more thoroughly shocked and angered some of his medical readers by his empirical investigations into his patients as they engaged in sexual intercourse. The theoretical umbrella for Sims's examinations of women, their vaginal fluid, and, concomitantly, the condition of the semen in the vagina, was his intention to make sterile couples fertile. By the protocol of many of his peers, Sims delved too far into the privacy of these couples. The starting point for Sims's investigations directly into sexual activity began with the treatment of female patients suffering "vaginismus."[91] These women, according to details provided by Sims, were hypersensitive in their sexual and reproductive areas, and unable to participate in copulation.

As in the case of Patient X, described at the beginning of this book, some of Sims's patients, although married, remained virgins for many years following marriage. Along with vaginal discomfort and rigidity, they also suffered from muscle spasms. Sims's initial therapy involved a surgery he developed in which he excised thickened tissue of the hymen and the surrounding area—that is, he surgically deflowered his vaginismus patients. He also made lateral incisions in the vaginal sphincter muscles to remedy the spasms. Sims did not always resort to this mode of surgery, however, and in his text he frequently admitted to its experimental nature. Sometimes, again as in the case of Patient X, he declined to operate because the woman was a member of the highest social stratum.

Many years later, Sims defensively published the case history of a woman who suffered from vaginismus among other symptoms. In this instance he felt surgery was a necessity regardless of her social status. She was "Mme. X, young, beautiful, and representing two of the first families of the aristocratic Faubourg St. Germain."[92] In writing about his concerns regarding sterility, he presented the world in terms of the social stratification of European royalty, to which he had grown accustomed. "Suppose a dynasty was threatened with extinction, and the cause of sterility was ascertained to be an enucleable fibroid; here the perpetuity of a good government and the welfare of the State might depend upon the result."[93] For Madame X, he operated not for a fibroid, but for vaginismus and also its corollary of sterility, slitting the lateral sphincter muscles of the vagina—and then performed further surgery for an "indurated cervical canal and a contracted cervix."[94] She became pregnant and suffered from an apparently fairly common nineteenth-century disorder accompanying pregnancy—uncontrollable vomiting.[95] She died under the care of an *accoucheur* (a midwife), whom Sims blamed for failing to perform the abortion he considered necessary to save her life.

Sims resorted to a different type of therapy for several other women. He utilized ether to render a patient unconscious and then asked or directed the husband to engage in intercourse with her.[96] Sims observed that the woman's sexual organs were, for the most part, greatly relaxed when unconscious. He was delighted to report several cases of pregnancy from such encounters. Unfortunately, Sims eventually determined that the vaginismus condition was unremitting, returning even after childbirth and often creating a painful pregnancy.

Sims described one couple under the care of another physician who engaged in etherized sexual activity for more than a year. Although they produced children this way, they ultimately abandoned the practice, distrusting the consequences of such a habit.

The practice of etherizing a woman in order to relax her during intercourse is particularly striking in contrast to the unanesthetized surgeries Sims practiced in Montgomery and at the Woman's Hospital. Although Emmet left ambiguity surrounding his own failure to use anesthesia, he puzzled over Sims's reluctance to employ anesthesia before the mid-1860s.[97] Sims seemed to have such an air of authority about him that few challenged him.

Sims never considered the possibility of a nonphysiological component in the vaginismus condition. In fact, his empirical and close-hand study of sexual activity confirmed for him a belief that "the act of copulation is purely mechanical. It is only necessary to get the semen into the proper place at the proper time. It makes no difference whether the copulative act be performed with great vigor and intense erethism, or whether it be done feebly, quickly, and unsatisfactorily, providing the semen be deposited at the mouth of the womb, everything else being as we would have it."[98] Although physicians routinely recognized false pregnancies as mentally induced, most physicians did not look at psychological origins of disease as a factor, particularly in sexual matters. Reflex theory worked in the opposite direction, positing that in women nervous and hence mental disorders most likely originated in the sexual organs. A formulaic approach to sexual intercourse, focused entirely on reproductivity, provided the underpinning for Sims's advocacy of surgical dilation of the cervix. If only the obstacle to menstrual flow were removed, then ovulation would proceed and the sperm and egg could unite in the uterus. These theories were inaccurate in terms of what we know today, but consistent with the scientific knowledge of the period. Along with other medical practitioners, Sims believed that ovulation accompanied menstruation, fertility was at its height during menstruation and the week that followed, and that fertilization took place directly in the womb, with the spermatozoa moving aggressively and the egg staying passive. Sims and others assumed that human fertility was analogous to the heat in other mammals.

Sims's interest in the mechanics of reproduction led him to discover something few had considered in examining cases of human sterility. Using a microscope, he studied semen to find cases in which the spermatozoa were dead after intercourse. Probably because of the vehement cultural sanctions against masturbation, the necessity of acquiring samples for this laboratory work led Sims to examine his patients, in particular to fetch a semen sample from the woman's vagina, immediately following intercourse, within minutes or even seconds. After identifying the vitality or lack thereof among the sperm, Sims went on to explore the positive or negative environment of the mucous in the vagina. These issues were his prime concern in promoting fertility.

Examination of semen following sexual exchange, although it rode the edge of social acceptability, was ahead of its time in many ways. In 1884, Sims's peer and rival practitioner of vesico-vaginal fistula surgery, Joseph Pancoast, employed Sims's technique, but added the donation of sperm from an outsider as part of his effort artificially to induce conception.[99] Sims's son, physician Harry Marion-Sims, carried on Sims's work in this area. The semen test was eventually named the Sims-Huhner test.[100]

The London *Medical Times and Gazette* disapproved wholeheartedly of Sims's research: "Still more we doubt whether many a one will be found to undertake the 'business' he describes. Fancy a respectable husband quitting his bed hastily, and leaving his palpitating spouse to be examined in less than a minute after the nuptial mysteries."[101] This exchange, Sims's investigations of sexual intercourse and therapies for sterility, and the newspaper's Victorian disgust for his intrusions and direct investigations of an unmentionable activity illuminate an important insight into Victorian society. Social approbria affixed to sexuality had two sides—that which was explicit and that which was silent.[102] In the end, Victorian culture, of which Sims was profoundly a part, was completely caught up in sexuality. The enforced silence on some fronts allowed a different articulation to emerge. Sims's explorations of sexuality, as shocking as they were, were nonetheless untouchable—somehow a protected part of his identity as a physician, perhaps in part because he employed elements of scientific method. Through his research and medical practices, Sims found a way to talk about sex and sexuality at great length, and many others joined in the exchange that followed.

Previous to the publication of *Clinical Notes*, at an unspecified date, Sims had attempted artificially to fertilize women who were barren. These women, he maintained, had refused to undergo the surgery he suggested—

the division of the cervical os—so in a sense, he punished them for their obstinance. They were probably patients in the Woman's Hospital, given Sims's avowed sentiment "the hospital being the legitimate field for experimental observation."[103] They were undoubtedly women of lesser social status, either by class or ethnicity: "The experiments . . . were made on half a dozen different patients. During the two years that I was engaged in them I made fifty-five uterine injections. I think I am entitled to subtract about half the number as having been badly done, or having been made with badly constructed instruments, or under injudicious circumstances."[104] Perhaps these cases were among those Emmet felt Sims remembered inaccurately, as Sims did not take actual records of the Woman's Hospital patients with him to Europe, nor had he kept them very carefully in the first place.[105] In any case, the experiments were fraught with difficulty and resulted in pain for the women involved. Sims had to experiment to identify the correct amount of fluid to use. The result when he injected too much fluid was dangerous and extremely uncomfortable for the patient. The only precedent he found in medical texts involved the use of dogs and pigs, in the context of the artificial insemination of domestic animals for breeding purposes.

Given the women's case histories, infertility, and refusal of cervical incisions, Sims felt his only alternative, and theirs, was experimentally to inject spermatozoa directly into the uterus (using a hypodermic needle). How much the women themselves sought pregnancy is never clear.[106] He was successful in impregnating one woman in this fashion, but she suffered a miscarriage. He was thus forced to revamp the procedure but never achieved consistent results. In this activity, Sims certainly foreshadowed modern obstetrical efforts to create life artificially. The *Medical Times and Gazette* was horrified, however, and claimed that Sims had divorced all morality from his medical practice.[107] Another journal, the *Southern Journal of Medical Sciences*, decried the experiments with ether during intercourse and also the attempts at artificial insemination, speculating as well on the class and suspect morality of the patients involved.

> And yet we have no right to conclude that those subjects on whom Dr. Sims thus exhausted his experimental genius belonged to the declared outcasts of their species, for in this sphere there does not exist that desire for children that could lead to such utter abandon. Indeed, the conviction is forced upon us that Dr. Sims must have found his victims in that other extreme of society, where at least real virtue has no home, but is only too successfully by the tawdry drapery that money throws around the sexes.[108]

This author felt no doubt that Sims's experimental work on fertility related to the richest stratum of society. One reason Sims had difficulty successfully fertilizing his patients was his erroneous concept of the menstrual cycle. What is startling to consider is the success Sims did have in carrying some of his patients into a pregnancy.

Sims's book provided a classic formula for the Victorian notions of sexual exchange. The text was premised on the desirability of fertility and childbirth for a married woman. Sims urged that intercourse take place in a prone position, with the man on top to ensure conception. He also worried that "too frequent sexual indulgence is fraught with mischief to both parties."[109] With excessive sexual exchange, the limited amount of sperm would be spent. Hence, Sims argued, "it is much better to husband the resources of both man and wife."[110]

He maintained boldly:

> God has given us appetites and desires, and endowed the act of copulation with a pleasurable erethism, simply that we might be forced to "multiply and replenish." . . . It matters not how awkwardly and unsatisfactorily the act of coition may be performed, so that semen with the proper fructifying principle be placed in the vagina at the right moment; and, on the contrary, it matters not how perfectly and satisfactorily it may be done, if the semen lacks this fecundating power.[111]

"Erethism," or simply an extreme sensitivity of the reproductive tissues, was Sims's verbal limit in describing the pleasure of intercourse. Still, frigidity on the woman's part or early ejaculation on the man's made no difference. Sims thought that if every young medical practitioner understood the simple and seemingly straightforward nature of intercourse and reproduction, the knowledge "may do much to render many families happier, by setting them right on a point of more vital importance to domestic happiness than many of us have ever dreamed of."[112] Sims apparently believed minimizing the standard of pleasure in intercourse would amplify what contentment a couple might feel in their home life.

Sims did, of course, recognize the importance of male excitement in the act of sexual intercourse, even with the limited goal of fertility in mind. Although he never mentioned female physical activity during coitus other than passively accepting the sperm, nor the historically suspected connection between female orgasm and conception, he frequently alluded to the youth and vigor of the male during the act.[113] Assessment of male activity was part and parcel of his evaluation of the cause of sterility in any given couple.

While Sims, on the surface of his text, engaged in what might be considered archetypical Victorian thought processes portraying gender roles of masculine strength and female passivity as physiological components of sexuality, certainly his reviewers found his efforts bold and radical. Carrying bedside therapies beyond the imaginable, Sims in his medical practice took empiricism into the private and most hidden side of his society's life. His explicit exposure of that life transformed its very qualities, rendering them at the very least self-conscious. In this fashion, Sims prescribed sexual activity for sterile couples on given days and at given times, with his presence to be promptly solicited. Yet at the same time he urged that "the sexual act should never be done except at the spontaneous prompting of nature."[114] While maintaining the absolute irrelevance of the quality of sexual encounter and the necessity of spontaneity, he turned his full attention to the matter—and the attention of others as well.

Although some of Sims's research in this area was done in New York, he wrote and published about it while abroad, and his works were among the many journal articles and published lectures of the four men who worked together as head surgeons at the Woman's Hospital. Each wrote and published texts used throughout the Western world as beginning guides to a new medical specialty. Sims's *Clinical Notes on Uterine Surgery with Special Reference to the Management of the Sterile Condition* described his therapies for the treatment of female reproductive disorders. Emmet wrote a book on vesico-vaginal fistulas, which was published in 1868, and Thomas also published a text on female disease in the same year. Edmund Peaslee published *Ovarian Tumors: Their Pathology, Diagnosis, and Treatment, Especially by Ovariotomy* in 1872.[115] Many praised Peaslee's essentially conservative presentation, and his text developed a topic of growing importance to medical practice and surgical gynecology.

Ovariotomy and a Shift in Paradigm

Ovariotomies were not publicly discussed in the *Bulletin of the New York Academy of Medicine*; their mixed reputation made them controversial even in the 1870s and a less likely focus for published Academy papers. What made ovariotomy particularly dangerous and highly morally freighted in the public eye (both medical and lay) was the accompanying mortality rate. In the first ten years of its more common, albeit tentative use, the chance of death associated with this "capital" or major surgery was exceedingly high: a patient had little chance to survive because of the risk of infection.

T. Gaillard Thomas and Edmund R. Peaslee, along with Sims, were the surgeons associated with the Woman's Hospital who first began to practice ovariotomies, Peaslee undoubtedly before Thomas and perhaps before Sims. By the time of his death in 1878, Peaslee's reputation was that of an accomplished ovariotomist. Thomas gained praise for his innovation of vaginally performed ovariotomy, first performed in 1870.[116]

Ovariotomy—or the surgery to remove both ovaries and especially initially, to remove tumors—as defined at this time marked for many, in retrospect, the first act of gynecology. Americans were keen to claim it for themselves. Ephraim McDowell performed the first recorded, publicized, and successful ovariotomy in rural Kentucky in 1809. Decades later, Samuel Gross, along with other prominent American medical men, lionized McDowell as a pioneer ovariotomist, the first of the new gynecological surgeons who emerged in the nineteenth century—the father of ovariotomy. McDowell's successes had been remarkable since he operated essentially without precedent and without the assistance of antisepsis or anesthetic.[117]

To the first generation of gynecologists, describing the first surgeon to perform an ovariotomy was tremendously important. To recognize McDowell as such sent a message to Europeans that Americans were in fact the original gynecologists. McDowell lived on the frontier in Kentucky; four out of five of the patients on whom he practiced this surgery in the second decade of the nineteenth century were African American.[118] However, after this until the 1840s, physicians, for the most part, eschewed the practice of ovariotomy, and even then they only tentatively acknowledged its viability. Nonetheless, those who performed the surgery eventually were known to be in the vanguard of medical practice.

England claimed its own father of gynecology in Spencer Wells. Wells began to practice ovariotomies in the late 1840s, was knighted by the queen for his achievements in 1866, and is still known as a master of the surgery. Also pivotal were Lawson Tait and Thomas Keith,[119] as well as Philadelphia surgeons and brothers Washington L. and John Atlee, who began practicing the surgery in the 1840s.[120]

Ovarian tumors were debilitating and often led to death. The growths attained phenomenal size, giving the patient a freakish appearance because of her huge abdomen. Cases like this were often portrayed in medical texts describing various therapies, including surgery. Other disorders included cysts on the ovary. Physicians designated cysts and tumors of the ovary as ovarian dropsy. In time, a variety of tumors, cysts, and other ovarian conditions came to indicate the need for an ovariotomy. At the same time, a physician's ability to diagnose ovarian disease ranged from precise to uncertain.

Before ovariotomies were performed in the 1840s and even during the first decades of its practice, medical practitioners frequently tapped tumors through the abdominal wall, using an instrument called a trocar. They then drained fluid from the growth out through the peritoneal cavity. This therapy was more effective than the use of medicines, which had little or no effect on the tumors and cysts. Often, though, the growths recurred. At times death would ensue as the woman weakened and her entire system suffered. As a rule, physicians allowed the tumors to reach maximum size before initiating any medical procedure. Sometimes they encouraged the woman to wrap her abdomen with a supporting belt. There were instances when the woman lived a long life in this fashion, with the tumor intact. Still, doctors commonly felt that the victim of ovarian dropsy was doomed to an early death. J. Y. Simpson described at length the process of tapping the ovarian tumor, though he reported that "the tapping requires to be repeated again and again; more or less frequently in different cases; but always as a general rule with shorter and shorter intervals as the disease lingers on, till finally the patient dies exhausted."[121] David Hayes Agnew, in his text *Surgical Diseases of Women*, stated tersely: "The progress of ovarian dropsy, when left to itself differs in different subjects. The drift of the disease is always to a fatal termination, and this, in a majority of instances, occurs within three or four years, produced by peritonitis, exhaustion, or organic disease induced by mechanical pressure."[122]

Even in the 1860s and early 1870s, ovariotomies were quite rare. Surgery offered hope for these women, but it also threatened their lives to a much greater extent than surgery for vesico-vaginal fistulas or cervical surgeries, which seldom resulted in death. Ovariotomies' eventual success would depend upon measurable changes in surgical procedure as well as its advocacy by medical practitioners. Peaslee was such an advocate; he wrote, for instance, about the many years of life that were saved by the surgeries of Spencer Wells.[123] In the past, scholars have generally credited these surgeries in the innovation and implementation of anesthesia and antisepsis or asepsis. In contrast, today's scholars suggest discarding facile portraits of a scientific revolution in which medicine sharply transmogrified from a time when doctors had no real therapies to physicians who were armed with superpowers derived from anesthesia and antiseptic methods.

Hindsight may make the transformations look sharper, but it also tends to shape the past as if it leads directly, in a straight line, to the present. What really happened is much more complex but profoundly significant for science and medicine today. As we have seen, early in the nineteenth century, the medical world in the West absorbed the perspectives, knowledge, and insights of French clinicians and heeded new understandings in pathology. Much of the impact in the United States of these imported ideas was to imbue a new generation of physicians, including Sims, Emmet, Thomas, and many others, with a strong skepticism about the use of purgatives, scarring, leeching, blistering, and bleeding. Diagnosis and definition began to change, but not all at once, and not by totally abandoning one method for another. The publications of most of the practitioners at the Woman's Hospital demonstrated shifts in position or moved to embrace different therapies over time, often practicing all at once.

Many physicians of the middle third of the nineteenth century drew their treatments from the theoretical ideas of fevers and inflammation. The practice of morbid pathology carried shifts in cosmology but essentially focused on lesions and tissues and the localization of disease. Technological innovation with auscultation and percussion, Laennaec's stethoscope, Récamier's metrodome, and the microscope also served to produce a more specific focus. Both pathology and diagnostic emphases enhanced the practice of surgery. There was a great deal still not understood, and in the face of epidemics of cholera, typhus, and yellow fever, physicians still had little with which to fight disease.

Abdominal surgery was introduced in the late 1860s, following the practices of Lister and initially involving the application of carbolic acid on the wound. Cleanliness of physicians and operating rooms, not to mention the use of gloves, were separate issues altogether.[124] Both Peaslee and Sims were very methodical about personal cleanliness for surgery, but as personal characteristics rather than drawing from theory. Certainly the success of surgery for each was vastly improved by these personal habits.[125] While Sims never gained the same acclaim as Peaslee specifically as a highly skilled ovariotomist, he did express an early interest in the surgical procedure and went on to perform the surgery many times, as did other physicians and surgeons.[126] In his first years at the Woman's Hospital in the 1850s, Sims petitioned the consulting physicians for permission to perform an ovariotomy. Not until 1860 did he gain permission.[127]

In the 1840s, surgeons and physicians alike had heard about or experimented with ether and chloroform. Besides the issue of the physiological effect of anesthesia, the size of a dose, and other questions concerning details of implementation, there were cosmological questions about pain and its meaning in sickness and in religion. There was a new tension between ministers and physicians about their respective roles at the bedside of the patient. A very central issue became the use of anesthesia during childbirth. Despite much disagreement about the right or wrong of removing pain from delivery, and its corollary in interpreting the biblical injunction connecting suffering with birth, it was not many years after Simpson had begun to use anesthesia for birth that Queen Victoria requested him to help her to escape the pain of labor and delivery. Anesthesia challenged the authority of the clergyman and the gender identification of suffering womanhood.

A discussion in the *Bulletin of the New York Academy* demonstrates the concern that accompanied the use of anesthesia throughout the midcentury. In conjunction with a paper presented by Fordyce Barker in the spring of 1862 on the use of anesthetics in childbirth, members of the Academy made several unreported proposals. But putting them aside to address later, a physician asked about a recently reported death from chloroform at Bellevue. A few months later, Barker reported to the Academy as chair of the committee investigating the death. The publication stated that Barker, John Metcalfe, and several other physicians testified that the cause of the woman's death was cardiac arrest. After some laboratory analysis, there was still no other explanation for what caused her death. Although the *Bulletin* presented nothing more, these sparse bones suggest the enigma that anesthesia represented in the early 1860s to physicians.[128]

Questions persisted about the causes of diseases and sickness. Some were reluctant to accept scientific theory as truth, yet they were eager to characterize the physician as morally superior. At the Woman's Hospital, the image of the surgeon as "the Great Physician" persisted throughout the 1870s. During an anniversary meeting of the Woman's Hospital in 1873, Reverend Ormiston described the entanglements of Christianity and science: "I can conceive no nobler or more Christ-like man than an able, pious physician or a skillful, saintly surgeon. Where religion, enlightened by science, and science sanctified by religion, unite, as they do in such a home as this, to glorify God in the relief of human suffering, we can hear the words and the works of the Great Teacher and Divine Healer."[129] On the same occasion, Dr. Alfred Post described bringing the "best gifts of science" to lie on the "altar of Christian love."[130] In 1870, at another anniversary meeting, a New York obstetrician declared in a similar vein, "We come here to-day to celebrate a crystal wedding—the union of science and Christian love."[131] Understanding and utilizing scientific law revealed the powers of God.

Sims's work on sterility symbolized the same union of science and Christianity in the workings of the Woman's Hospital. When he first used the microscope, his mentor placed the Lord's Prayer under the lens to gain Sims's attention and approval.[132] Sims was delighted. He identified with the physicians who sought new scientific knowledge and its concomitant change in cosmology and understanding of sickness and health, yet he saw science still primarily as an expression of the power of God, and he saw himself primarily as His steward.

In the late nineteenth century, physicians in the West accepted bacterial theory as an explanation for the origins of sickness at varying rates. Post-Franco-Prussian War Germany in the 1870s became a center of activity in research of micrococci and a related theory of infection. Many physicians were more favorably drawn to this work than to Lister's germ theory of putrefaction, and Germany in some ways supplanted the medical authority previously held by France.[133] Lister's theories did not include a recognition of micrococci or bacteria until after others began to publish on their presence in the 1870s. The discovery of anthrax, the tubercle bacillus, by Robert Koch in 1882 also led to amendments of Lister's practices.[134] In 1865, however, Joseph Lister introduced his antiseptic technique of carbolic acid applied during surgery. A key difference between Lister's ideas and German theory was that Lister continued for a long time to consider pus as sometimes beneficial—"laudable pus," as it was known—and as negative only in association with inflammation, not as the seat of disease.

Evaluation of putrefaction was important for those who were surgeons operating in the abdominal cavity. Exchange among these physicians focused on various forms of infection—erysipelas, peritonitis and septicemia—came to include discussion of what was the best treatment for the pedicle or stump left from removal of the ovaries following ovariotomy. Peritonitis was an inflammation of the peritoneum, the lining of the abdominal cavity. Septicemia was a form of blood poisoning that could combine with peritonitis and was almost always fatal. Erysipelas had characteristics of skin inflammation. Physicians debated the etiology of erysipelas, which was in fact a distinct and separate infection but might have occurred as a result of abdominal surgery; we know now that erysipelas is caused by streptococcus. Streptococci and staphylococci were identified in the 1870s by the German physician Theodor Billroth but not widely accepted as scientific fact.[135] Peaslee was particularly thorough in writing about postsurgical treatment of the pedicle, urging physicians to keep it external to the body as the best way to avoid the patient's death. Sims and others also joined in discussing this topic. Both

Thomas and Peaslee were particularly attuned to refined issues in pathology and to understanding specific states of tissue and their relationship to sickness. Morphology, or addressing the structure rather than the origins of disease, dominated physicians' perspectives until the acceptance and breakthrough of germ theory in the late nineteenth century.

Most American physicians were notoriously slow in their acceptance of the German scholarship and somewhat reluctant to employ that of Lister. Although many thought of the origins of disease as airborne, the product of atmospheric miasma and animalicules, some sanitation measures and changes in medical therapeutics began to gain public support. Surgeons at the Woman's Hospital, however, were for the most part in the mid-sixties readily engaging antiseptic measures, and sometimes also using Lister's methods. Sims, for instance, had his own methods of cleanliness and procedure in the operating room. At one point he wrote about the benefits of clean cotton-wool and its lesser expense than the carbolized dressing espoused by Lister. Many other physicians wrote letters to the *British Medical Journal* in positive response to Sims's ideas.[136] The worldwide web of connections with Europe, both through Sims's travels and his life there and through individual networks left them very aware of the scholarship in medical theory and practice.

Closely linked to issues of sanitation and the origins of disease, and foremost in the minds of hospital administrators and physicians in the 1850s and 1860s were hospital architecture and structural planning. Following her experiences in the Crimean War in 1859, Florence Nightingale published her manual, *Notes on Hospitals*. This work articulated many of the ideas already afoot among health reformers, advocating ventilation and the circulation of fresh air as pivotal in combating disease. Somewhat similar to Lister, Nightingale subscribed to theories of putrefaction and fermentation as explanations for the origins of disease.[137] By the end of the nineteenth century, these theories were outmoded and cast aside with a surge of appreciation and recognition for the significance of laboratory science and the concomitant implementation of the discovery of bacteria—the paradigm for scientific medicine.[138]

Doctors and hospital staff, reformers and administrators, patients at the Woman's Hospital and elsewhere in New York City at midcentury and through the 1860s and 1870s held more closely to the ideas expressed by Nightingale. In fact, Sims's last child was born in the late 1850s and was given the name Florence Nightingale Sims. In the early 1860s, Sims himself went to England and met Florence Nightingale and sought ideas for the architecture of the new Woman's Hospital to be built during the 1860s.

Understanding disease and deriving medical techniques to prevent it in a hospital context was of enormous import for all medicine, especially surgery. Practitioners were not likely to talk about disease per se but they did address issues of sepsis and, throughout the middle third of the century, sought to stem the mortality associated with abdominal surgery. On the other hand, at the Woman's Hospital, Sims, Emmet, Thomas, Peaslee, and the hundreds of associated doctors rapidly increased the practice of ovariotomy. Issues of high mortality rates pressed hard on the people of the institution and on the institution itself.

CHAPTER 6

Power, Politics, and Profession

                      *I*n 1868, the Woman's Hospital Association merged with the Board of Governors to become the Board of Governors and the Board of Lady Supervisors of the Woman's Hospital of the State of New York. After years of fund-raising and preparation, the first pavilion of the new hospital was completed and ready to open in October with seventy-five beds. The event marked a watershed in the institution's history and a new chapter in early gynecology. Moving the Woman's Hospital from 83 Madison Avenue to 49th St. and Lexington Avenue, in addition to situating the institution in a new neighborhood further uptown, brought many changes.

    Leading up to the opening of the Wetmore Pavilion, as the first building was named, was a series of political and financial maneuvers set in the years immediately preceding, during, and immediately following the Civil War. As a visual comparison of the two buildings demonstrates, the institutional costs rose precipitously with construction of buildings and hospital ownership. In 1856, in conjunction with the memorial presented to the state legislature, an all-male Board of Governors convened to oversee the construction of the buildings. After various failed negotiations, Sarah Doremus convinced the city in 1858 to grant land for the institution. With the stipulation that the hospital provide twenty-five free beds for city patients, the city donated a lot the size of a city block, a pauper's graveyard. In the summer of 1859, workers removed 47,000 dead bodies, a mass grave eighteen bodies deep of impoverished victims of the cholera epidemic of 1832.[1] The bodies were reburied on Ward's Island along with those from other reclaimed potter's fields in the city. Such an inauspicious and repugnant, not to mention unsanitary, task often preceded the establishment of a new institution in nineteenth-century urban America. In *Moby Dick*, for instance, Melville described a

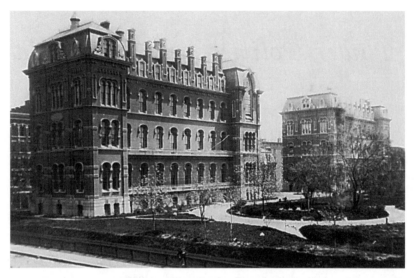

FIGURE 12. Baldwin and Wetmore Pavilions between Park Avenue and Lexington. *(Courtesy of the Bolling Medical Library, St. Luke's–Roosevelt Hospital Center, New York.)*

similar ground-breaking in Boston.[2] Parts of Bellevue Hospital also required the relocation of a potter's field.

In 1859 the state legislature granted $50,000 in matching funds. The hospital would have access to this money only if it could raise $100,000 from private sources. James Beekman worked with other members of the Board of Governors to find funds—not an easy task after April 1861 and the beginning of the Civil War. For the most part, the Woman's Hospital Association and the Board of Governors kept their funds separately, but distinctions in fund-raising and occasionally the purpose of bequeathed funds were not always clear. According to the constitution and the structure of the institution, the funds for the new hospital building represented a completely different mission from the maintenance of the Madison Street hospital. On one occasion in 1862, Sarah Doremus, as the assistant treasurer for the women, sought a loan of $5,000 to meet expenditures. While she felt strongly that the governors' money should be safeguarded in order to acquire the state grant, she also disputed the acquisition of some of their funds. Sims, she claimed, had usurped funds for the Governors that had been bequeathed to the Woman's Hospital Association.[3] Although the managers sustained the hospital through trying times, the women dutifully paid back money borrowed, and the lay-

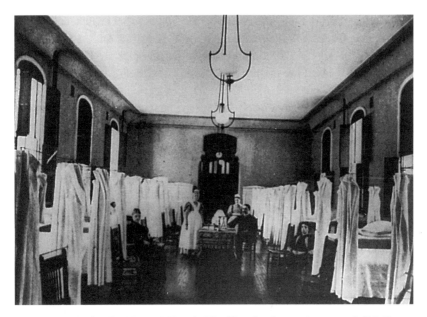

FIGURE 13. Ward at the Woman's Hospital Pavilion, Lexington Avenue and 49th Street, New York. *(Courtesy of the Reynolds Historical Library, University of Alabama at Birmingham.)*

men became its governors with the completion of the Wetmore Pavilion in 1868.[4]

The onset of war combined with Sims's departure for Europe to precipitate a failure of confidence among both the women managers and the patients (all of whom left the hospital). Only by convincing some of his private patients to reside at the Woman's Hospital was Emmet able to regain the support of the managers.[5]

Building the Wetmore Pavilion demonstrated the immediate success and growth of the original Woman's Hospital endeavor. Many of the original supporters, physicians and lay people alike, made the acquisition of land and construction of the new buildings a central mission, yet the enormity of the fund-raising task challenged the managers' ability to maintain authority. During the first decade of the hospital, when much of the most significant history of the hospital occurred, the managers had undisputed claim to hospital management. This is the history celebrated for more than one hundred years.[6] During the late 1860s and through the 1870s, conflict and controversy occurred in running the hospital.

Money was often tight. Whenever the rent could not be met, the women knocked on Beekman's door and asked for a "loan." In August 1865 Sarah Doremus wrote a note to Joseph Collins, the treasurer for the Governors' funds. "Will you do me the favor to speak to the Board [of Governors]?"[7] She needed fifty more dollars.

In 1863 the foundation was laid for the new hospital, but only through intense political lobbying were laymen such as Beekman able to keep funds available for the building of the first pavilion. Throughout these years there was much give-and-take among Beekman, the politicians, and the civilian population about the goals of the hospital. As late as 1867, Beekman was lobbying for one pavilion to house lying-in patients and the other to house those with what now would be designated as gynecological disorders.[8] Before he died in 1861, Dr. John Francis also envisioned two pavilions, one for lying-in cases and the other for females diseases. Although Beekman, Francis, and others still connected female health directly with giving birth, the hospital continued to move toward the specialization we now know as gynecology, which is related to but exclusive of birth.

In addition to Beekman's tenacity, not to mention his expertise and political connections, in acquiring state grants for hospital construction, he led fund drives and exchanged personal letters with wealthy citizens to gain large donations. Eventually he collected the entire $100,000 necessary to gain the state's commitment of $50,000 for the new pavilion. When the new hospital pavilion opened in 1868, however, the Lady Supervisors found their budget burdened with $1,530.30 of expenses in surgical supplies and instruments, among other debts.[9]

The Wetmore Pavilion brought a new bureaucratic structure. The Board of Governors with its president (Beekman), its vice-president (Appollos R. Wetmore, a previous vice-president of the Association for Improving the Condition of the Poor and a wealthy Protestant reformer, for a substantial period), and its treasurer (who changed often) presided over the institution.[10] Wetmore, a New York merchant, was undoubtedly an early friend and associate of Doremus in her evangelical labors throughout the antebellum period in New York City. The Board of Governors had three groups of nine governors, including J. Marion Sims briefly as the sole physician member of an otherwise lay board, with terms ending at one-year intervals, totaling twenty-seven. (In the late 1860s and early 1870s Sims continued to travel frequently back and forth across the Atlantic. He maintained a presence at the Woman's Hospital but his position was redefined.) Under this board, at least in the description presented in the annual reports, was the newly renamed Lady Board of Supervisors—within which there was also a president (Sarah Doremus), a vice-president (Caroline E. Lane for several years, until she replaced Doremus as president), and other executive officers—and a thirty-eight-member Board of Managers made up of six members, twenty-six Lady Supervisors, and six honorary members. The Medical Board was made up of Emmet, who was the Surgeon-in-Chief and headed the Board, and four assistant surgeons, six attending surgeons, one senior consulting surgeon, nine consulting surgeons, and eight consulting physicians, with three House Surgeons, one of them serving as the House Surgeon and the others serving under him—a total of thirty-two medical practitioners. Although women physicians and surgeons practiced in New York City and elsewhere, none were on the staff of the hospital during its first two and one-half decades of existence. After John Francis's death, James Beekman became the titular head of the institution.

The women managers, now Lady Supervisors, struggled over the new bylaws as they sought to define the limits of their authority.[11] The women were particularly concerned that they would lose their power to appoint medical staff. They reached an agreement with the governors whereby they were to run the internal aspects of the hospital, including the matrons, supervisors, nurses, and house physician as before. Through the Board of Governors, the women retained a voice in medical appointments, particularly an ability to voice complaints and to veto nominees for staff positions.

Under the new arrangement, the women kept their own treasury. They were in charge of the dispersal of funds for internal organization, while the governors supervised the building funds and the grounds. They also audited the supervisors' treasury. Such a distinction between internal and external realms was difficult to keep and led to conflict between the two boards. The women filed at least one lawsuit to regain control of an estate. This legal conflict was an embarrassment to the organization and was resolved out of court. A new committee was created with two members from each of the boards—governors, supervisors, and medical personnel.

While the committee allowed for some negotiation, disagreement persisted over the mission of the hospital. J. Riddle Goffe, a senior surgeon at the Woman's Hospital in 1918, recalled the opening of the Wetmore Pavilion in this way:

> At the laying of the cornerstone . . . Mr. James W. Beekman . . . said: "to practise and to teach this surgical discovery, the cure of vesico-vaginal fistula—is the object of our hospital." [Goffe found in the Acts of Incorporation, Section IX], . . . All the professors and

matriculated students of any regular medical college in the State, and all other members of the medical profession and students of medicine may be admitted to the privilege of visiting said hospital. . . . The primary object of the hospital is the direct relief of suffering humanity; the second object is the extension of their relief to the widest possible degree by using it as a school of practical instruction of the medical profession.[12]

Although the medical practice at the hospital was changing, its mission was now specifically the treatment of vesico-vaginal fistulas. Most important, the Woman's Hospital was to serve as a school, open to all who practiced "regular" medicine. During the time of Sims's medical education, sectarian medicine abounded, as we saw in the first chapter. Although diversity of medical practice continued, the idea of a standard for medical practice and education was gaining momentum, and the Woman's Hospital saw itself as part of such a shift toward science or regular medicine. Those who practiced any of a number of alternative medical therapeutics, from the Thomsonians and advocates of water cures to homeopathists, were not invited to visit the institution.

Not surprisingly, the aftermath of the Civil War influenced the lives of many who were associated with the hospital and helped to create changes in the personnel. Sims was slow to move back to New York from Europe, missing the opening of the Wetmore Pavilion. He kept his Paris residency for several years after the war. From a political point of view, Sims was naturally disenchanted with the Civil War and its military assault on slavery and on his homeland, the South. United States Secretary of State William Seward had Sims watched during his residence in Paris because of Sims's fierce loyalty to the Confederacy. In the name of diplomatic relations, Seward also convinced the Belgian government to withhold a medal from Sims during the war.[13] One of Sims's sons died as he tried to join the Confederacy during the war, succumbing to yellow fever. Following the war's end, Sims traveled frequently back and forth across the Atlantic. His willingness and ability to travel extensively reflected both his wealth and his attachment to his wealthy, noble, and royal patients, abroad as well as in New York. He became actively involved in the Ambulance Committee during the Franco-Prussian War. Financial success on the Continent did not obliterate Sims's feeling of exile and frustrations with the outcome of the war in the States. In a letter to a South Carolina physician and friend, Sims confided, "What a dreadful mistake it was to give the negro the franchise."[14] Thomas Emmet felt some of the same dissatisfactions, as in many ways he stood in for Sims at the Woman's Hospital. In 1861 Emmet was named Surgeon-in-Chief, but he had ongoing tensions with the women managers.

In 1867, with the postwar devastation of the South all around him, Josiah Nott, a New Orleans surgeon and writer on polygenism, went north to New York. His antebellum practice made him a respected obstetrician and known scientist; he was particularly respected for his surgery of the coccyx. Drawing from ideas of reflexive action, he practiced the procedure for neuralgic symptoms.[15] Sims practiced and consulted with Nott at the Woman's Hospital and in private practice several times in the late sixties.[16] T. Gaillard Thomas befriended Nott as well. In 1870, Emmet too made Nott's acquaintance and as a result gained respect for his medical capabilities. Emmet offered him an appointment at the Woman's Hospital. Emmet and Nott published articles together in the 1870 *American Journal of Obstetrics and Diseases of Women and Children*.[17] The Lady Supervisors objected to the plan but relented in time, apparently overruling objections to Nott's Southern allegiance and political writings. However, Emmet recalled that "espionage" drove Nott out after a few months.[18]

Although Nott no longer held an appointment at the Woman's Hospital, he stayed in New York City, looking for a way to establish a career after the devastation of the Civil War. Both Emmet and Thomas continued to practice medicine with Nott. Emmet and Thomas each perceived race as a critical distinction among humans and puzzled on its meaning. Emmet, for instance, felt strongly about the Irish and argued that the English had diluted its purity—the inverse of the prejudices of the larger society. In fact, Emmet feared at times that female invalidism was a sign of human weakening through racial mixture. Thomas too looked to women as he considered the implications of race, writing about women of the so-called lower order "rising" during labor, by which he meant African American women and Native American women who gave birth easily and then stood up and walked during birth and immediately afterward. In a dualistic mode, Thomas wrote, "In the lower walks of life women rise after labor."[19] Normal and predominant were European Caucasian males, and women of various makeups formed the "other" group.

Following the war, racial feelings ran high. Those of the Confederacy were only strengthened in their conviction of a racial hierarchy of humans, while Union loyalists were united more in their anger and hatred over the casualties and losses inflicted by the Southerners than in a belief in racial or ethnic hierarchies. Tensions increased between the Protestant and Catholic

Irish, leaving Emmet somewhat isolated. Social categories were shifting and society moved toward consolidation and a strengthened class structure emerging out of racial distinctions.[20] People associated with the Woman's Hospital also lived out these newfound differences.

The actions of the Lady Supervisors against Nott angered and frustrated Emmet, but later he wrote of it as just one of many encounters with the women administrators. During that same period the women had refused to appoint Emmet's nephew, Bache McEvers, an experienced staff physician at the hospital, to the Medical Board, thus further angering Emmet.[21]

In 1868, Sims's temporary return to America was not the hero's welcome he likely had hoped to enjoy. But he kept relative peace at the Woman's Hospital. Emmet had become accustomed to singular authority at the hospital, but nonetheless offered Sims his original position as head surgeon. Sims, undoubtedly to Emmet's relief, turned down the offer, continuing to operate at the Woman's Hospital but deferring to Emmet's tenure. Sims instead became head of the Medical Board, an arm of the administration of the hospital.[22] Sims's address before the anniversary meeting of the hospital was optimistic and expressed his pleasure with the institution. "Unity of purpose has bound us together by ties as strong and as indissoluble as are those of the family itself. Indeed, we are one great united family."[23] He referred to himself as a brother or a son, returning after a long absence. In this anniversary address, Sims restated his desire to include upper- and middle-class women among the hospital patients, influenced in part by his European practice, which was highly affluent.

Yet these episodes were small compared to the imbroglios precipitated by J. Marion Sims. In the spring of 1870, he received the first formal rebuke of his medical career from fellow physicians—a rare occurrence among practitioners of his stature. New York State had a relatively high incidence of legal action filed by the lay populace against physicians, but physicians chastising one another publicly and formally was a much less likely occurrence.[24] The New York Academy of Medicine—the same association that published the *Bulletin* reviewed in the last chapter, the same organization that invited Sims to give an honorary lecture in 1857, his "Silver Sutures" address, so soon after he had moved to New York City and so soon after the Woman's Hospital had begun—took him to task. On November 11, 1869, the Ethics Committee charged him with soliciting publicity for himself by openly discussing a matter that they felt should have remained private.

Charlotte Cushman (1816–1876), the real object of the furor, was a fabulously successful actress from Boston.[25] At this time, females on stage were considered very risqué, and by some, akin to prostitutes. In contrast, Charlotte Cushman's acting career reached tremendous heights in the Western world, and, first acclaimed in London, she rose from humble origins to become a member of the elite while maintaining a high degree of social probity. She was, for instance, friendly with the Peabody sisters of Boston and with Louisa May Alcott.[26] Her challenge to social expectations included her great wealth as an independent woman. Despite her daring life and because of her talent, playing such parts as Lady Macbeth, she won the hearts of many on both sides of the Atlantic.

Early in 1869, she had found a small lump on her breast and feared cancer, since she had watched her grandmother die of breast cancer. Living in Rome, with numerous contacts throughout Europe, Cushman sought medical advice from physicians in Paris, including J. Marion Sims. Returning to England, physicians there, particularly J. Y. Simpson, urged her to undergo a mastectomy. Objecting, Sims and the others advised her to let the disease progress before seeking surgery, not recognizing the condition as life-threatening while also distrusting Simpson's technique.

Cancer was little understood, with diagnosis deriving from recognition of its physiological destruction. Usually medical treatment involved surgery and came very late in the disease's progression. Some cite the end of the nineteenth century as the time in which cancer became more prevalent, because people began to live longer. Throughout much of the nineteenth century tuberculosis was one of the most common killers; tuberculosis, or phthsis, thus somehow won a measure of cultural approval. Those who died of it had an aura of sensitivity and cultivation. Cancer patients, on the other hand, suffered opprobrium.[27] In the eyes of many, they were rank and miserable in the throes of death. Furthermore, rarely mentioned aloud, female breasts remained highly private yet celebrated symbols of femininity and motherhood. Their powers as the source of infant nutrition were key issues in public health, infant mortality, and the role of wet nurses.[28]

Breast surgery was quite uncommon. In 1857 Sims proudly boasted of having operated for breast removal three times, in 1849, 1852, and 1853.[29] Although by this time there was some availability of anesthesia, particularly following the leadership of J. Y. Simpson in the use of ether, mastectomies were a difficult new procedure and were rarely performed early in the disease. Their success was very limited. In 1867, very close to the time of this incident, a British surgeon, Charles Moore, laid out the principles for the practice of radical mastectomy, arguing that it was necessary "to remove the whole breast, including the skin, lymphatics, fat, pectoral muscles, and diseased axiliary (under the arm) glands."[30] Simpson's text on female diseases published in 1868 does not describe mastectomies.

Textbooks on female diseases mentioned cancers, citing uterine cancer as the most common and breast cancer as the next most common. In fact, T. Gaillard Thomas suggested that uterine cancer was quite common among his patients.[31] Unlike uterine, cervical, and vaginal details, descriptions of surgeries and therapies for breast cancer were not included in these texts. No one liked to talk about breast cancer. In a famous painting of 1889, *The Agnew Clinic*, the daring artist, Thomas Eakins, portrayed David Hayes Agnew in a Philadelphia surgical amphitheater demonstrating a mastectomy before his students. Although the patient had one visible bare breast, that breast was not the object of surgery.[32] The physicians are operating on the other breast.

Instead of heeding Sims's advice, Cushman witnessed the exacerbation of her symptoms and decided to undergo surgery in Edinburgh with Simpson in the fall of 1869.[33] Following the operation, Cushman experienced difficulty in restoring her health. Rumors then ran rampant about her health and her fans demanded information. Relying on the speed of transatlantic cables when he was abroad, Sims was already in the habit of relaying news releases through the press in Paris. He depended regularly on the expertise of a Paris physician and journalist, W. E. Johnston, to submit stories on Sims's behalf. Although removal of a breast was a taboo topic, even in a medical text, Sims, not one to be reticent, wired the *New York Daily Times* to reassure the public that "our countrywoman is now convalescent."[34] In his assessment of her health, he reasoned that because she had survived a reasonable number of days following surgery, her postoperative relapse would either have killed her or run its course; Sims was not Cushman's physician and most likely had not examined her directly for this information. Given Cushman's status as an unmarried woman, violating her privacy with news releases and transoceanic cables seemed even more violent to some, particularly the members of the Academy's Ethics Committee, including E. R. Peaslee.

In the short term, Charlotte Cushman did rally from surgery, but Thomas Finnell, a member of the N.Y.A.M. Ethics Committee, proceeded to press charges. First, he maintained, Sims betrayed the privacy of the patient, *especially* one so accomplished and well known as Charlotte Cushman. The code read as follows: "The obligation of secrecy extends beyond the period of professional services; none of the privacies of personal and domestic life should ever be divulged by the physician, except when he is imperatively required to do so."[35] Furthermore, Finnell argued, and his committee agreed, no physician should use his connections with a celebrity to advertise his practice.

Apparently stories narrating Sims's European surgical accomplishments frequently appeared in New York papers during his prolonged European absence. Upon Sims's return in 1868, "paragraphs with like nature without number" appeared in New York papers to "set forth the great skill of Dr. Sims; the important operations he had performed, and particularly the distinguished persons he had attended."[36]

In this setting of discomfort and tension, Sims's part in the publicity surrounding Cushman's surgery evoked anger from the Ethics Committee. After the committee moved to bring the charges to Sims, they summoned him to meet with them on December 11, 1869. Sims not only missed the meeting, but left New York instead and sailed to Paris. On December 13, a story appeared in the London *Medical Times and Gazette* defending Sims's letter to the *New York Daily Times* and maintaining his innocence. The committee strongly suspected Sims had wired the medical sheet with the information, even as he refused to answer directly to the committee. At the same time, to the dismay of Finnell and his associates, some New York papers further acclaimed Sims's medical prowess, and one in particular affixed a disclaimer "that Dr [*sic*] Sims was a very modest man, and would not allow himself to be brought to the notice of the public."[37]

In June 1870, Sims presented his written defense to the committee and immediately left for Europe without waiting for a response. He fervently maintained in his defense before the committee that he had in fact simply answered the demands of a panicked public regarding Charlotte Cushman's health. He reiterated his high connections among European surgeons and physicians and protested his innocence of violation of any ethical standards whatsoever. At this point, the Ethics Committee found him guilty of the charges and imposed their most severe punishment, to reprimand Sims as a fellow in the Academy, for violating the ethical codes of the association.

While this punishment seems mild and even out of place in the context of the other medical activities engaged in by Sims and others, the New York Academy of Medicine Ethics Committee was passionately involved in pursuing the case. In the creation of medical organizations and the articulation of ethical codes at mid-nineteenth century, medical practitioners were attempting to establish acceptable and professional patterns of demeanor. Their sense of what was appropriate moral behavior for a physician was changing for many reasons. Sims had challenged many physicians' sense of propriety with his bold reliance on the speculum. Now that he was a member of the medical elite, his public gestures in this case were a matter of concern.

Among physicians there was a growing effort to erect and maintain internal standards of professional behavior. Many practitioners felt in the early efforts to establish a peer-driven collective identity that disputes regarding medical therapies or details of practice should stay within the medical community, and not be aired publicly.[38] Finnell and the others also believed that public advertising of medical skills was beneath the dignity of the profession, and that proclaiming the secrets of and association with members of the social elite violated standards of decency.

In the case of Charlotte Cushman and in other conflicts regarding the practice of medicine, J. Marion Sims acted as a self-governing individual and refused to take the standards established by an organization of physicians as his personal regulation. He practiced medicine under his own private set of ethics, which did not answer to peer review. In this regard, he embodied the Jacksonian and perfectionist perspective that sanctioned the autonomy and moral agency of the individual in maintaining social order. For many, Sims invoked the panache and daring of a manly hero, using his moniker of surgeon to rally public support.

Conflict over the health of Charlotte Cushman went beyond the establishment of professional codes, however, to contain hostilities washed up from the storm of the Civil War. Here tension between the geographic and cultural regions of the North and South came to play. Thomas Finnell, the man whose strong feelings precipitated the accusations by the Academy against Sims, was a former surgeon with the Union Army. Another member of the Ethics Committee, E. R. Peaslee, was also a Northerner who had participated in the military side of the war. Throughout the 1870s Peaslee and Sims grew testier with one another, yet continued their association. After all, they were members of the same Presbyterian Church on Madison Square. Charlotte Cushman herself was a friend of William Seward, and gave benefit performances on behalf of the Union during the war. In Washington, D.C., she appeared several times to raise money for the U.S. Sanitary Commission, bringing more than $8,000 to the Civil War organization.[39] Her adopted son served as foreign consul.

To some, Sims, an avowed Southerner with adopted residence in the North, was attempting to reestablish a medical reputation in New York, in the wake of the divisiveness caused by the war, evoking the good name of Charlotte Cushman among others. Among his peers and New York City colleagues, the Academy's Ethics Committee voiced objection and acted on it. Undoubtedly Sims also harbored resentment against a female professional who had garnered much fame and public acclaim while supporting the Union cause during the war. She challenged all that Sims recognized as the virtues of womanhood and yet won cultural acclaim. Unfortunately, Charlotte Cushman's cancer spread to her other side not long after the death of J. Y. Simpson in 1870, and further surgery failed to save her life. She was greatly mourned upon her death in 1876, at the age of sixty-two. Sims and Peaslee remained at odds for the rest of Peaslee's life.

Sims remained largely undaunted by the Academy's reprimand, angered by the event and defensive in the face of what seemed to be American, or at least Northern, disrespect for his achievements. When he returned to Europe the year following the Cushman incident, Sims presented a speech ruminating on the political situation in the States. He declared, "I am proud of my country abroad, but ashamed of it at home. The humiliation of the South is inexcusable. The ruin is unjustifiable."[40] Nonetheless, Sims felt the affirmation of union was for the best. As he defended the South, he also urged it to accept its defeat and move toward restoration of its politics and economy.

In September 1871, in Paris, Sims precipitated a physical and unprovoked altercation with an American dentist living in Paris, Dr. Thomas W. Evans. Sims assaulted the man during a meeting of the American Sanitary Committee. They had met to determine activities for wartime ambulances and to organize the surgeons. Evans had refused to make Sims a member of the committee for the organization of ambulance surgeons. Sims than grabbed him by the neck and dealt him a blow to the face that bloodied his nose and knocked him to the floor. Sims had to be pulled off the man.[41] By the time Dr. Evans pressed charges against Sims, he had already left Paris, returning now to New York. In the years following the Civil War, Sims's Southern origin stood in stark relief, and his sense of honor was ever on display.

Thomas Addis Emmet too experienced moments of crisis. In the spring of 1871, Emmet experienced a nervous collapse. Following the habits of many in his time, Emmet set sail to restore his equilibrium. He traveled to Russia and Ireland for six months, and then returned to the hospital and to New York.[42] Undoubtedly he was influenced by the return of J. Marion Sims to New York and the accompanying fireworks. Emmet learned the foundations of his surgical technique from Sims, but he made his career through a much more conservative approach. By 1871 he was very well established as a surgeon and came to be known as a "conservative" surgeon, meaning that he premised his techniques on the conservation of tissue.[43] However, he, like Sims, had experimented extensively on women's bodies and Emmet had become a surgeon treating female disorders.

Emmet had suffered political reversals as well. The South had lost the Civil War. In New York City the Tweed Ring that had long run Tammany Hall and city government was crumbling and fell along with the long-term reign of Democrats in 1872. Disorder and chaos ruled. In Paris, the French suffered a loss in the Franco-Prussian War and soon came the bloodbath of the Paris Commune, which occurred in 1871. Emmet had been a loyal follower of the French medical school that now lost its position as the leading authority in medical theory.

The status of the Irish shifted in postwar New York. The massive emigration had greatly slowed and the domestic environment seemed to suffer. Not long after Emmet returned to New York, things really began to fall apart. In 1872, the Orange Riot occurred—a St. Patrick's Day Parade turned violent, with the Protestants attacking Catholics. This tension touched deep family roots for Emmet and added further weight to his troubles. At the same time, Emmet had not only to deal with the irascibility of J. Marion Sims, but also the tendentiousness of the Lady Supervisors in their distaste for the Irish, the Catholics, and Emmet's politics. The responsibilities of the medical governance of the hospital grew in proportion to the construction and the new buildings. There was now a high mortality rate to reckon with. In 1872, the Board of Governors and the Board of Lady Supervisors created a replacement for Emmet's position as chief surgeon. There were now four surgeons-in-chief, Emmet, Sims, Peaslee, and Thomas.

To make matters worse, the Medical Board overruled Emmet's Turkish-bath arrangement for the new pavilion in favor of a waiting room.[44] By this time, Thomas Emmet had become a strong supporter of the use of hydropathy, the use of Russian and Turkish baths in medical therapies. The other chief surgeons apparently did not share his loyalty to the use of water therapies.

At the other end of the spectrum was James Beekman, who was deeply involved in the Union side during the Civil War. Recall that Beekman was vice-president of the New York Hospital and director of the New York Dispensary, in addition to his executive position with the Woman's Hospital. During the war, both New York Hospital and Bellevue treated wounded soldiers under a federal contract.[45] He gained knowledge of hospital construction and was influenced by the concept of "hospitalism" as articulated by J. Y. Simpson. The idea was that building many small buildings rather than one large pavilion would provide the ventilation and fresh air many saw as the key to good health, and this would also stem contagion. In 1871, Beekman published an address he gave to the New York Hospital Society with an appendix on the building of hospitals.[46] Here he revealed his dissatisfaction with any extant hospital buildings (throughout the Western world). Although he was careful to choose examples from Paris of the high rate of mortality in hospitals,

Beekman thinly veiled his distrust of New York City hospital structures. Coming too late to change the plans for the Wetmore Pavilion, the war combined with Beekman's elite social status and political prowess to make him an expert on the administration and building of hospitals. He now saw there was more involved than raising funds.

Thus the postwar era and changes in the atmosphere of the hospital accompanied the completion and opening of the Wetmore Pavilion. Sims's reputation was now international, and his new status was sometimes rebuffed.

The Lady Board of Supervisors and Crisis in the Hospital

Just as doctors and administrators found their world changing in the wake of the Civil War, so too did women find new roles in health care. Nursing practices developed during the war would do much to reshape treatment at the Woman's Hospital in the years after. In the months just following the beginning of the Civil War, several women from New York City got together to create an organization that would centralize relief for regiments throughout the country and would establish the recruitment and training of nurses.[47] Under the leadership of Elizabeth Blackwell and her sister, Emily Blackwell, the women founded the Women's Central Relief Association. Usurping Elizabeth Blackwell's leadership and vision in the devising of a nursing corps, the U.S. government appointed Dorothea Dix as superintendent of women nurses for the U.S. Army.[48] The Women's Central Relief Association remained a part of relief efforts during the war and provided a way for several elite women philanthropists to participate in the war—including Caroline Lane. Several other women later connected with the Board of Lady Supervisors were involved in the volunteer effort, including members of the Howland and Woolsey family. Adumbrating the early history of the Woman's Hospital, the enthusiasm and significance of the effort led to the involvement of two well-known New York men, Frederick Law Olmsted and the Reverend Henry Bellows, and their initiation of the United States Sanitary Commission. There were many similar regional women's relief organizations, but the New York City group was responsible for catalyzing the U.S. Sanitary Commission.[49]

The history of this organization is fascinating, albeit separate and significant in and of itself. As a member of the Union League Club, Beekman was an associate of Frederick Law Olmsted, who had been instrumental in the creation of Central Park and became the head of the United States Sanitary Commission. For our history, the engagement of the Woman's Hospital in the formalization of nursing and nursing education begins here with direct

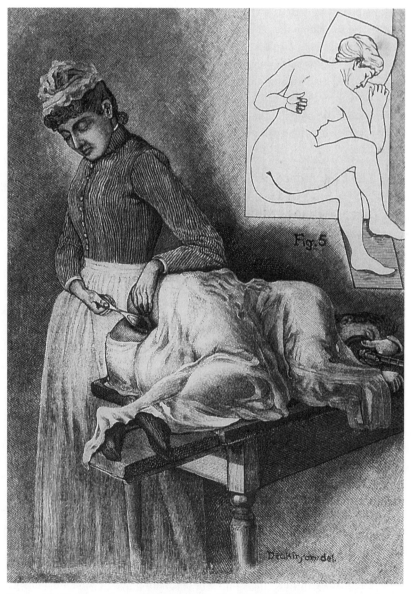

FIGURE 14. Uniformed nurse with patient in Sims's Position, receiving anesthesia. In Alexander J. C. Skene, *Treatise on the Diseases of Women* (New York: Appleton, 1888). *(From the Special Collections, Southern Illinois University School of Medicine.)*

involvement in the Civil War. For the most part, nursing prior to this time was a loosely defined area. In the 1840s, for instance, prisoners from Blackwell Island served as nurses at Bellevue Hospital. With the war effort, the influence of Florence Nightingale, and the actions of several leaders throughout the Western World, nursing emerged as a closely defined profession. Among those involved was New York doctor and associate at the Woman's Hospital, Edward Delafield, who joined other physicians at Bellevue Hospital to oversee training of the nurses before they were sent to military zones.

After about a year with the U.S. Sanitary Commission, Olmsted chose a group of fifteen women from among an inexperienced elite to serve aboard transport ships during the peninsular campaign, which included the Battle of Shiloh. Among those chosen, Caroline E. Lane went into the experience enthusiastic but naive. She and the others came back with hands-on memories of caring for desperately wounded soldiers and a new sense of themselves as women in relation to health care. Lane and her peers weathered conflicts with authorities, especially Olmsted about the parameters of their activities, bearing on the limits of womanhood. One author symbolized the changes in terms of apparel, contrasting the women's newfound taste for flannel shirts to the complicated and confining dress of Victorian upper-class women.[50] Others, nurses and women physicians alike, had to confront limitations imposed by Dix.

The New York women now saw skills involved with nursing as important in healing. Not only did Florence Nightingale's theories of nursing include sanitary conditions in hospitals, but also a definition of nursing that had never before existed. Nursing became increasingly a female vocation. Nurses were women because their tasks fit the culturally designated division of labor by sex and gender, leaving women in charge of creating an efficient domestic order, a moral atmosphere and a well-run, healthy environment. Nurses, according to Nightingale, were not medical professionals per se, but rather subordinates to doctors. In many ways analogous to the role of domestic servants, their task was to serve the physician.[51] Character and discipline became key qualities.

Olmsted's designated group of elite women were not serving as nurses, but rather as supervisors. During their time on the ships, Lane and the others maintained an elite position of authority and depended on the strictures of social hierarchy to run the medical services. This included overseeing working-class nurses as well as the work of contrabands, the slaves who followed Union soldiers to escape during the war. What came from this adventure paralleled Beekman's ideas for hospital building—a new reformist vision of scientific philanthropy, moving away from moral and religious be-nevolence toward a class-based science of giving.

In the early 1870s Louisa Lee Schuyler, a leader from the war days and the Sanitary Commission, began to organize women who had participated in the war relief and to make a felt presence in the governmental bureau-cracy that oversaw hospitals in particular. Appalled by the filth and disorder at Bellevue Hospital and stymied by physicians' unwillingness to organize nursing, Schuyler and her companions, including Lane (who was undoubt-edly also motivated by problems she saw at the Woman's Hospital), set about to establish the State Charities Aid Association. This association gained au-tonomous powers for the women's committee to engage in inspecting and vis-iting hospitals to oversee their condition. They had direct input into the State Board of Charities, which was the state's umbrella organization overseeing various state-run institutions and asylums.

In 1873 these women, using the State Charities Aid Association as a vehicle, were directly responsible for the founding of the Bellevue Nursing School. Two others were established that year; the three were the first in the country.

Medical professionals were deeply caught up in arguments about wom-anhood and what women could or should do. Throughout the early 1870s, social controversy flourished regarding the role of women in medicine. Fol-lowing the ideas presented by E. H. Clarke—ideas that were widely held—many physicians and others argued that education was detrimental to female health. Women's bodies and their purpose in reproduction, the argument went, simply could not bear the loss of energy to their brains.

The contradictions were there, with women so central in the hospital's organization yet excluded from executive governance and medical practice—within the realm of the institutional walls. Rare indeed was the voice sup-porting the work of women as physicians. Mary Dixon Jones, a young physician, did observe surgery at the hospital, but only as a visitor.[52] Neither did physicians rally behind establishing training schools for nurses at anni-versary meetings of the Woman's Hospital, yet speakers extolled Dorothea Dix and Florence Nightingale as exemplary models of womanly behavior. The Lady Supervisors and the laymen governors and physicians dwelled in sepa-rate worlds to a degree—with the women developing a kind of resistance af-ter the war to their subordination, but never fundamentally challenging the framework that held the hierarchy in place.

Early years of the professional organization of the American Medical Association, founded in 1848, touched on issues of women and medicine, with an emphasis on women as the objects of surgery and health care. Within the first years of its existence, the American Medical Association acted to define the role of physicians vis-à-vis abortion. From 1860 to 1880, the AMA. and its members first identified abortion as criminal and worked throughout the country to establish state laws criminalizing it.[53] Moving further to remove the practice of midwifery, physicians acted to make themselves the only prescribers of abortifacients—an area once occupied by herbalists, midwives, and various other practitioners.

In 1872 the first of the Comstock Laws was passed in Congress, outlawing the dissemination of information about birth control and abortion.[54] T. Gaillard Thomas and Thomas Addis Emmet each became increasingly engaged in identifying what they called criminal abortion. They were distrustful of women who came to them as patients seeking medical care. Emmet suggested that many of the women he identified as "sterile" were women who had undergone abortions.[55] Thomas also thought women were often childless because they had interfered in reproduction by using contraception or abortion. He presented a dramatic and tragic story in his class to demonstrate the horrors of abortion—a case of a woman who had tried to abort herself with a coat hanger who died of hemorrhage. Thomas maintained he found a piece of the hanger in her abdomen.[56]

Perhaps because of the efforts to contain women and to define their bodies as the provenance of medicine, nursing education emerged without the engagement of the AMA in setting curricular standards.[57] While nursing was a new field for women and represented a kind of economic independence, the door was not wide open to all applicants. Statistical evidence shows that at the Bellevue Hospital Nursing School, there was a preponderance of Episcopalian and Presbyterian women who succeeded in becoming nurses, and a high proportion of dropouts who were Catholic.[58] At the Woman's Hospital, the original Irish Catholic nurse Margaret Brennan, particularly well remembered by Emmet but without formal training, left the Woman's Hospital in the 1870s after nearly forty years of nursing practice. She had originally come to the hospital as a patient.[59] Although Emmet found her work to be invaluable, the Lady Board of Supervisors saw it differently. In 1875, Mary Jay Edwards recorded notes on nursing for the minutes of the Board of Lady Supervisors. The women sought change in the nursing staff, hoping to enhance "the comfort and welfare of the patients by replacing careless and incompetent nurses by persons of a much better stamp and character, possessing also the advantage of being Protestant."[60]

After the opening of the Wetmore Pavilion, new rules (from the Lady

Board of Supervisors) governing the behavior of the house staff were imple-
mented. Nurses often had been patients and came from lower economic
groups than the Lady Supervisors. Their status was closer to that of domestic service than to the occupation of nursing as it is now understood. In fact,
in 1870 a rule for patients stated that "those patients in the Free Ward who
are able shall assist in nursing, and render such other services as the matron
may direct."[61]

Typical of institutions in which women supervised, the rules were re-
strictive and parental.[62] Patients were only given limited hours with visitors,
and men were given very little time in the hospital, never after dark. Alcohol
was also forbidden, except through the matron. The supervisors and the house
matron had the authority to make patients leave. By 1875 several rules governing the lives of nurses delineated reasons for expulsion. One rule forbade
the nurses to accept gifts; a nurse could lose her position for violation of this
rule, or for insubordination. Not only did the structure of hospitals, governance, and staffing change in the postwar period, but at the Woman's Hospital the nature of surgery changed as well, as "capital" operations or major
surgery—surgeries of most significance—became more common. Ovariotomies, which were the most frequent such operations, grew in number, and
the number of mortalities associated with surgery increased rapidly. Added
to the practice was a new variation called "normal ovariotomy." Robert Battey,
a Georgian, published a series of articles, beginning in 1872, on a form of
ovariotomy he invented to treat conditions much more difficult to diagnose
than ovarian tumors,[63] known as "Battey's Operation" or "normal ovariotomy."
The procedure removed the ovaries, but not in response to any organic disease of the organs: the ovaries themselves were normal, except that they supposedly elicited one or several nervous symptoms, such as insanity, epilepsy,
or dysmenorrhea. The symptoms prompting this procedure were rather fluid
and ill-defined.

While the practice was controversial among surgeons, it was widely
performed by the 1880s. Certainly Battey's Operation derived from the practice of ovariotomy itself. By the turn of the century, the designations separating the two operations were hopelessly confounded: oophorectomy, female
castration, spaying.[64]

Sims took up the practice of Battey's Operation in the early 1870s. As
was the case in so many of the newly devised operations, Sims experimented
with the surgical treatment for a variety of symptoms even though the practice was attended by great risk of death.

Writing later in the decade, Sims recalled a period of extremely high mortality in 1873. Just as the practice of cervical surgery had spread like wild-fire in the first years of the Woman's Hospital, the practice of abdominal surgery, including uterine surgery, grew quickly. He described a patient who needed surgery for an intra-uterine fibroid: "When Mme. de—— arrived in New York, we were passing through the epidemic of puerperal fever, which will long be remembered for its great mortality."[65] Sims moved this patient out of New York City to perform surgery.

Puerperal fever was associated with childbirth. Although the Woman's Hospital had no lying-in wing, physicians who operated at the hospital, most notably T. Gaillard Thomas and Fordyce Barker, were also active in attending childbirth. The latter two had appointments at Bellevue as well. Sims noted that puerperal fever's contagion might spill over into other surgeries and moved his place of surgery out of town. Thomas, Barker, William Lusk, and other obstetricians in New York were loath to see that puerperal fever's contagion came through the physician's hands. By this time, despite their inexplicable reluctance, material was already circulating in medical journals that identified the simple routine of cleanliness and hand washing by physicians as the method to stop the spread of puerperal fever.

In 1868, Bellevue's mortality rate from the fever began to climb with periodic, veritable epidemics. Maternal deaths from septic origins, which included puerperal fever, in New York City between 1870 and 1880 were well over 50 percent.[66] The epidemic of 1873 peaked in 1874. Between January and June 1874, at the height of the epidemic at Bellevue, of 166 women who delivered, 31 died—nearly 19 percent.[67]

Adding to the problem of their failure to wash up between patients after visiting different wards and hospitals or performing autopsies, physicians became increasingly interventionist in their obstetrical methods. Tears in the perineum, vesico-vaginal fistulas, and other so-called accidents of childbirth gained attention and were identified as the result of the physicians' failure actively to guide labor and delivery.

T. Gaillard Thomas became even more expert on childbirth and developed medical strategies for addressing various situations during labor. In 1870, Thomas published an essay, "The Induction of Premature Delivery as a Prophylactic Resource in Midwifery," describing various "morbid states," including a deformed pelvis, that dictated an induced labor. Thomas's method of determining a medical technique included the use of pelvimetry in making a choice between Caesarian section and induced delivery. His delivery method followed several steps, beginning with bathing the woman's birth canal in warm water, then using a cervical dilator, and finally introducing a catheter through the bag of waters. Next he gave the patient an enema, checking throughout the process to see if labor had begun. If labor still had not begun in earnest, Thomas anesthetized the patient, passed his hand into the vagina and two fingers into the uterus. In the specific case he described as an example, the medical therapies resulted, he announced proudly, with the delivery of a baby boy. Even before reaching into the uterus and pulling out the infant manually, Thomas did not wash his hands to prevent the possible introduction of disease directly into the patient's system. Given the right sequence of events, such an induction of labor could easily have led directly to a woman's death, and undoubtedly it did in more than a few cases.[68]

Thomas and his associates practiced in a web flung among several hospitals, traveling from patient to patient and carrying various organisms with them. Because they were concerned about other issues, medical practitioners could not see how they contributed to the deaths of patients. In the early nineteenth century, physicians articulated their distrust of midwives by referring to "meddlesome midwifery," which made physicians themselves afraid to meddle in birth for a time.

By the 1870s, Thomas and others were beginning to play a more active role in delivery, not always to the patient's benefit. Unaware of his own contribution to an extraordinarily high maternal mortality, along with that of colleagues including Fordyce Barker, John Metcalfe, and William Lusk, Thomas argued stridently against the practice of female midwifery in a speech advocating the further development of a science of gynecology.[69] His discovery of vesico-vaginal fistulas helped to fuel his embrace of medical intervention in birth. Paradoxically, the problems of patient morbidity and mortality did not stymie the growth of the specialty. In 1872, at Bellevue Hospital Medical College, the year of Thomas and Peaslee's new appointments to the Woman's Hospital as chief surgeons, E. R. Peaslee became the first American professor of gynecology.[70]

High rates of mortality motivated women reformers and hospital administrators to take an active part in the provision of health care and medicine in their hospitals. Part of the authority of membership in the State Charities Aid Association was overseeing hospital conditions throughout the city. Members of the Bellevue Visiting Committee became very alarmed at the soaring number of deaths in the Bellevue maternity ward. Having gained authority and forthrightness in their ability to supervise health care, the women of the committee requested from the Bellevue Medical Board that they be put in charge of the maternity patients and that they be allowed to move them out of the hospital. When the doctors refused their offer, the committee went to the State Charities Aid Association, over the heads of the Medical Board, with the same request. Putting pressure on the doctors to comply, the women threatened to publicize, in specific newspapers, the likely role physicians played in the spreading of puerperal fever from patient to patient.[71] One physician called the women "spies."[72] Although the doctors complained about the inconvenience of visiting patients elsewhere, in June the lying-in department at Bellevue Hospital was closed and the patients were relocated in the Charity Hospital on Blackwell's Island. Nightingale training in many ways precluded acceptance of the antiseptic methods of Listerism and the scientific explorations of the origins of disease, which would become known as germ theory; yet this episode demonstrated that the Bellevue Visiting Committee and the State Charities Aid Society were attentive to the current discourse on contagion and addressed the high maternal mortality from puerperal fever.

Trouble was brewing at the Woman's Hospital as well. In the early 1870s, alarm grew among the Lady Supervisors as the very character of the institution seemed to have altered. During the next two years, conflict and frustration increased. They objected to many aspects of the medical practice during this time. Recorded in the letters, minutes, and reports of the managers of the hospital are comments lamenting patients' lack of privacy, as well as the increasing number of cancer patients.

Periodically the Lady Supervisors gained the approval of the Board of Governors to add new buildings and private rooms for treatment of patients who were exceedingly ill or had undergone serious surgery. Isolation was one solution, particularly for the postoperative recovery of tumor patients, which meant primarily but not exclusively those undergoing ovariotomies. The vision of the original Woman's Hospital, as the Lady Supervisors understood it, was shaken. They had lost authority with the newly active role of the Board of Governors and the strengthened Medical Board.

Over a period of two years, the supervisors repeatedly complained about the growing number of breast cancer patients treated in the wards and argued against admitting them. W. Gill Wylie, Sims's son-in-law and a young resident surgeon at the hospital in 1872 (who later became an author and noted physician in his own right), described the women's perspective as follows: "At that time the use of antiseptics was not so well understood, and some of these patients, when tamponed after being curetted, occasionally caused offensive odors in the wards."[73] Many people identified "miasma," or qualities of the atmosphere, as the source of a disease—hence the preoccupation with proper ventilation, the fetor of cancer, and the fear of sickness gone this far.

Cancer and various tumor cases were challenging to the women in the hospital administration, and the Board of Governors seemed to stand behind them. The seriousness of the sickness accompanied by difficult and slow recovery created problems. This situation became an integral part of the first significant disagreement between the women and the medical staff.

Of course, many patients treated for ovarian tumors also suffered from cancer. Although the women administrators labored at great length to maintain tumor rooms for these cases, they saw breast cancer as separate and not fitting under the rubric of female disorders that originally defined the hospital. The underlying logic maintained that the Woman's Hospital was an institution only for diseases *peculiar* to women. Cancer, of course, was not gender-specific, and why breast cancer was unacceptable and uterine and ovarian cancer at least somewhat acceptable is difficult to comprehend. In part, mastectomies were new and virtually untried; but probably, most importantly, breasts, or mammae, were an overwhelmingly powerful symbol for female sexuality and femininity and their disease became taboo. The connection of the practice of surgical gynecology with the treatment of breast cancer was evident to many, but not to the Board of Lady Supervisors.

Laboratory science was beginning to appear at the institution and among the associated medical personnel, E. R. Peaslee and Edward Delafield could identify cancer through the microscope. By the early 1870s the hospital also had a staff physician, a pathologist, in charge of autopsies. Among them was William Welch, who worked for several years with pathology at the Woman's Hospital in conjunction with an appointment at Bellevue before taking a position at Johns Hopkins in the 1880s. The potential groundwork for laboratory science was well underway, but its benefits seemed ambiguous at best to lay administrators.

In the early years of the hospital, the women managers had been loyal to J. Marion Sims. He was, after all, the person who made the hospital possible. One foreboding came in 1862 when the Lady Supervisors noted in their minutes that some writers had rebuked Sims, but they themselves chose to shield him from criticism.[74] After the end of the war, the women grew less sympathetic to Sims's point of view and became more jaded in their view of the hospital.

The smell was terrible, the women argued, and damaging to the well-being of the other patients. The presence of breast cancer victims among the other patients was but another example of the lack of privacy given the patients. For instance, doctors failed to use a screen to provide privacy for women being treated in the outdoor clinic, and also for the women in the wards of the hospital. When the Wetmore Pavilion first opened, the women of the Inspecting Committee for the hospital reported, "The screen is scarcely ever, if ever, used in the operating room, and all of the patients feel most unpleasantly about it. Sometimes they are placed on the table, which is dragged in front of the screen, facing all the doctors, some of the patients feel that the embarrassment retards their recovery."[75] In 1872, the Lady Supervisors resolved, that "the nurse is ordered to place the screen between the table and the surgeons before the entrance of each patient."[76]

In fact, the new hospital facility had many drawbacks, including the nerve-wracking sound of the railroad—"the ceaseless and discordant screeches of engines. . . . rendered night hideous."[77] Grand Central Station was but a few blocks away. The problem of noise was unsettling because there was little that could be done to remedy the situation. Meanwhile, efforts were underway to complete the second pavilion.

In January 1873, the minutes of the meeting of the Board of Lady Supervisors reported that "the principal event in the month had been the admission of 2 cancer patients by the Medical Board to the open ward of the Hospital, thereby creating great discomfort and danger to the other patients in the ward."[78] One of the patients suffered from breast cancer, and the supervisors found her presence in the ward completely unacceptable. T. Gaillard Thomas, as the spokesman for the Medical Board, sent Sims to the Lady Supervisors. Sims's unsatisfactory response to the women's complaints was to read what the secretary characterized as a paper on treating cancer. The Medical Board, however, or the collective representation of the four chief surgeons, offered to limit admissions to those "curable cases of Cancer of the uterus, or those susceptible of decided amelioration." They also offered not to admit patients with breast cancer. In a conciliatory tone, the Medical Board agreed to consider the comfort and well-being of the other patients in the process of admissions.[79]

At the same meeting, after hearing from Sims and from the Medical Board, the women resolved completely to exclude cancer patients from care at the hospital. They argued that "no cancer cases known to be such can be received in the present arrangement of the Hospital without *detriment or discomfort to the other patients*."[80] They sent the resolution to the Medical Board and the Board of Governors.

In June of the same year, the minutes of the Lady Supervisors' meeting noted two cases of cancer—one of them breast cancer—admitted to the open ward. Irately, they sent a note to Thomas, the secretary of the Medical Board, requesting the patients' removal before surgery. There was no response from the doctors, who proceeded to operate on the patients. The women patients began a slow recovery. "In the mean while [*sic*] the Ward was made so very offensive from the nature of the disease that two or three patients actually left and others complained bitterly of the discomfort to which they have been subjected."[81]

Given a hand in the establishment of nursing education, the Lady Supervisors demanded more control over the wards and policies of admission. The women refused to accept Sims's resolution to include the cancer patients in the new pavilion. The construction of the Baldwin Pavilion had begun in February 1873, and all parties in the administration of the hospital sought to influence its design.

By the end of the year, the frustrations and anger of the women peaked. After a further incident on December 6, they sent a special report, dated December 31, to the Board of Governors. The Medical Board, they argued, persistently violated mutually accepted regulations of the three boards. "Within . . . *three days* of our strong remonstrance in person to Mr. Beekman . . . and within a *week* of the time in which a death occurred from cancer—which case caused extreme annoyance and suffering to all other patients in the Ward—so much so that they could not eat their meals—(for it must be remembered that all meals are set in the Wards) yet . . . within this short time Dr. Sims brought in another case and operated the next day, before any of the managers were cognizant of the facts."[82]

Sims apparently rejected the position of the Lady Supervisors and refused to heed the urgings of the Board of Governors as well. The women's ideas of an organization of nursing at the institution also became formalized. They explained their position, returning to a complaint they had frequently voiced. The nursing staff was shorthanded. There simply were not enough nurses to perform their tasks. The seriously ill patients, plus the increased number of "capital" surgeries, taxed the staff beyond their limits. The cancer cases made their work impossible.[83]

Demands to maintain the institution internally grew with the new facilities. The number of patients grew as well. The outdoor department was open daily now with a rotating staff, rather than just a few days a week. The medical staff now included an electrician, who used electrotherapy. A new elevator malfunctioned at one point, and fell to the bottom floor, injuring a patient.[84] In 1873, in an apparent suicide, a patient fell out a window to her death. The house physician was moved by the incident to impose the injunction that patients remain only on the floor of their residence.[85] This latter regulation was difficult to administer, since the women often stayed in the hospital for two or three months.

Furthermore, the women maintained, the number of spectators attending surgery was far too high. In December 1873 the women estimated that seventy observers had attended one of Thomas's surgeries. They objected to the large number, stating that "both coming in and going out, the noise of the tramp upstairs and the loud talking of such a crowd confuses and unecessarily [*sic*] alarms the patient."[86] The great number of physicians led the supervisors to ask, "Is the Woman's hospital to be made a Public School,—or is it a Private Hospital where our afflicted Sisters can come without fear?"[87] Unlike the physicians, the Lady Supervisors did not give priority or even accept fully the role of the hospital as a center of medical education.

The excitement and innovation that accompanied the beginnings of surgical gynecology did not apply to the Lady Supervisors. In the spring and summer of 1873, more patients died in a month than had previously died in a year. The women, since the beginnings of the hospital, envisioned an institution for women patients as a retreat, as a private experience, and as a hospital free from the great mortality rates of other hospitals. The practitioners, however, were caught up in a burgeoning new medical field and in the dissemination of technique and knowledge, if not also in a degree of self-adulation and pride. The medical men *defined* the hospital as a public school and took pleasure in the many visitors who attended surgery there. In the annual report for the year 1873, Thomas had described the many physicians who had visited the hospital. He wished to "extend the clinical advantages of the Hospital to as many physicians as could be instructed without detriment to the patients," demonstrating with his words an attentiveness to the discontent of the women, yet heeding the resolve of the Medical Board.[88]

In January 1874, the Medical Board and the Board of Governors both resolved, first, to refuse malignant cases; second, to limit spectators to fifteen at operations, and only on invitation.[89] A conference committee was organized to consist of members from each wing of the hospital administration. The group met monthly in an attempt to smooth the difficulties. The Lady Supervisors maintained an assertive stance and fired a physician on the staff, apparently overruling and therefore displeasing the Medical Board.[90] In the winter months of 1874, an outbreak of postoperative infection spread throughout the institution, paralleling the epidemic of puerperal fever at Bellevue. Patients died at the rate of three a month in January and February, and Thomas reported that "all serious operations were suspended . . . on account of a pernicious epidemic influence."[91]

According to the records of the Lady Supervisors, the hospital had run smoothly for most of the past year with little overt conflict. After spearheading fund-raising and architectural plans for a very expensive building that proved

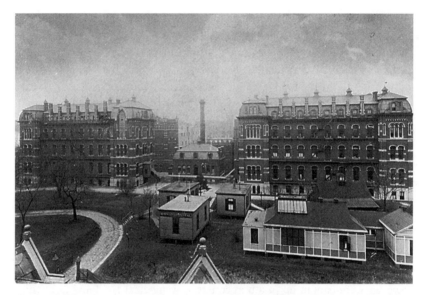

FIGURE 15. Cottages around the Wetmore Pavilion built to prevent contagion and hospitalism. *(Courtesy of the Bolling Medical Library, St. Luke's–Roosevelt Hospital Center, New York.)*

almost uninhabitable upon opening, Beekman himself somewhat distrusted the physicians' ability to apprise their environment and their own role in it.

Perhaps the resignation of Sarah Doremus in October 1874 contributed to the buildup of tension. After she quit her directorship of religious activities at the hospital, her participation in hospital administration was no longer tangible. As the time neared for the anniversary meeting of the institution, November 19, 1874, the surgeons met to prepare statements. Sims remembered having met in the previous January with the other three chief surgeons to discuss the regulations pertaining to the exclusion of cancer patients and limitations on the number of spectators.[92] By November Sims still strongly objected to the restrictions pertaining to cancer patients but resolved to object to the limited number of spectators. His understanding after meeting with the Medical Board was that the group would act in concert and voice objection to adding the two new regulations to the bylaws of the hospital's constitution.

During the annual meeting of the Woman's Hospital, Beekman expressed optimism over the hospital's future but concern over raising the funds to support the new pavilion. He brought the bad news that the Baldwin Pavilion, like the Wetmore (which would be closed upon the completion of the Baldwin), had no appropriate area for surgery. Worrying about ventilation and the presence of permeable surfaces, Beekman submitted that cottages built on a temporary basis would provide the proper arena.[93]

Most suggestive of the pressing internal tension during the annual meeting was Thomas's report from the Medical Board. He asserted that there were patients in the wards of the hospital who could afford treatment elsewhere, but who chose instead to exploit the less expensive services of the Woman's Hospital. "Let it be remembered that every woman whose resources enable her to procure treatment elsewhere, and who occupies a bed here, does so to the exclusion of another who lacks the very advantages which she usurps, and for want of which she may suffer and die."[94] Thomas also referred to "a slight but passing misunderstanding between it and the two lay Boards of the Hospital. . . . The Medical Board desires, and has ever desired, in the interests of the patients and of themselves, that the number of spectators should be limited."[95] Thomas declared a Medical Board preference for a limit of twenty-five spectators, but a willingness, nonetheless, to comply with the regulation.

A physician not associated with the institution, a Dr. Potter, delivered an address in which he berated the hospital for slighting the role of women. He exhorted those present to find a role for female medical practitioners.[96] Perhaps this presentation combined with aggravation at Thomas's submission drove Sims to brash behavior. Sims violently condemned the lay administration of the hospital. He called the new regulations of medical practice "tyrannies," and protested the authority of the governors and supervisors, dramatically and publicly submitting his resignation from the hospital as an act of protest.[97]

After the anniversary meeting for the institution, Sims felt utterly betrayed by his colleagues, and they in turn voiced little sympathy for him. A few days later, Colonel George Davis (who had been in the Union Army, and pursued railroad endeavors) spoke for the Board of Governors. Sims, he said, "evinced a spirit of insubordination and an avowed determination on his part."[98] The women administrators referred to the "*outrage* of their [Sims's words] utterance at such time and place."[99] Sims had perpetrated a "public attack."[100] After resigning from the Woman's Hospital, Sims never regained the primary association with the institution he had once had as its founder.

Class and Sex

What had become a conflict between Sims and the rest of the hospital administration did not address any of the interconnections of class and sex in medicine and in society directly. Besides the few already-noted exceptions, the Lady Supervisors never entered into discussions of womanhood or specific medical therapies. Perhaps recognizing the tenuous nature of administrative/medical cooperation at the hospital as well as the utility of his ties to the institution and maybe having second thoughts about the strength of his public demands, Sims attempted to withdraw his resignation. As head of the Board of Governors, George Davis—despite Thomas's pleas on Sims's behalf—in effect expelled Sims from practice in the Woman's Hospital. Thus J. Marion Sims, the chief instigator and founder of the Woman's Hospital in the State of New York, was no longer affiliated with the institution and no longer had a hospital appointment.

There was not a great deal of publicity or media commotion about Sims's resignation and subsequent failure to be reinstated. Although Sims felt betrayed by his fellow chief surgeons, there was no outright professional conflict.

Like the Board of Governors, the women administrators were more than happy to accept Sims's resignation. They were not completely sanguine, however, about their relations with the remaining members of the Medical Board. Mary Jay Edwards, as secretary for the Board of Supervisors, voiced displeasure at the nature of the remarks made by T. Gaillard Thomas during the anniversary meeting. She argued that the Medical Board ought to communicate directly with the supervisors instead of using the occasion of the gathering to complain. Edwards denied any intent on the women's part to privilege the more economically sound patient over the charity case.[101]

Denials from the Lady Supervisors to the contrary notwithstanding, other evidence suggests that Thomas had identified a source of conflict in the management and in the admission of patients. Caroline Lane, as president of the Executive Committee of the Board of Supervisors, wrote an additional letter to the Board of Governors. She lamented "the ease with which a Hospital like 'the Woman's' can be changed from its original object & intent, if not most carefully watched. A Medical Board looks upon a Hospital in a very different light from the builders and founders."[102] She complained of the difficulty the women met in collecting funds for the institution, arguing that a change in purpose of the hospital made money-raising impossible.

Lane relayed the story of a woman, referred by a Lady Supervisor, who sought treatment for a tumor at the hospital. "The Woman was met by many of the patients saying 'do not come here to be operated upon unless you are willing to be made a subject for a great crowd of Dr's [*sic*] & students.'"[103] Another woman, in a private room, was advised by a member of the Medical

Board "to leave at once, it was no place for a lady, her associates would be of the most common sort."[104]

Mary Jay Edwards wrote yet another letter to the Board of Governors on January 9, 1875, regarding Sims's resignation and affairs of the hospital. She voiced for the supervisors an ongoing concern about the mortality statistics and the high rate of death. Once again in the context of money raising, Edwards asked for an investigation, reporting that she often heard the criticism, "we kill more than we cure."[105] To a degree, the women distrusted the efficacy of capital surgery, and the controversy surrounding Sims's resignation gave them the opportunity to express displeasure at the "bill of mortality." Earlier in a separate manuscript, Caroline Lane had described a case of interest to her. A woman on the first floor, a private patient, was convalescing from surgery but was still very feeble. Lane hoped to get her home to Maine so she might "die among her own people. She was too delicate for any treatment when she came to us, and was subjected to *the same violent remedy* as the others" [my emphasis].[106] In this quote, Lane suggests the women objected not necessarily to the disease of cancer and other serious sickness, so much as to the treatments the surgeons delivered.

Dissonance grew in part out of questions concerning class. Generally in this period, ailing individuals who had economic wherewithal avoided hospitals at all cost.[107] Women and men of wealth or with middle-range income could find medical treatment, including surgery, at home. Usually they did. Hospitals were not healthy; recovery from surgery was safer at home. Doctors saw hospitals differently from patients and sought positions there so that they might enhance their private practice outside the hospital by gaining reputations and by making contacts through the lay boards that supervised institutions.

Marion Sims and Thomas Emmet both had private clinics where they earned income from practicing medicine. After the Woman's Hospital moved to Lexington Avenue and 49th Street, Emmet moved into 83 Madison Avenue, the site of the original hospital, and established his own private hospital there. Here he treated paying patients who sought a more exclusive and private care.

In addition to making up the private practice of both physicians, women of means became patients in the Woman's Hospital. The administration and structure of the Woman's Hospital were arranged to accommodate a different level of ability to pay on each floor, with the most wealthy patients and the most private accommodations on the first floor. The poorer women were in the Wetmore Pavilion, just as in the original arrangement. On the middle floors were patients who could pay small boarding fees. The top floor housed the outdoor department for the most destitute.

The women fought for the inclusion of wealthier patients partly because they brought in money from boarding fees. In the original hospital, the annual expenditures had been low enough so that the boarding fees made a strong contribution. Still, the treasury was forced to rely heavily on state and private donations in order to keep supplies stocked and patients fed and sheltered. In 1857 the hospital had a total annual income of $474 from boarding, with monthly expenditures averaging $500 a month. After 1868, with the new building and a larger capacity, the income from boarding grew. In 1870, the reported annual total income was $11,926, and expenditures were more than $95,000. The number of patients admitted had more than doubled, but the hospital costs grew at an even greater rate. The possibility of sustaining the hospital on patient boarding fees was small. The next year, boarding income decreased to $11,192, but the expenditures climbed to an average of $700 a month.[108] When the Baldwin Pavilion of the Woman's Hospital opened in 1877, the administration, with the blessing of the Board of Governors, advertised the luxury and comfort of the best rooms on the first floor and openly sought the interest of upper-class women.

In the context of the hospital and the postwar period, how did the women administrators and others, especially male philanthropists and doctors, perceive "class" and its relevance to sickness and medicine? Class was a new social category and many often denied, or failed to see, their own status.[109] In the postwar era, class became a predominant issue. Signs of a class of workers or laborers were everywhere. In New York City, the working class operated from one of its strongest positions in history, leading up to the railroad strike of 1877. From the perspective of the upper and middle classes in the 1870s and 1880s, Herbert Spencer's adaptation and revisions of Darwinian evolution to explain social systems resulted in the popularity of "survival of the fittest" as a justification for the diverse economic standings of people, an idea Spencer gleaned from Malthus. Class and race merged and created a new language to justify the rise of sudden great wealth among a few.

A close look at the words used by those associated with the hospital and published in hospital publications reveals some specific ways in which the textual meaning of the word "class" differed from present-day usage. Rather than gaining a self-conscious identity from what we see today as their class, at this time the middle and the working classes were just emerging, taking shape as an element in the process of industrialization.[110] Individuals could not refer to themselves or to others as middle class if they did not know what the term denoted. Both hospital-associated physicians and the women managers, however, considered the question of medical care for women with little or no economic underpinning as central to their institution, drawing from the antebellum concept of the "worthy poor."

The word "class" sometimes meant something other than economic status. For instance, "class" appeared as a referent in the published annual reports of the Woman's Hospital to a category of diseases associated with women. Some saw women then as a class that shared common reproductive disorders. At the hospital's first anniversary meeting, New York physician John Francis referred to "the particular class of diseases" treated at the hospital. He went on to mention "the imperative need of a hospital for women afflicted with complaints peculiar to the sex, and aggravated by poverty and neglect."[111] Erastus Benedict, a prominent citizen and supporter of the hospital, spoke at the same occasion. He too referred to "the class of cases" the Woman's Hospital attended.[112] Benedict took the definition further by expanding this "class of cases" to include "treatment of all the disease peculiar to suffering woman."[113]

From this perspective, sex transcended economic status. The notion of "suffering woman" is noteworthy. The gender definition implied suffering as a quality of womanhood. David Hayes Agnew demonstrated a further association with this specific meaning of womanhood in his conflation of class and gender in the treatment of vesico-vaginal fistula cases. "If there is any class in this world, more than another, placed under unbounded obligations to cherish and respect our art [surgery], it is the mothers of the land."[114]

Later ambiguity and conflict among hospital administrators were evident over the purpose of the hospital and over the importance of the economic status of the patient. The Medical Board in particular was wont to chastise the Lady Supervisors for indulging patients of their own class too much. Thomas Emmet argued in 1865 that the mission of the Woman's Hospital was to "ask for the poor—she who in affluence can, by proper rest, and with the comforts of life around her, so far mitigate her suffering . . . but for the woman depending on her daily labor, there is a point beyond which nature refuses longer to be taxed."[115] Emmet and others expressed concern that the hospital catered too much to the middle and upper classes and failed to treat those who were more fundamentally in need of medical care.

With time, the women managers of the Woman's Hospital changed from being somewhat unaware of their class standing to a strong and defensive identification with the middle and upper classes.[116] Notions of womanhood were changing toward a model of greater independence—the new woman;

benevolence was not so tightly connected to femininity as philanthropy became scientific and systematically organized.

In the 1850s benevolent activity began with an emphasis on the unity of women and their bonds as mothers, and the hospital in fact treated women of all classes. By 1868, Sims was proud to describe the hospital as a place where "educated and cultivated women could go for relief when they had not the means to command it. . . . No lady is degraded by entering the Woman's Hospital as a patient."[117] Many of the Lady Supervisors seemed to adopt or share Sims's perspective. Sims's own practice by this time was devoted to the care of European royalty and aristocracy, and to a lesser degree elite American women.

By the 1870s, other physicians, most notably Thomas and Emmet, and some hospital governors saw the hospital more as a medical refuge for the destitute and took issue with the Lady Supervisors who demanded accommodations and special considerations for women of the upper and middle classes as well. Although the debate had all the appearance of a focus on the class status of patients treated by the hospital, beneath the surface was tension over the role of women in society and of the Lady Supervisors. As these women took the initiative to speak for their peers, the men now in charge of the institution felt the need to urge them into deference.

Overlap between class and sex created further confusion. Class derived its meaning most often from the economic status of the head of the household—the man. It was difficult sometimes to ascribe class to women who had no independent economic status or were independent. Independent working-class women, for instance, were in a world of their own.[118] In the immediate years following the Civil War, the Fifteenth Amendment passed, excluding women specifically from citizenship and suffrage (which had never been explicit) because of their sex, and at the same time married women were declared not to have the right to the wages they earned.

As members of the elite, the Lady Supervisors of the Woman's Hospital, led by Caroline Lane, were conscious and protective of their class. While they engaged in the benevolent work of helping in the hospital administration, they lacked the sacrifice and selfless devotion to the poor shown by Sarah Doremus.

When Thomas Emmet later wrote his autobiography, he perceived the cause of his conflict with the Lady Supervisors as purely the duality of manhood and womanhood. "Women are not qualified for making medical appointments," he said. "There are certain positions for which women are not fitted, for experience teaches they are by nature partisan." In fact, Emmet maintained, from the perspective of 1911, "I have never yet met a woman who, in my judgment, should have a vote. . . . I cannot recall a single instance in my experience where the opinion of a sensible woman was at fault on any subject relating to everyday life if she gave it offhand on being asked, and yet she would be unable to reach any conclusion based on logical reasoning."[119] Although Emmet's appointment did not end in 1874, he and Sims shared a disdain for the authority of women in the hospital. This was an element of superiority that both placed women on a pedestal and robbed her of personhood, cutting across class lines. This view was evident in the medical practice among physicians associated with the Woman's Hospital.

In the London *Lancet*, publishing part of the *Clinical Notes* text in the mid-1860s, Sims clearly stated his view of female rationality. When remarking on cases of cervical incision, he argued that at times he did not advise women as to the nature of the surgery they would receive: "I am opposed to operating on any rational being without first explaining what is to be done, and the wherefore. In the cases [cervical incision for sterility] alluded to the operations were performed at the suggestion and earnest wish of the husbands, who feared that they might not be submitted to if fully explained."[120] Clearly these patients were less than "rational," due to their lower social status or possession by a husband, not their frailty. Later, in 1878, Sims repeatedly used a metaphor of holding the woman patient prisoner as a key part of her recovery from surgery.[121]

Other women left clinical situations out of embarrassment and fear of successive therapies. In T. Gaillard Thomas's clinic, Thomas Savage, his student, recorded the ridicule and laughter that followed women who fled on foot.[122] Without a doubt, economic class, and also race, were powerful agents of discrimination. Women whose diagnoses and presences were part of clinical lectures were poor patients receiving charity. Education for medical students was the fee exacted from them. Emmet, in a rare moment, disparaged the poorer patients at the Woman's Hospital, calling them less intelligent and less reliable than those in his private practice.[123] Women in all economic situations, however, received surgeries.

Physicians noted that working women and those struggling to survive were more likely to suffer reproductive disorders for prolonged periods, and to seek medical help only after symptoms were already incapacitating. There were many cases, for instance, of extreme uterine prolapse at the Woman's Hospital, also described in medical texts, in which the uterus inverted and became external. Of course, there were many patients in the middle class who also complained of a variety of female disorders, including prolapse.

Although not exclusively, complaints of dysmenorrhea, sterility, and difficulty in adolescence, especially chlorosis, seemed to occur among the more privileged.[124] Therapies for disturbances in adolescence were symbolic of Victorian culture and its relation to early gynecology. Puberty was an immensely difficult time for young women of the middle and upper classes. Just as they were maturing, their parents often closed them off from "stimulation," including the active pursuit of education, and urged them to rest. For young men, the opposite happened, as they prepared to begin careers and to enter the public world. At the same time, the female adolescents were ignorant of physiology and the biological cycle of reproduction. They experienced menarche with little or no previous knowledge about it. Some thought they were bleeding to death.[125] Health reformers sought to make knowledge of sexuality and reproduction public and accessible. They directed their efforts to adults, however, and not young people.

The prevalence of chlorosis, a form of anemia in which the patient turned green, indicates the difficulties experienced by female youth in the nineteenth century. The disease caused problems in digestion and a variety of other symptoms, including rapid heartbeat and fainting. Medical practitioners turned their attention to the condition in the Victorian period.[126] Once again, physicians sought to identify the normal from the abnormal, in this case in the development of human female sexuality and fertile reproductivity.

Thomas's clinic for medical students included one chlorotic patient. As with most chlorotic patients, the woman was young—eighteen years old—and single. She had visited three different doctors previously. Her major discomfort came from a headache of eight to ten months' duration. Her other symptoms of chlorosis included a pain around her heart, vomiting, swollen breasts, and a lack of her period. To make matters worse, her face was paralyzed on one side. Thomas prescribed a rich diet—fatty food and a pint of cream every twenty-four hours. He included a dosage of iron, which is also important in the treatment of anemia today. Thomas thought that the young woman's lack of a menstrual period caused many of the symptoms she described. He sent the woman to the hospital, where doctors would pass a uterine sound through her cervical canal twice a day. At the same time, in keeping with the presence of an electrician at the Woman's Hospital, Thomas prescribed the daily application of an electric probe on the cervix. Savage's notes did not detail the results of this treatment.[127]

In his lectures, T. Gaillard Thomas also described a young women who reached the age of seventeen without the onset of menstruation. She came with her mother, who described symptoms of chills and fever. Thomas diagnosed a small undeveloped uterus and "undeveloped state of the patient's mind." This, Thomas said, was his first case of problematic female adolescence. He prescribed the use of anesthesia and the introduction of graduated sponge tents. In addition he described administering electricity, with one pole of the battery in the vagina, and one over each ovary. This treatment, he thought, would cause the uterus to grow.[128] Thomas devoted the last chapter of his gynecology text to the treatment and diagnosis of chlorosis, especially distinguishing chlorosis from anemia.

Thomas Addis Emmet became very interested in the process of female sexual maturation and addressed much energy to the treatment of adolescent complaints. Just as Sims had met many cases of menstrual discomfort in the first years of the hospital, so Emmet, in the first years of his private hospital, met many cases of disorder in puberty: "When I had gotten my private hospital in working order, as early as 1862, I was surprised to find so large a proportion of my patients were anaemic women in their adolescence, undersized, and with their nervous systems in a shattered condition from overstudy."[129]

Emmet shared E. H. Clarke's ideas that too much education and stimulation (typified by the pursuit of higher education) among young women atrophied the uterus and threatened healthy reproduction, which, of course, the argument went, was the be-all and the end-all of female existence. Emmet associated hysteria also with many of his private patients' afflictions.

Emmet devised what he felt was an innovative and beneficial treatment for these patients. He argued that microscopic analysis of blood samples demonstrated the minimal importance of iron treatment. The problem lay not so much in too few red corpuscles but rather in the lack of sunlight. Emmet did urge nutritional changes on his patients, both private and at the hospital. Above all, in these cases of "vapors" and adolescent disorder, he kept "patients, in a nude condition . . . hour after hour, for days and sometimes for weeks, with the skin exposed to the action of sunlight, receiving no other treatment than frequent rubbing of the body."[130] The hospital was the fourth floor of Emmet's home. The activity and prolonged nakedness must have been radical for the young Victorian women, who put so much stake in their physical modesty.

Emmet felt that his private hospital, in its first years, "had much in common with a lunatic asylum." The hospital made it possible, he argued, "to get a patient sufficiently isolated for her to become as a child in my hands."

> In some respects the power gained was not unlike that obtained over
> a wild beast, except that in one case the domination would be due
> to fear, while with my patient, as a rule, it would be confidence in

my skill, with the desire to please me and to merit my approval from the effort she would make to gain her self-control. I have at times been depressed with the responsibility attending the blind influence I have often been able to gain over nervous women under my care.[131]

Emmet had other more conventional and more physiological therapies for hysteria, which he described in his text on gynecology. One was a method he devised to embarrass a woman in the midst of a hysterical fit. He used catheters to release a woman's intestinal gas, and thus, he maintained, to shock her back to rationality with the rude sounds of her own body.

Emmet was unusual in his belief that hysteria was a separate condition that did not call for the use of surgery. He did maintain nonetheless that education caused flexure of the uterus among young women. He, of course, treated that condition with surgery. He was also quite convinced that he could trace ante-flexion and cervical disorder back to adolescence and early menstrual patterns in his patients. Adolescence among females was a time of physical growth, and to introduce mental exertion was to threaten the health of the woman, according to the medical thought of these early gynecologists.[132]

Surgical therapies at the Woman's Hospital assumed a connection between the biological process and cycle in females and the appearance of nervous disorders. In this time, before the development of psychiatry, doctors assumed that they might heal hysteria and uncontrolled emotional outbursts, convulsions, and various other symptoms with specifically delineated surgical procedures. Thomas, Emmet, and Sims all assumed a weakness and subordination in women due to their gender and biology, regardless of class.

Gynecology Becomes a Profession

In 1876 Sims was named president of the American Medical Association (AMA). In the same year, Sims, Emmet, Thomas, Peaslee, and several others founded the American Gynecological Society. E. R. Peaslee was the first president of the newly formed national professional group (before England had established an analogous organization).[133] Gynecology was now a medical specialty, and the practitioners from the Woman's Hospital, including J. Marion Sims, were at its core. Disagreement and past history among the men was in scant evidence for a few years after Sims's resignation and, for the most part, never played an obvious role in its unfolding. The surgeons engaged in a discussion of cervical surgeries. An examination of the original assumptions attending the birth of gynecology had begun.

When, as president of the organization, Sims spoke before the AMA, he gave a rather loosely connected presentation. His focus was the establishment of a code of ethics, and he began by acknowledging that African Americans and women could now participate in the American Medical Association. At this meeting, following new AMA policy, Sarah Hackett Stevenson of Chicago took the first seat held by a woman. Representing a new generation of women physicians, she had graduated from the Woman's Hospital Medical College, established in 1865 and modeled after the New York State Woman's Hospital but run by a woman. Sims acknowledged the moment but had very little to say about it.

Sims was concerned about the changes and growth in medicine and the guidelines that were needed to define its practice. His intent was to argue for the establishment of state boards of health and the mobilization of medicine and the public to fight syphilis. He essentially argued for medical control of contagion and epidemics and urged the legislation of medical inspection and supervision of syphilis-infected prostitutes and also of those on board ships coming into port. To his way of thinking, syphilis was analogous to contagious diseases such as yellow fever. He sought quarantine of the sick individual and medical supervision of the situation. The AMA itself never officially advocated the legislation against syphilis, but did distribute a pamphlet that supported the state regulation of prostitution, with medical personnel in charge. Sims and David Hayes Agnew came to the common position that "it is the duty of the State to protect not only the lives and liberties of its citizens, but their health as well."[134]

Sims's voice joined others in a conversation that became a conflict about the AMA Code of Ethics issued back in 1847. The point of contention was a consultation clause that prevented physicians from consulting with anyone or any institution except those practicing regular or mainstream orthodox medicine. The exchange over the Code of Ethics became particularly heated in New York State in the early 1880s. Those who looked to science, especially laboratory science, as the medical standard argued for the end of the consultation clause and developed the idea of science as the ultimate arbiter of truth in medical practice. Though he was not necessarily deeply involved in this latter debate, Sims devoted energy to advocating the patent right of physicians to claim instruments and other techniques as their own. By 1878 he wrote articles in which he used the first person throughout, except when he cited his various positions and surgeries, which he referred to in the third person—"Sims's operation," for instance. There is no evidence from the publication of the records of the AMA meeting of the collegiality and peer exchange that characterized the participation of Woman's Hospital physicians that had been evident earlier.

Emmet and Peaslee took part in an extensive exchange over cervical surgeries. Emmet read a paper at the American Gynecological Society's first meeting entitled "The Etiology of Uterine Flexures, with the Proper Mode of Treatment Indicated."[135] In this paper, Emmet set out the parameters of what he considered his own cervical surgeries to treat uterine flexure. He analyzed 345 cases from his private practice and argued that the private patients "from the higher walks of life" gave more telling evidence for the American Gynecological Society audience.[136] Continuing his previous examination of the connection of sterility with female disorder, Emmet argued for the importance of uterine flexure in the creation of childlessness. He was emphatic about the recklessness that had accompanied the use of cervical incisions and described in great detail his modifications of the practice. Discussion followed the recognition of the absence of T. Gaillard Thomas, who was supposed to chair the session. Fordyce Barker took over, announcing the additional absence of Sims from the audience. Peaslee then dominated the discussion, amplifying his perceptions of the uses and misuses of cervical incisions, and establishing his own set of criteria for surgery. He forcefully stated the dangers of too great a reliance on cervical surgery.

In June 1876 Peaslee gave a paper entitled "Incision and Discussion of the Cervix Uteri" before the New York Academy of Medicine. True to his medical approach, Peaslee systematically reviewed the surgeries, gave them a new name derived from the Greek, "trachelotomy," and argued persuasively for reform in their practice. In effect, Peaslee asserted that there was only one situation that called for such surgery: stenosis of the cervix, or narrowing of the os. All other rationales, from dysmenorrhea to sterility, were without basis as an argument for surgery. He suggested that patients experienced a high degree of misfortune because of what he called indiscriminate use of surgery. Peaslee went on, drawing from an earlier article published by Emmet, to specifically criticize Sims's choice of instruments and his methods. He proposed a much more narrowly confined rationale for the surgery and advocated his own technique of a lesser incision.

An American obstetrician, Dr. James White of Buffalo, in 1877 addressed members of the AMA concerning cervical surgery. White was well known in medical circles and the lay world for his participation in clinical instruction for childbirth during which he exposed male medical students to an actual delivery, an activity that does not seem out of the ordinary today but challenged cultural standards in 1850. The celebrated Loomis trial, which brought White to court, publicized his activities and brought an end to these clinical lessons.[137] He referred to the surgery as "free division of the cervex [*sic*] uteri as a means of curing stenosis of the canal of the neck, often present in dysmenorrhea and sterility. . . . These operations were for some years resorted to without much discrimination, became very *fashionable*, and it is to be feared, many practitioners resorted to them recklessly or as a matter of routine, without much reference to the indications or requirements of the individual case under treatment" (White's emphasis).[138] Earlier, Emmet had argued forcefully against these same violent therapies: "But few of the many physician [sic] who undertake to treat these diseases fully realize there is a natural limit to this tolerance [by the womb]. No portion of the body has suffered more from the overzealous interference of ignorant practitioners, and from the carelessness of those, who though not ignorant, fail to make . . . a thorough investigation."[139] He went on to include surgery in his castigations. "Under the guise of surgery, the uterus has been subjected to a degree of malpractice, which would not be tolerated in any other portion of the body. Its cavity has been, and is to this day made the receptacle for agents so destructive."[140]

Two years after Sims's exit from the Woman's Hospital, enmity, or at least distaste, among the four surgeons had grown. On May 7, 1877, Montrose A. Pallen, a New York physician, gave a paper before the New York County Medical Society on "Dysmenorrhoea and the Operation for Its Cure."[141] Although minutes and records of these meetings were regularly published in various periodicals, no record was published to describe the fracas that followed the paper presentation. As we have seen, there was by now a professional tradition of lively exchange among the audience regarding the paper's subject. This particular paper sparked a memorable outburst that pitted Peaslee and Sims against each other and drew its fire from the surgical practice of cervical incisions.[142] Only upon Sims's death did the *New York Medical Journal* recapitulate the ferocity of the exchange and the veritable standoff—the cavalier and the Yankee—that ensued. "The two men shook hands, and the paper never saw the light."[143]

Although Sims, Emmet, Thomas, and Peaslee published their exchanges widely, the critical stimulus to the explosion was carefully excluded from the public record. The collective effort of physicians to establish a specialized medical field of gynecology grew out of the experiments and medical network and education at the Woman's Hospital. Its development represented submersion of conflict and uncertainty and relied on mutual respect and a collective identity as gynecologists. Even those who took issue with some of Sims's methods recognized him as a forerunner in the field.

Echoes of Sims's resignation from the Woman's Hospital reverberated as the controversy took shape. On May 18, 1877, anger and a collective reaction from Thomas, Peaslee, and Emmet appeared in the form of a pamphlet addressed to Sims.[144] Sims was leaving the country and so did not respond until the fall. All publicly reviewed the topic of the anniversary meeting in December 1874 and Sims's resignation.[145]

The intense whirl of words came in the wake of a biography of Sims written by his agent, Henri Stuart. The underlying animosity and tension are evident in the pamphlets. The substance of the exchange shows that other aspects of the medical conflict stand out. This exchange pinpointed specific surgical procedures and the relative skills of the four men.

The *Virginia Medical Monthly* solicited Sims's biographical sketch from Stuart and published it in the spring of 1877. The journal was an eclectic magazine, written for irregular, rather than allopathic or orthodox, physicians. Sims argued that the nature of the publication alone was enough to rile Sims's former colleagues.[146] Emmet, Thomas, and Peaslee were also outraged at the content of Stuart's piece, which dwelled on Sims's strong sense of manhood, honor, and honesty, casting doubt on the integrity of the others. Stuart suggested that the three surgeons had deserted Sims, using lies and cowardice to maintain their own positions. The three responded in kind and jointly issued a defense of their actions, which they published as a circular in May.

Thomas, Peaslee, and Emmet outlined the rules regarding spectators and cancer patients and described what they saw as Sims's initial acceptance of the rules, followed by an outburst and his resignation during the anniversary meeting. In early June, Sims, in turn, responded to this description of the meeting with his own history. After complaining that he had received the circular just as he left for Europe, Sims denied responsibility for Stuart's description of the event. He claimed a personal interest in defending the "interest and honor" of the medical profession in standing up to the rules of the hospital. He believed he had a right, as a citizen and as a spokesman for medicine, to deny the regulation of spectators in surgery and the admission of cancer patients. Sims went on to cite some statistics of disputed origin, describing surgeries and mortality rates. Using his own numbers, he demonstrated his own abilities and the manipulations of Davis and the Medical Board as he interpreted them.

In late June, the three surgeons again responded in concert, denying the validity of Sims's story, questioning the source of his statistics, and asserting their previous loyalty to him as a colleague. In their examination of his record at the hospital, they listed his use of certain surgeries, that is, slitting the cervix and Battey's Operation, as questionable. They remarked, using italics, "It appears upon the records *that 64 of Dr. Sims' operations consisted in slitting the cervix uteri,* a procedure which was not practiced one-third as often by any one of his colleagues as by him, and which was resorted to by Dr. Sims nearly twice as often as by the other three surgeons combined."[147] Emmet suggested in other publications that the number of cases was much higher and that he worked with Sims on many of them.

Unlike Sims, the other surgeons yielded to the administrative boards concerning the treatment of cancer. "The contamination of the wards and the inconvenience to patients, arising from the odors created by cases of uterine cancer" was given as the reason to exclude such cases.[148] The doctors also argued that Sims often filled the operating room with spectators and that he had sometimes placed his cancer patients in the hospital beds governed by other surgeons, to draw the disapproval of the women away from himself. Although all of the surgeons involved had practiced a variety of experimental surgeries, Thomas, Emmet, and Peaslee, using hospital records, identified Sims as culpable for some questionable medical practices. Even as they used statistics from the hospital to demonstrate their point, the surgeons wondered why Sims attacked them and not the Board of Governors or the Lady Supervisors as the source of his problems with the hospital.

Knowing on which side their bread was buttered, the three surgeons developed their most extensive rebuttal as a "Tabular Statement" addressed to the Board of Governors of the Woman's Hospital. Responding to what they obviously knew to be a point of concern for the governing bodies, the surgeons prepared statistics on the mortality rate accompanying ovariotomies. The mortality rate associated with Peaslee's ovariotomies was low, nearly as low as that of Thomas Keith, who was considered by many to be the safest practitioner of the surgery during this period. Peaslee, in fact, took issue with Sims's ovariotomy procedure. During the pamphlet exchange of 1877, a comparison of the mortality rates for ovariotomy was a central issue in the conflict. Table 2 was presented by Peaslee, Thomas, and Emmet in their pamphlet and rebuttal of Sims. They isolated the statistics for complete ovariotomies (including Battery's Operation) from 1872 through 1875 at the Woman's Hospital, as shown in the table.

These statistics show that Sims lost more patients than anyone else in absolute numbers. Sims himself was quick to point out, however, that

TABLE 2. *Complete Ovariotomies at the Woman's Hospital, 1872–1875*

Surgeon	Number of Operations	Number of Deaths
Dr. Sims	11	7
Dr. Thomas	11	4
Dr. Peaslee	6	4
Dr. Emmet	2	0

Source: E. R. Peaslee, T. A. Emmet, and T. G. Thomas, *Reply to Dr. J. Marion Sims's Pamphlet* (New York: Trow's Printing, June 1877).

proportionally others fared still more poorly than he. He argued in his defense: "Mr. Spencer Wells has more than once lost in succession seven or eight cases of ovariotomy. Suppose he had had these unfortunate results at the outset of his brilliant career? Why, he might have been denounced as a reckless and unsuccessful surgeon. But he has had more than twenty successful ovariotomies under the same general plan pursued in his unsuccessful cases."[149]

While Sims may have been under fire for his practice of Battey's Operation, the conflict rested more on his arrogance than his performance of the surgery. Peaslee, Thomas, and Emmet each operated with Battey's procedure, and all lost patients during the surgery.[150]

Among gynecologists, there was widespread use of statistics and jockeying of information in an attempt to measure the safety and the success of all forms of ovariotomy. Numerous references appeared in professional journals pointing to inaccurate mortality records. Many felt the statistics were a smoke screen. While the medical practitioners sought to avoid public exposure of the extensive conflict among themselves, numbers offered a safe way to examine their procedures.

For the surgeons, the question of survival from the surgery did not apply to the question of whether or not to use the surgery. The quest, as W. L. Atlee and others saw it, was one for truth and science: "A victory has been achieved, not alone by the prowess of the friends of ovariotomy, but because they labored for a cause which bore the seal of truth. No human effort can sustain an operation that has no merit in itself, and no human influence can put down an operation intrinsically good. Ovariotomy has triumphed because 'truth must prevail.'"[151]

While Sims was correct in his determination of the importance of treating cancer patients, his arrogance and strong notion of self-review—

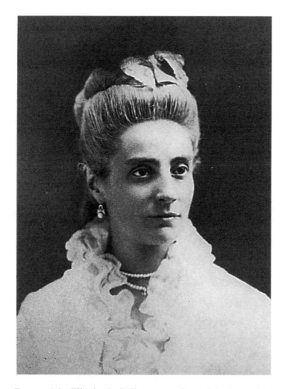

FIGURE 16. Elizabeth Cullum, member of the Board of Lady Supervisors at the Woman's Hospital. She campaigned for the inclusion of cancer patients at the hospital, then died of cancer herself. *(Courtesy of the Reynolds Historical Library, University of Alabama at Birmingham.)*

responsibility to answer only to his own standards—led him to ignore the concerns of other associates of his hospital. Hospitals specializing in the treatment of cancer soon appeared in New York City. His impetuousness and easily ignited temper cost him the affiliation of his own hospital.

When the second pavilion was ready for occupancy in September 1877, the first pavilion was emptied of patients and declared unfit for use, for reasons never made public. An outbreak of infection apparently forced the administration to shut it down.[152] Contagion was still not completely understood. Not until 1884 did Thomas publicly acknowledge the likely link between a physician's antiseptic practice and the spread of puerperal fever.[153] One physician described the basement of the first pavilion as malarial, with contaminated

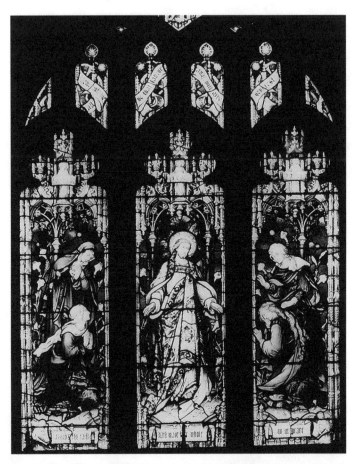

FIGURE 17. Stained glass window in the chapel of the Woman's Hospital on 110th Street, New York, c. 1911. This window is now in place at the Reynolds Historical Library at the University of Alabama in Birmingham. *(Courtesy of the Reynolds Historical Library, University of Alabama at Birmingham.)*

air infecting the patients. Perhaps the earth from the evacuated cemetery held infectious material that caused sickness in the hospital. Sims claimed, however, that none of the workers who actually dug up the bodies ever got sick. Some quietly protested the loss of more than $100,000 in the construction of a now worthless pavilion.[154]

In 1884 the New York Cancer Hospital opened. Women volunteers and members of the Board of Lady Supervisors, Elizabeth Cullom and her cousin

Mrs. John Jacob Astor, donated generously to its fund. Elizabeth Cullom died of uterine cancer four months after the hospital opened. These two women fought unsuccessfully for the admission of cancer patients to the Woman's Hospital.

The pioneering days were nearly over. Right on the heels of the pamphlet exchange, Edmund R. Peaslee died in January 1878. In 1879, T. Gaillard Thomas became Professor of Gynecology at the College of Physicians and Surgeons; from his previous position, a total of three chairs were created with the addition of two other appointments, one in pediatrics and the other in obstetrics. These provided a model for the newly separated professional specialties of gynecology, obstetrics, and pediatrics.[155] Thomas's active involvement at the Woman's Hospital of the State of New York ended in 1887.[156]

J. Marion Sims lived a gypsy existence in his final years, traveling from place to place. In 1880 he was named president of the American Gynecological Society. His many awards and honors, international as well as American, go beyond the scope of this book. He was reappointed as a consulting surgeon to the Woman's Hospital shortly before his death in 1883.

The Woman's Hospital outgrew its facilities in 1900, when Thomas Addis Emmet operated for the last time there. The new hospital opened in 1906 at 110th Street and Amsterdam Avenue where it is today, part of St. Luke's Hospital. A two-story open chapel was part of that new building, containing a stained-glass window designed by the Board of Lady Supervisors in 1878; Margaret Sage unveiled the window, a biblical scene in French leaded glass, in 1901.[157] Emmet died in 1919 at the age of ninety-one.

Conclusion

⟨—➤◆⟫⟶

$\mathcal{T}$o conclude this history, let us go back to considering the perspective of the women who were patients.[1] Race, class, and gender were all integral to their experience of sickness and disease. What follows is the case of a woman of the early 1870s, one of several cases of ovariotomy described in an article by J. Marion Sims. She exemplifies enduring themes well worth emphasizing, and her case is unusual in the extent of its documentation.

Among the patients at the Woman's Hospital, this patient, whom I shall call Patient L, had some distinguishing characteristics. Sounding like an early anthropologist, Sims wrote, "[She was] for this region a rare type of the human species. She was a mulatto, with straight hair, a cross between the negro and Indian."[2] Her race was her identity, what Sims saw as her central quality. Detail suggested that her mixed racial background influenced her behavior. "She was one of the most obstinate and self-willed patients I have ever had."[3]

In 1872, W. T. Walker, a new assistant surgeon at the Woman's Hospital of the State of New York, admitted a thirty-seven-year-old married woman suffering from an ovarian tumor. J. Marion Sims recorded her name as Mrs. Burley L. She had given birth to one child and had had several abortions (which may or may not mean she had miscarriages) before she was twenty-four.[4] After that time, off and on over twelve years, she was treated for the ovarian tumor. Following the standard procedure of the time, doctors used periodic tapping to drain fluid as necessary.

When she was admitted to the hospital, she was given a choice between a further tapping of her abdomen or ovariotomy. Apparently she elected to undergo an ovariotomy. W. T. Walker performed the surgery on November 8, with the help of two other physicians. Walker's operation lasted one hour and twenty minutes, during which time one of his associates administered the ether.

Walker called upon Sims to insert a drainage tube in the vagina as part of the measures used to promote healing. As was typical of his method, Sims was intent upon developing a signature surgical technique for ovariotomy. In an article concerning ovariotomy published in the *New York Medical Journal* of 1873—an article that included a discussion of Patient L—he detailed his technique in preventing septicemia. Unlike E. R. Peaslee and other ovariotomists of this time, Sims abandoned his preoccupation with the pedicle following extirpation of the woman's ovary.[5] Rather, he determined to drain constantly and completely any fluid collecting in the peritoneal cavity, periodically flushing water through the area with tubes. His interest and practice in abdominal surgery and the treatment of septicemia was largely influenced by his wartime experience in the Sudan with the Ambulance Corps during the Franco-Prussian War.[6]

For five days following the surgery, Patient L's recovery was uncertain. In the daily log of her postsurgical recovery, her willfulness and disobedience were noted specifically in her rising up out of bed on the second day after surgery. Sims was emphatic, however, that this behavior did no harm to her recovery. However, he remarked, "It would be very difficult to convince any of the nurses . . . that this poor woman did not sacrifice her life by her own imprudence."[7]

She gradually weakened, grew feverish, suffered vomiting and diarrhea, and died on the fifth day. The hospital pathologist completed a thorough autopsy on the woman, as was routine. The Lady Supervisors and members of both other administrative boards worried about the need for a separate building for the pathologist and his museum. They feared disease spread from his work. Still, the work continued: "Every case that dies in the Woman's Hospital is subjected to postmortem examination. It is nothing but just that the patient who has the benefit of our attendance and treatment should repay us by the use of her body to search out means for the relief of humanity."[8] In this quotation, the role of the patient who died at the hospital came through clearly, "It was nothing but just . . . ." "Just" meant "justice served." As part of being a patient in such a teaching hospital, Patient L's death served medical education.

For Patient L, Sims's drainage system through the Douglas cul-de-sac had failed. Bloody infected fluid collected in the peritoneal cavity. Microscopic inspection of fluids from the autopsy revealed the presence of putrefaction and, in association, septicemia. Now Sims felt he knew that adequate drainage placed properly in the cul-de-sac behind the cervix would prevent septicemia by completely draining the fluid from the abdominal cavity.[9]

In his article, Sims argued that Patient L's decease validated his preferred technique for the prevention of postsurgical septicemia. Following Patient L's operation, this technique merely malfunctioned, or so he theorized. Sims felt that if the drainage had occurred properly, she would have recovered; her surgery had been "a successful operation, though the patient died."[10]

Parallels exist between early surgeries of appendectomy, which began at the turn of the century, and ovariotomies. While some might argue for the importance of practicing ovariotomy in recognizing and treating the specific pathology of ovarian tumor, in the case of Patient L and other early gynecological surgeries, medical willingness to proceed with experimentation varied by individual status, by race and class.[11]

> While I lament and regret the death of our patient, I have great comfort in feeling that she has not died in vain: that her death leads to the establishment of a principle . . . that may be the means, [sic] of saving *valuable* lives, and many . . . *more valuable* than this one sacrificed on the altar of science. The case as it stands proves more, I think for the truth of my views than if she had recovered. (Emphasis mine)[12]

Through the window of the case of Patient L, the medical hierarchy of the Woman's Hospital and J. Marion Sims comes clear. Sims disputed the accuracy of the nursing staff's perception that the patient had caused her own demise by refusing their orders. On the one hand, Sims described the patient as unruly, but on the other, he insisted that his medical therapeutics determined her health. The patient in this case was at the lowest social rung. The nursing staff distrusted her determination to move about and take matters into her own hands. Sims treated this woman as he treated other patients who were not middle- or upper-class women of European stock. Judging from the words he used, there was no doubt that Patient L had a lesser status. In fact, Sims maintained that in her death she would give a greater service than she had in life, saving what he called more valuable lives. Patient L's corpse belonged to the institution.

Sims stood at the top of the social hierarchy encapsulated by Patient L's case. He viewed the hospital staff, both the assistant surgeon and the nurses, as auxiliary at best. As a younger physician gaining clinical experience, Walker had merely operated for him. The nurses were overly concerned servants. Sims patiently explained that Patient L had been simply sitting peacefully in an easy chair when she rose out of bed, suggesting that the concern among the nurses stemmed from too much emotion. Of course, at the bottom of this social pyramid lay the patient, who died.

Several other cases Sims described in connection with the article were surgeries *he* performed—often in Newport, Rhode Island, where he took refuge from the fevers, gangrene, and contagion of the urban hospital setting ("hospitalism" as it was called).[13] Patients treated in Newport were private cases and undoubtedly came from a higher stratum of society. Emphasizing Sims's authority, discussion of these cases focused exclusively on his medical technique. He was the central figure who, through his surgery, could save lives.

Not usually speaking indirectly or through metaphor, Sims simply stated what he saw. Though he did not intend to do so, Sims revealed in his description of Patient L the debt he owed to his patients. In the long run, she became a victim but she was far from passive. She sought out medical care and she elected daring surgery. The presence of her story in Sims's article brings the issue of the lives of patients into relief. Class and race combined with gender to provide a framework and meaning for the medical therapies Sims elaborated.

While women experienced a wide variety of health needs, mainstream medicine intervened and prevailed, defining a narrow series of surgical therapies that became essential medical practices. Few seemed to notice that death continued to take women during childbirth; instead, a specialized system of treatment grew up around the investigation of female reproductivity. Cancer became a pressing issue.

More serious "capital" surgeries quickly supplanted the preponderance of minor surgeries, especially for vesico-vaginal fistulas. The number of vesico-vaginal fistula patients seems to have peaked at about the time of Sims's death in 1883. Several factors may have contributed to the apparent rise and subsequent fall in the incidence of these fistulas. Most important, Sims's operation, combined with the publicity given vesico-vaginal fistula patients, probably made the prevalence of the condition more apparent. Patients came forward once a treatment was available. Surgeons and physicians operated to remedy the fistulas, recorded the surgery, or published the fee bill.

In the second half of the nineteenth century, slavery ended and the ethnic origins of immigrants changed, while the historical context for immigration altered. These changes probably included shifts in diet that may have lowered morbidity from rickets. Also, by the end of the century, medical practitioners grew more adept and experienced in the area of childbirth, including gaining facility with the instruments at their disposal. All these factors contributed to the decline in the numbers of vesico-vaginal fistula patients. Physicians interpreted the decline as a major victory for J. Marion Sims and surgical gynecology. The devising of a surgical closing for the fistulas coincidentally spelled an end to the condition itself. At the Wetmore Pavilion in 1868, Thomas Addis Emmet was in charge of a ward of patients who suffered from vesico-vaginal fistulas.[14] By the 1930s, vesico-vaginal and recto-vaginal fistulas most commonly resulted from accidents in gynecological surgery. Caesarian sections, hysterectomies, and bladder stone removal, as well as surgery for cancer of the cervix all contributed victims of vesico-vaginal fistula.[15]

Vesico-vaginal fistula surgeries paved the way for further medical intervention in the lives of women by virtue of their success. The cure for vesico-vaginal fistulas deflected attention from an accompanying increase in the practice of ovariotomy, with its attendant high rate of mortality. Ovariotomies were another step in medical specialization. The debate among physicians regarding the proper use of the surgery was in many ways a soul-searching enterprise.

By 1872 "the altar of science" had become a metaphor for Sims.[16] Set in the context of the regular practice of high-risk-taking experimental surgery, more life threatening than what he practiced in his earlier career, his language symbolized the blending of Christian morality with deference to the authority of science. As earlier in his life, science for Sims represented revelation from God. The physicians' sacrifice sanctified the altar; science was the instrument. For Sims and some of his associates, this science included a wide range of medical practice, from inoculation to the use of the microscope to the inspection of prostitutes. Sims, along with Fordyce Barker and doubtless others, was not as ready as T. Gaillard Thomas to declare science the only authority in the practice of medicine.[17] Sims, and his colleagues to a lesser or greater degree, came to see the physician as steward, as the one to make choices of sacrifice, of life and death. T. Gaillard Thomas agreed with Sims that the physician, the agent of God through science, was the final arbiter. Thomas Addis Emmet and Edmund Peaslee were perhaps less sure.

Today much has changed, but diverse threads of consistency hold strong. Beginning in 1855, the Woman's Hospital of the State of New York became a central and significant institution in laying down the foundations of gynecology. The early small and pioneering hospital offered unique opportunities for innovation. In 1883 Sims wrote a letter to Protheroe Smith reminiscing about Smith's Soho Square Hospital: "Without a special hospital you and I could not have done the work we have done. Without a special hospital Sir Spencer Wells could never have accomplished the great work that makes his name immortal. Nor could Lawson Tait have done so much for abdominal surgery."[18] Here Sims acknowledged the power of his experiences in small women's hospitals, starting in Montgomery, and in this his common ground particularly with the English ovariotomists.

Following the early practitioners, surgery became central to the specialty.[19] The idea of female cycles as pathological provided an anatomical map of the surgical approach. Influenced by this early framework, today Caesarian sections and hysterectomies are extraordinarily common.

Gynecology as the specialized treatment of women has a mixed reputation. Although the terms and nature of experimentation have shifted, willingness to pursue previously untried procedures without adequate research and study of female health continues.[20]

In the 1940s, '50s, and '60s, women took untried drugs such as DES (a synthetic estrogen to stop morning sickness and prevent miscarriage) only to discover their children inflicted with various forms of serious reproductive disorders as adults.[21] Dalkon shields, Norplant, breast implants, and thalidomide are further horror stories of women's health and their iatrogenic origins. There are countless accounts from the recent twentieth century of women of Latina, Native American, and African American heritage who have without knowledge or consent undergone sterilization following birth.[22] The epidemiology of breast cancer, AIDS, and many other conditions disclose a high incidence among those living in poverty and those whose lives are defined as "other" because of the color of their skin. They experience a high incidence of sickness but a low rate of access to medical treatment.[23] The central themes continue, but persistent failure to acknowledge the complexities of historical experience reinvents issues, making real change very difficult to effect. Essentially the elements of bias, stereotype, and discrimination were and are profoundly embedded in the social systems of the industrialized world.

Bioethics and medical ethics rarely treat these issues.[24] Focusing on specific cases and conditions leads to the denial of a bigger picture in which race, class, and gender are key ethical issues in the practice of medicine.[25] The history of the Woman's Hospital demonstrates how hard it is to break through the confines of what Ronald Takaki describes as the iron cage of our culture and ideology.[26] Because of his own blinders of discrimination, T. A. Emmet was driven by a passion for the Irish people but was unable to create a medical system that treated people equally. As a woman, Caroline Lane gained a powerful sense of potential when she traveled on the *Daniel Webster* to transport soldiers, yet she failed to implement a system to deliver health care to women across social boundaries.[27] Although Lane and the Lady Supervisors ultimately succeeded in removing Sims and the radical therapies he represented from their hospital, in the long run their efforts came too late. Their voluntarism was more than anything else a contribution to the medicalization of female bodies. The supervisors were fettered by personal allegiances and failures to pursue higher ends of health reform. They were as much victims as agents. At the same time, at an institution that has been remarkably self-conscious of its history, the history of the post-Civil War Board of Lady Supervisors was completely buried. Little record or recognition of Lane and her part in efforts to establish nursing education or to address issues of high mortality has surfaced until now.

Telling the story straight includes examining all the players and acknowledging the misuse and exploitation as well as the triumphs. All too often, medical history as part of the larger society has resisted including examination of the relevance of social hierarchy and the biases that keep people categorized: how they are at least as much at work in the medical world as they are elsewhere.

In the nineteenth century, race, class and sex were the key categories for understanding sickness and medicine. By investigating the influence of subjectively perceived differences among people in the past on the framework of medical care, new approaches can emerge to more effectively contribute to health and healing throughout society.[28] Exploring and contextualizing the narrative of a profession that carries so much authority in our society today reveals the depth and interconnectedness of medicine, society, health, and healing in the past.

NOTES

Prologue

1. J. Marion Sims, "On Vaginismus," *Bulletin of the New York Academy of Medicine* 1 (April 1862): 428.
2. Ibid., 428.
3. Ibid., 429.
4. The members of the lay boards governing the hospital insisted on its proper name as the Woman's Hospital of the State of New York. For its history and the history of gynecology in America see Seale Harris, *Woman's Surgeon: The Life Story of J. Marion Sims* (New York: Macmillan Co., 1950); James Pratt Marr, *Pioneer Surgeons of the Woman's Hospital* (Philadelphia: F. A. Davis Co., 1957); Matthew Mann, ed., *A System of Gynecology by American Authors*, 2 vols. (Philadelphia: Lea Bros., 1887); Ely Van De Warker, "The Personal Factor in the Work of the American Gynaecological Society," *The American Gynaecological and Obstetrical Journal* 17 (July 1900): 3–9; James V. Ricci, *One Hundred Years of Gynaecology, 1800–1900* (Philadelphia: Blakiston, 1945); Lawrence D. Longo, "Obstetrics and Gynecology," in Ronald L. Numbers, ed., *The Education of American Physicians* (Berkeley: University of California Press, 1980), 205–225; and Fielding H. Garrison, *An Introduction to the History of Medicine* (Philadelphia: W. B. Saunders & Co., 1929). See Judith M. Roy, "Surgical Gynecology," in Rima D. Apple, ed., *Women, Health, and Medicine in America: A Historical Handbook* (New Brunswick, N.J.: Rutgers University Press, 1992), 173–195.
5. See Martin Pernick, *A Calculus of Suffering: Pain, Professionalism and Anesthesia* (New York: Columbia University Press, 1985), for social history of anesthesia.
6. On diversity and women's history, two excellent essays are Evelyn Brooks Higginbotham, "African-American Women's History and the Metalanguage of Race," in Darlene Clark Hine, Wilma King, and Linda Reed, eds., *'We Specialize in the Wholly Impossible': Essays in Black Women's History* (Brooklyn: Carlson Publishing, 1995), 3–24, and Nancy A. Hewitt, "Beyond the Search for Sisterhood: American Women's History in the 1980s," in Vicki Ruiz and Ellen

Dubois, eds., *Unequal Sisters: A Multi-Cultural Reader in U.S. Women's History*, 2d ed. (New York: Routledge, 1994), 1–19.

7. Hasia Diner, "'The Most Irish City in the Union': The Era of the Great Migration, 1844–1877," in Ronald Bayer and Timothy Meagher, eds, *The New York Irish* (Baltimore: Johns Hopkins University Press, 1996), 87–106.

8. For biographies of J. Marion Sims, see James Pratt Marr, *James Marion Sims: Founder of the Woman's Hospital in the State of New York* (privately published); Harris, *Woman's Surgeon*. See also J. Marion Sims, *The Story of My Life*, ed. H. Marion-Sims (New York: D. Appleton, 1886; reprint edition, New York: DeCapo Press, 1968). For a thoughtful appraisal, see Irwin H. Kaiser, "Reappraisals of J. Marion Sims," *American Journal of Obstetrics and Gynecology* 132 (December 1978): 878–882.

9. See Paul Starr, *The Social Transformation of American Medicine: The Rise of a Sovereign Profession and the Making of a Vast Industry* (New York: Basic Books 1982); and John Haller, *American Medicine in Transition: 1840–1910* (Champaign-Urbana: University of Illinois Press, 1981). The rise of laboratory science is best described by John Harley Warner, *The Therapeutic Perspective: Medical Practice, Knowledge, and Identity in America* (Cambridge, Mass.: Harvard University Press, 1986). See also Russell Maulitz, *Morbid Appearances: The Anatomy of Pathology in the Early Nineteenth Century* (Cambridge, U.K.: Cambridge University Press, 1987).

10. There are many books and articles about Victorian society and the rise of gynecology. A few publications include John S. Haller and Robin M. Haller, *The Physician and Sexuality in Victorian America* (Urbana: University of Illinois Press, 1974); Mary Hartman and Lois Banner, eds., *Clio's Consciousness Raised: New Perspectives on the History of Women* (New York: Octagon Books, 1976); Ornella Moscucci, *The Science of Woman: Gynaecology and Gender in England* (Cambridge, U.K.: Cambridge University Press, 1990); Mary Poovey, *Uneven Developments: The Ideological Work of Gender in Mid-Victorian England* (Chicago: University of Chicago Press, 1988); and Jane Sewall, "Bountiful Bodies: Spencer Wells, Lawson Tait, and the Birth of British Gynecology" (Ph.D. diss., Johns Hopkins University, 1991). See also Regina Morantz-Sanchez, *Sympathy and Science: Women Physicians in American Medicine* (New York: Oxford University Press, 1985).

11. On gender, see Joan Walloch Scott, *Gender and the Politics of History* (New York: Columbia University Press, 1988). For some of the vast literature on the topic of gender roles and the origins of gynecology, see the following: Poovey, *Uneven Developments*; Moscucci, *Science of Woman*; and Cynthia Russett, *Sexual Science: The Victorian Construction of Womanhood* (Cambridge, Mass.: Harvard University Press, 1989). See also Ben Barker-Benfield, *Horrors of the Half-Known Life: Male Attitudes toward Women and Sexuality in Nineteenth-Century America* (New York: Harper and Row, 1976). See also Regina Markell Morantz, "The Perils of Feminist History," *Journal of Interdisciplinary History* 4 (Spring 1974): 649–660; Carl Degler, "What Ought to Be and What Was," *American Historical Review* 79 (December 1974): 1467–1490. See Haller and Haller, *The Physician and Sexuality*; Carroll Smith-Rosenberg, *Disorderly Con-*

duct: Visions of Gender in Victorian America (New York: Oxford University Press, 1985).

12. See Morantz-Sanchez, *Sympathy and Science.* See also Thomas Neville Bonner, *To the Ends of the Earth: Women's Search for Education in Medicine* (Cambridge, Mass.: Harvard University Press, 1992). See Mary Roth Walsh, *Doctors Wanted, No Women Need Apply: Sexual Barriers in the Medical Profession, 1835–1975* (New Haven: Yale University Press, 1977). See Regina Morantz-Sanchez's forthcoming history of Mary Dixon-Jones's medical career and litigation; also, Regina Morantz-Sanchez, "Making It in a Man's World: The Late-Nineteenth-Century Surgical Career of Mary Amanda Dixon Jones," *Bulletin of the History of Medicine* 69 (Winter 1995): 542–568. See Ruth J. Abram, ed., *'Send Us a Lady Physician': Women Doctors in America, 1835–1920* (New York: W. W. Norton, 1985).

13. See Carl Degler, *At Odds: Women and the Family from the Revolution to the Present* (New York: Oxford University Press, 1980); Stephen Marcus, *The Other Victorians: A Study of Sexuality and Pornography in Mid-Nineteenth Century England* (New York: Basic Books, 1966). Nancy Cott, "Passionlessness: An Interpretation of Victorian Sexual Ideology, 1790–1850," in Judith W. Leavitt, ed., *Women and Health in America: Historical Readings* (Madison: University of Wisconsin Press, 1984), 57–69.

14. See Regina Morantz, "The Lady and Her Physician," 38–53, and Carroll Smith-Rosenberg, "Puberty to Menopause: The Cycle of Femininity in Nineteenth-Century America," 23–37, in *Clio's Consciousness Raised.*

15. For some of the extensive material on Victorian women, see Mary P. Ryan, *Women in Public: Between Banners and Ballots, 1825–1880* (Baltimore: Johns Hopkins University Press, 1990); Linda K. Kerber, "Separate Spheres, Female Worlds, Woman's Place: The Rhetoric of Women's History," in *Toward an Intellectual History of Women: Essays* (Chapel Hill: University of North Carolina Press, 1997), 159–199; Nancy Theriot, *Mothers and Daughters in Nineteenth-Century America: The Biosocial Construction of Femininity* (Lexington: University Press of Kentucky, 1988; rev. ed., 1996).

16. See Howard Kelly, *Medical Gynecology* (New York: D. Appleton, 1909); John F. Steege, Deborah A. Metzger, and Barbara S. Levy, eds., *Chronic Pelvic Pain: An Integrated Approach* (Philadelphia: Saunders, 1998).

17. See the introduction in Judith R. Walkowitz, *City of Dreadful Delight: Narratives of Sexual Danger in Late-Victorian London* (Chicago: University of Chicago Press, 1992).

18. Catherine Scholten, *Childbearing in American Society: 1650–1850* (New York: New York University Press, 1985).

19. See Robert V. Wells, "Family History and Demographic Transition," *Journal of Social History* 9 (Fall 1975): 1–19, and Daniel Scott Smith, "Family Limitation, Sexual Control, and Domestic Feminism in Victorian America," in Nancy Cott and Elizabeth Pleck, eds., *A Heritage of Her Own* (New York: Simon and Schuster, 1979), 222–245, for two among many interpretations of population and rate of reproduction in the nneteenth century. See Jan Lewis and Kenneth Lockridge, "'Sally Has Been Sick': Pregnancy and Family Limitation among

Virginia Gentry Women, 1780–1830," *Journal of Social History* 22 (1988–1989): 5–19.

20. Londa Schiebinger, *Nature's Body: Gender in the Making of Modern Science* (Boston: Beacon Press, 1993); Judith Barrett Litoff, "Midwives and History," in *Women, Health, and Medicine*, 435–450; Laurel Thatcher Ulrich, *A Midwife's Tale: The Life of Martha Ballard Based on Her Diary, 1785–1812* (Boston: Beacon Press, 1990); Janet Carlisle Bogdan, "The Transformation of American Birth," Ph.D. diss., Syracuse University, 1986; Richard Wertz and Dorothy Wertz, *Lying-In: A History of Childbirth in America* (New Haven: Yale University Press, expanded ed., 1989); Judith Walzer Leavitt, *Brought to Bed: Childbearing in America, 1750–1950* (New York: Oxford University Press, 1986); Jane B. Donegan, *Women & Men Midwives: Medicine, Morality, and Misogyny in America* (Westport, Conn.: Greenwood Press, 1978); Barbara Ehrenreich and Deirdre English, *Witches, Midwives, and Nurses: A History of Women Healers* (Old Westbury, N.Y.: Feminist Press, 1973).

21. *Compact Edition of the Oxford English Dictionary*, vol. 1 (Oxford: Oxford University Press, 1971).

22. Ibid.

23. See Warner, *Therapeutic Perspective*.

24. Leslie Reagan, *When Abortion Was a Crime: Women, Medicine, and Law in the United States, 1867–1973* (Berkeley: University of California Press, 1997); Janet Farrell Brodie, *Abortion and Contraception in Nineteenth-Century America* (Ithaca, N.Y.: Cornell University Press, 1994); Linda Gordon, *Woman's Body, Woman's Right: Birth Control in America* (New York: Grossman, 1976; rev. and updated, New York: Penguin Books, 1990).

CHAPTER 1   *Peoples and Places*

1. Russell C. Maulitz, in his *Morbid Appearances*, discusses at length the importance of the medical press in the nineteenth century. See also Thomas Neville Bonner, *Becoming a Physician: Medical Education in Britain, France, Germany, and the United States, 1750–1945* (New York: Oxford University Press, 1995).

2. For a valuable discussion of the naming and meaning of heroic therapies, see Robert B. Sherman "Sanguine Practices: A Historical and Historiographic Reconsideration of Heroic Therapy in the Age of Rush," *Bulletin of the History of Medicine* 68 (Summer 1994): 211–234.

3. See Ronald Takaki, *Iron Cages: Race and Culture in Nineteenth-Century America* (Oxford: Oxford University Press, 1979), 23. See also David J. Rothman, *The Discovery of the Asylum: Social Order and Disorder in the New Republic* (Boston: Little, Brown and Company, 1971).

4. See Richard Shryock, *Medicine in America: Historical Essays* (Baltimore: Johns Hopkins University Press, 1966); Alex Berman, "The Heroic Approach in 19th-Century Therapeutics," in Judith Walzer Leavitt and Ronald L. Numbers, eds., *Sickness & Health in America: Readings in the History of Medicine and Public Health* (Madison: University of Wisconsin Press, 1978), 77–86.

5. Thomas Malthus, *An Essay on the Principle of Population*, first published in

1798, ed. Antony Flew (London: Penguin Classics, 1970). For interesting analyses and abstractions of Malthus's argument, see Irene Diamond, *Fertile Ground: Women, Earth and the Limits of Control* (Boston: Beacon Press, 1994); Gordon, *Woman's Body, Woman's Right*; and Rosalind Petchesky, *Abortion and Woman's Choice: The State, Sexuality, and Reproductive Freedom* (Boston: Northeastern University Press, 1985).

6. See Petchesky, *Abortion*, 35–37.
7. See Alfred W. Crosby, *Ecological Imperialism: The Biological Expansion of Europe* (New York: Cambridge University Press, 1985); Charles E. Rosenberg, *The Cholera Years* (Chicago: University of Chicago Press, 1962); William H. McNeil *Plagues and Peoples* (New York: Doubleday, 1977).
8. Many cite population as significant in tracing historical change. See, for instance, Michel Foucault, *The History of Sexuality: An Introduction*, vol. 1, trans. Robert Hurley (New York: Vintage Books, 1990).
9. See Mary Poovey, *Making a Social Body: British Cultural Formation, 1830–1864* (Chicago: University of Chicago Press, 1995). See also Michel Foucault in his *History of Sexuality*.
10. See James H. Cassedy, *Medicine and American Growth, 1800–1860* (Madison: University of Wisconsin Press, 1986), 3.
11. See Kerber, "Separate Spheres, Female Worlds"; Mary Ryan, *Cradle of the Middle Class: The Family in Oneida County, New York, 1790–1865* (Cambridge, U.K.: Cambridge University Press, 1981); Jeanne Boydston, *Home and Work: Housework, Wages, and the Ideology of Labor in the Early Republic* (New York: Oxford University Press, 1991); Sarah Elbert, *A Hunger for Home: Louisa May Alcott and* LITTLE WOMEN (Philadelphia: Temple University Press, 1984). There is a great deal more material on this topic than I can present here.
12. There is a vast amount of literature on this topic. For an excellent place to start, see Anne Fausto-Sterling, *Myths of Gender: Biological Theories about Women and Men* (New York: Basic Books, 1985; rev. ed., 1992); Londa Schiebinger, *"The Mind Has No Sex?" Women in the Origins of Modern Science* (Cambridge, Mass.: Harvard University Press, 1989); Thomas Laqueur, *Making Sex: Body and Gender from the Greeks to Freud* (Cambridge: Harvard University Press, 1990); and Stephen Jay Gould, *The Mismeasure of Man* (New York: Basic Books, 1985).
13. See Nancy Stepan in the preface to her book, *The Idea of Race in Science: Great Britain, 1800–1960* (London: Macmillan, 1982).
14. See Winthrop Jordan, *White over Black: American Attitudes toward the Negro: 1550–1812* (Baltimore: Penguin, 1969), and Stepan, *The Idea of Race*.
15. See Stepan, *The Idea of Race*, chapter 1. See also Stephen Jay Gould, *Wonderful Life: The Burgess Shale and the Nature of History* (New York: W. W. Norton, 1989) and Londa Schiebinger, *Nature's Body: Gender in the Making of Modern Science* (Boston: Beacon Press, 1993).
16. See Donna Haraway, *Primate Visions: Gender, Race and Nature in the World of Modern Science* (London: Routledge, Chapman and Hall, 1989).
17. See Nancy Leys Stepan, "Race and Gender: The Role of Analogy in Science," in Sandra Harding, ed., *The "Racial" Economy of Science: Toward a Democratic*

Future (Bloomington: Indiana University Press, 1993), 359–376, for a discussion of the intertwining of race and sex in this debate.

18. See Stepan, *The Idea of Race,* and Gould, *The Mismeasure.* See also John S. Haller, *Outcasts from Evolution: Scientific Attitudes of Racial Inferiority* (Champaign-Urbana: University of Illinois Press, 1971; 2d ed., Carbondale: Southern Illinois University Press, 1995), and William Stanton, *The Leopard's Spots: Scientific Attitudes toward Race in America, 1815–1859* (Chicago: University of Chicago Press, 1960).

19. See Ronald Numbers, "Science and Religion," *Osiris* 1 (1985): 68, and Ronald Numbers and Todd Savitt, Introduction to Part I, *Science and Medicine in the Old South* (Baton Rouge: Louisiana State University Press, 1989), 6.

20. See George Fredrickson, *The Black Image in the White Mind: The Debate on Afro-American Character and Destiny, 1817–1914* (Middletown, Conn.: Wesleyan University Press, 1971).

21. See Schiebinger, *Nature's Body,* and Laqueur, *Making Sex;* see also Russett, *Sexual Science.*

22. See Stepan, *The Idea of Race* and "Race and Gender"; see also Gould, *The Mismeasure.*

23. See Cassedy, *Medicine and American Growth,* and Warner, *Therapeutic Perspective;* see also James Cassedy, *American Medicine and Statistical Thinking, 1800–1860* (Cambridge, Mass.: Harvard University Press, 1984).

24. See Ronald Takaki, *Iron Cages.* See also Leslie A. Falk, "Black Abolitionist Doctors and Healers, 1810–1885," *Bulletin of the History of Medicine* 54 (Summer 1980): 258–272.

25. Russell C. Maulitz presents the history of pathology in the early nineteenth century, comparing in particular England and France; see his *Morbid Appearances.*

26. John Harley Warner, *Therapeutic Perspective,* has an outstanding and in-depth exploration of empiricism in medicine.

27. Warner, *Therapeutic Perspective;* Cassedy, *Medicine and American Growth.*

28. Berman, "The Heroic Approach."

29. Maulitz, *Morbid Appearances,* 210.

30. Laqueur, *Making Sex,* is thought-provoking on the meaning and implications of mind and body separations in the history of science and medicine.

31. See William G. Rothstein, *American Physicians in the Nineteenth Century: From Sects to Science* (Baltimore: Johns Hopkins University Press, 1972), on licensing and regulation of hospitals and physicians.

32. See Susan Cayleff, *Wash and Be Healed: The Water-Cure Movement and Women's Health* (Philadelphia: Temple University Press, 1987); Jane B. Donegan, *'Hydropathic Highway to Health': Women and Water-Cure in Antebellum America* (Westport, Conn.: Greenwood Press, 1986). See also Rothstein, *American Physicians.*

33. See Guenter B. Risse, Ronald L. Numbers, and Judith Walzer Leavitt, eds., *Medicine without Doctors: Home Health Care in American History* (New York: Science History Publications, 1977).

34. See Cassedy, *Medicine and American Growth,* 10.

35. See ibid.

36. See Barbara J. Fields, *Slavery and Freedom on the Middle Ground: Maryland during the Nineteenth Century* (New Haven: Yale University Press, 1985).

37. There is extensive literature on this topic. A good place to start is with these two volumes of many excellent essays: Ronald L. Numbers and Todd L. Savitt, eds., *Science and Medicine in the Old South* (Baton Rouge: Louisiana State University Press, 1989); Todd L. Savitt and James Harvey Young, eds., *Disease and Distinctiveness in the American South* (Knoxville: University of Tennessee Press, 1988). See also Richard Shryock, "Medical Practice in the Old South," *South Atlantic Quarterly* 29 (1930): 160–178; John Harley Warner, "The Idea of Southern Medical Distinctiveness: Medical Knowledge and Practice in the Old South," in Judith Walzer Leavitt and Ronald L. Numbers, eds., *Sickness and Health*, 2d ed., rev. (Madison: University of Wisconsin Press, 1985), 53–70.

38. See James O. Breeden, "States Rights Medicine in the Old South," *Bulletin of the New York Academy of Medicine* 52 (March-April, 1976): 348–372.

39. See Todd L. Savitt, "Slave Health and Southern Distinctiveness," in Savitt and Young, eds., *Disease and Distinctiveness*.

40. See Lacy K. Ford, Jr., *Origins of Southern Radicalism: The South Carolina Upcountry, 1800–1860* (New York: Oxford University Press, 1988), for an interesting description of Sims's environment during his youth.

41. See Sims, *Story of My Life*, 40, and Harris, *Woman's Surgeon*.

42. Records of the State of South Carolina, South Carolina Department of Archives and History, Columbia.

43. See Ford, *Origins of Southern Radicalism*, and also Randolph B. Campbell, "Planters and Plain Folks: The Social Structure of the Antebellum South," in John Boles and Evelyn Nolen, eds., *Interpreting Southern History: Historiographical Essays in Honor of Sanford W. Higginbotham* (Baton Rouge: Louisiana State University Press, 1987), 48–77.

44. Sims, *Story of My Life*, 56.

45. Ibid., 69.

46. Ibid., 70.

47. See Elliott J. Gorn, "Black Magic: Folk Beliefs of the Slave Community," in Numbers and Savitt, *Science and Medicine*, 295–326.

48. Sims, *Story of My Life*. See also Harris, *Woman's Surgeon*, 18. See John Duffy, "The Impact of Malaria in the South," in Todd Savitt and James Harvey Young, eds., *Disease and Distinctiveness*, 33–34.

49. Sims, *Story of My Life*, 113–114. *Story of My Life*, and Harris, *Woman's Surgeon*, are rich with details and storytelling from Sims's life.

50. See William W. Freehling, *Prelude to Civil War: The Nullification Controversy in South Carolina, 1816–1836* (New York: Harper and Row, 1965).

51. Harris, *Woman's Surgeon*, 16.

52. See the manuscript of a draft of *The Story of My Life* by J. Marion Sims, held by the State of Alabama Department of Archives and History.

53. Sims, *Story of My Life*, 116.

54. Typed and edited manuscript of *Story of My Life*, subtitled "A series of little Life Stories, chronologically arranged." This manuscript was donated to the Alabama State Archives by Sims's son-in-law, John A. Wyeth, in 1902.

55. See Bonner, *Becoming a Physician*, and Maulitz, *Morbid Appearances*. Bonner is particularly clear in his intent to right previous assumptions of the simple and inadequate nature of medical education in the United States in the 1830s.

56. See John Harley Warner, "The Selective Transport of Medical Knowledge: Antebellum American Physicians and Parisian Medical Therapeutics," *Bulletin of the History of Medicine* 59 (Summer 1985): 213–225.

57. See also Dale Smith, "The Emergence of Organized Clinical Instruction in the Nineteenth-Century American Cities of Boston, New York and Philadelphia," Ph.D. diss., University of Minnesota, 1979.

58. See William Norwood, *Medical Education in the U.S. before the Civil War* (Philadelphia: University of Pennsylvania Press, 1944; reprint ed., New York: Arno Press, 1971); John Harley Warner, "Southern Medical Reform: The Meaning of the Antebellum Argument for Southern Medical Education," *Bulletin of the History of Medicine* 57 (Fall 1983): 364–381; Martha Carolyn Mitchell, "Health and the Medical Profession in the Lower South, 1845–1860," *Journal of Southern History* 10 (1944): 424–446; William D. Postell, *The Health of Slaves on Southern Plantations* (Baton Rouge: Louisiana State University Press, 1951); and Joseph Waring, *A History of Medicine in South Carolina, 1825–1900* (Columbia: South Carolina Medical Association, 1967).

59. See Norwood, *Medical Education,* and Waring, *Medicine in South Carolina.*

60. See Sims, *Story of My Life*, 128.

61. See Ruth Richardson, *Death, Dissection and the Destitute* (London: Routledge and Kegan Paul, 1987), for a valuable exploration of the use and availability of bodies for medical science in England in this period.

62. Shryock, *Medicine in America.* See the final chapter, "The Interplay of Social and Internal Factors in Modern Medicine," for a description of the stigma attached to autopsies.

63. See Sterling Stuckey, *Slave Culture: Nationalist Theory and the Foundations of Black America* (New York: Oxford University Press, 1987). See also Eugene D. Genovese, *Roll, Jordan, Roll: The World the Slaves Made* (New York: Pantheon Books, 1974); John W. Blassingame, *The Slave Community* (New York: Oxford University Press, 1972), and many many other books too numerous to mention.

64. Norwood, *Medical Education*, chapter 22.

65. Ibid., 91; Samuel D. Gross, *Autobiography with Sketches of His Contemporaries* (edited by his sons), vol. 2 (Philadelphia: George Barrie, 1987), 28.

66. M. E. Darrach, "Memoir of George McClellan, M.S.: A Lecture Introductory to the Theory and Practice of Physic in the Medical Department of Pennsylvania College for the Session of 1847–1848" (Philadelphia: King and Baird, 1847), 27 (Holdings of the Library of the Philadelphia College of Physicians and Surgeons.)

67. Ibid., 14.

68. Sims, *Story of My Life*, 136.

69. Gert Brieger, "Surgery," in Ronald L. Numbers, ed., *Education of American Physicians: Historical Essays* (Berkeley: University of California Press, 1980), 188.

70. Maulitz, *Morbid Appearances*, 215.

71. Reginald Horsman, *Josiah Nott of Mobile: Southerner, Physician, and Racial*

Theorist (Baton Rouge: Louisiana State University Press, 1987). See also Sims, *Story of My Life.*

72. See Bonner, *Becoming a Physician*, 204.

73. See Sims, *Story of My Life*, and Harris, *Woman's Surgeon*. See also E. Brooks Holifield, *The Gentlemen Theologians: American Theology in Southern Culture, 1795–1860* (Durham, N.C.: Duke University Press, 1978), and "Science and Theology in the Old South," in Ronald Numbers and Todd Savitt, eds., *Science and Medicine in the Old South* (Baton Rouge: Louisiana State University Press, 1989), 127–143. See also Thomas G. Dyer, "Science in the Antebellum College: The University of Georgia, 1801–1860," in Numbers and Savitt, eds., *Science and Medicine*, 36–54, and Ronald Numbers and Janet Numbers, "Science in the Old South," in *Science and Medicine*, 9–35.

74. Sims, *Story of My Life*, 82–83. See also Horsman, *Josiah Nott*, on T. Cooper and his influence on Nott.

75. See Holifield, *Gentlemen Theologians*.

76. See Sims, *Story of My Life*, for details of his friendship and acquaintance with Thornwell. See also Harris, *Woman's Surgeon*. On Thornwell, see Holifield, *Gentleman Theologians*, and "Science and Theology." See also Drew Gilpin Faust, *A Sacred Circle: The Dilemma of the Intellectual in the Old South, 1840–1860* (Baltimore: Johns Hopkins University Press, 1977).

77. See Suzanne Lebsock, *The Free Women of Petersburg: Status and Culture in a Southern Town, 1784–1860* (New York: W. W. Norton, 1984), for an exploration of the role of women as widows in the governance of estates and on the topic of men marrying up in Southern society.

78. J. Marion Sims, letter to Theresa Jones, December 31, 1835, in *Story of My Life*, 372.

79. Frank L. Owsley, *Plain Folk of the Old South* (Chicago: Quadrangle Books, 1949), 183.

80. Sims, *Story of My Life.*

81. J. Marion Sims to Theresa Jones, May 11, 1836, in *Story of My Life*, 380. All of the letters published in Sims's autobiography are held in the original by the Southern Historical Collection. Cross-checking revealed careful accuracy in the reproduction of the letters in the book.

82. See Takaki, *Iron Cages*, 78.

83. See John Duffy, "Medical Practice in the Ante Bellum South," *Journal of Southern History* 25 (1959): 53–72, and Savitt and Young, eds., *Disease and Distinctiveness*; John H. Ellis, *Yellow Fever and Public Health in the New South* (Lexington: University Press of Kentucky, 1992).

84. John Duffy, "Medical Practice," and "The Impact of Malaria," in Savitt and Young, eds., *Disease and Distinctiveness*, 29–54.

85. Seale Harris, in *Woman's Surgeon*, diagnosed Sims's sickness as chronic dysentery. Sims may have suffered from a disease similar to that which killed his mother, a combination of malaria and some other strain such as typhoid fever.

86. Letter from J. Marion Sims to Theresa Jones, October 10, 1836, reprinted in *Story of My Life*, 387.

87. See Steven M. Stowe, "Religion, Science, and the Culture of Medical Practice

230   *Notes to Pages 25–29*

in the American South, 1800–1870," in James Gilbert, Amy Gilman, Donald Scott, and Joan Scott, eds., *The Mythmaking Frame of Mind: Social Imagination and American Culture* (Belmont, Calif.: Wadsworth, 1993), 1–24.

88. J. Marion Sims to Theresa Jones, December 31, 1835 in *Story of My Life*, 373. Stowe quotes from the same passage in his "Religion, Science and Culture."
89. DeBow's *Review* 4 (November 1847): 402–403.
90. The Scrapbook of F. F. Michel, 1877, Alabama State Historical Society.
91. See Sims, *Story of My Life*, and Harris, *Woman's Surgeon*.
92. J. Marion Sims, "Double Congenital Hare-Lip-Absence of the Superior Incisors, and Their Portion of Alveolar Process," *American Journal of Dental Science* 5 (1844–1845): 51–56.
93. J. Marion Sims, "Removal of the Superior Maxilla for a Tumour of the Antrum; Apparent Cure. Return of the Disease. Second Operation. Sequel," *American Journal of the Medical Sciences* 13 (April 1847): 310–314; "Osteo-Sarcoma of the Lower Jaw," *American Journal of the Medical Sciences* 11 (1846): 128–132.
94. Sims, *Story of My Life*, 140–141.
95. One of John Eberle's texts was *A Treatise on the Practice of Medicine*, 2d ed. (Philadelphia: John Grigg, 1831). Sims also mentioned a text by Eberle on diseases of childhood.
96. Charles Rosenberg, "The Practice of Medicine in New York a Century Ago," *Bulletin of the History of Medicine* 41 (1967): 223–253.
97. Todd L. Savitt, "Slave Health and Southern Distinctiveness," in Savitt and Young, eds., *Disease and Distinctiveness*, 130.
98. J. Marion Sims, "Trismus Nascentium—Its Pathology and Treatment," *American Journal of the Medical Sciences* 11 (April 1846): 363.
99. Kenneth Kiple and Virginia H. King, *Another Dimension of the Black Diaspora: Diet, Disease and Racism* (Cambridge: Cambridge, U.K.: University Press, 1981); Michael Johnson, "Smother Slave Infants: Were Slave Mothers at Fault?" *Journal of Southern History* 47 (November 1981): 493–520; Todd Savitt, *Medicine and Slavery: The Disease and Health Care of Blacks in Antebellum Virginia* (Champaign-Urbana: University of Illinois Press, 1978); Robert Fogel, *Without Consent or Contract: The Rise and Fall of American Slavery* (London: W. W. Norton, 1989); Richard H. Steckel, "A Peculiar Population: The Nutrition, Health, and Mortality of American Slaves from Childhood to Maturity," *Journal of Economic History* 46 (September 1986): 721–741, and "A Dreadful Childhood: The Excess Mortality of American Slaves," *Social Science History* 10 (Winter 1986): 429–463.
100. See Steckel, "A Dreadful Childhood."
101. See John Duffy, ed., *The Rudolph Matas History of Medicine in Louisiana*, vol. 2 (Baton Rouge: Louisiana State University Press, 1962), 65–71; Richard B. Sheridan, *Doctors and Slaves: A Medical and Demographic History of Slavery in the British West Indies, 1680–1834* (Cambridge, U.K.: University Press, 1985). See also Savitt, "Slave Health."
102. J. Marion Sims, "Further Observations on Trismus Nascentium, with Cases Illustrating Its Etiology and Treatment," *American Journal of the Medical Sciences* 16 (July 1848): 59–79. The last article was "Further Observations on

Trismus Nascentium, with Cases Illustrating Its Etiology and Treatment," *American Journal of the Medical Sciences* 16 (October 1848): 255–366.

103. Sims, "Further Observations," July 1848, 74.

104. Sims, "Trismus Nascentium," and "Further Observations," July 1848.

105. Sims, "Further Observations," July 1848, 74.

106. Sims, "Further Observations," October 1848, 359.

107. Federal Census, City of Montgomery, December 5, 1850.

CHAPTER 2 *Anarcha, Betsey, and Lucy*

1. See James V. Ricci, *The Genealogy of Gynaecology: History of the Development of Gynaecology throughout the Ages, 1000 B.C.–1800 A.D.* (Philadelphia: Blakiston, 1943), 521.

2. Reagan, *Abortion Was a Crime*, and Brodie, *Contraception and Abortion*.

3. Johann Dieffenach, as quoted in Moritz Schuppert, *A Treatise on Vesico-Vaginal Fistula* (New Orleans: Daily Commercial Bulletin, 1866), 7.

4. Laqueur, *Making Sex*; Russett, *Sexual Science*. See Schiebinger, *"The Mind Has No Sex?"*

5. Katherine Ott, *Fevered Lives: Tuberculosis in American Culture since 1870* (Cambridge, Mass.: Harvard University Press, 1996), is excellent in its discussion of the social construction of tuberculosis. See also Charles E. Rosenberg, "Disease in History: Frames and Framers," in *The Milbank Quarterly* 67, Suppl. 1 (1989) (special issue, "Framing Disease: The Creation and Negotiation of Explanatory Schemes,"1–15).

6. Naomi Zack, "The American Sexualization of Race," in Nancy Zack, ed., *Race/Sex: Their Sameness, Difference, and Interplay* (New York: Routledge, 1997), 145–155.

7. There are many sources on this topic. See Robbie E. Davis-Floyd, *Birth as an American Rite of Passage* (Berkeley: University of California Press, 1993); Robbie E. Davis-Floyd and Carolyn Sargent, eds., *Childbirth and Authoritative Knowledge: Cross-Cultural Perspectives* (Berkeley: University of California Press, 1997); Brigitte Jordan, *Birth in Four Cultures: A Crosscultural Investigation of Childbirth in Yucatan, Holland, Sweden, and the United States*, 4th ed., rev. and expanded by R. Davis-Floyd (Prospect Heights, Ill.: Waveland Press, 1993); Pamela S. Eakins, ed., *The American Way of Birth* (Philadelphia: Temple University Press, 1986); see also Sheila Kitzinger, ed., *The Midwife Challenge* (London: Pandora Press, 1988).

8. See Leavitt, *Brought to Bed*; Barbara Katz-Rothman, *In Labor: Women and Power in the Birthplace* (New York: W. W. Norton, 1991).

9. Renate Blumenthal-Kosinski, *Not of Woman Born: Representations of Caesarean Birth in Medieval and Renaissance Culture* (Ithaca, N.Y.: Cornell University Press, 1990).

10. See Walsh, *Doctors Wanted*, on Samuel Gregory's school for midwives founded in Boston in 1848. See also Janet Carlisle Bogdan, "Aggressive Intervention and Mortality," in *American Way of Birth*, 60–103.

11. On Martha Ballard, see Ulrich, *Midwife's Tale*. On Patty Sessions, see Chris

Rigby Arrington, "Pioneer Midwives," in Claudia Bushman, ed., *Mormon Sisters: Women in Early Utah* (Salt Lake City: Olympus Publishing, 1976), 43–65, and Claire Noall, "Mormon Midwives," in *Utah Historical Quarterly* 10 (1942): 84–144.

12. Irvine Loudon, *Death in Childbirth: An International Study of Maternal Mortality, 1800–1950* (Oxford: Clarendon Press, 1992).

13. Sally G. McMillen, *Motherhood in the Old South: Pregnancy, Childbirth, and Infant Rearing* (Baton Rouge: Louisiana State University Press, 1990), 81.

14. Sylvia Hoffert's *Private Matters: American Attitudes toward Childbearing and Infant Nurture in the Urban North, 1800–1860* (Champaign-Urbana: University of Illinois Press, 1989), is good in its consideration of demographic changes as they connect with changes in childbirth practices.

15. Reynolds Farley, *Growth of the Black Population: A Study of Demographic Trends* (Chicago: Markham, 1970), 21, 34, as cited in Deborah Gray White, *Ar'n't I A Woman? Female Slaves in the Plantation South* (London: W. W. Norton, 1985), 69.

16. Valerie Lee, *Granny Midwives and Black Women Writers: Double-Dutched Readings* (New York: Routledge, 1996). See, for instance, Linda Janet Holmes, "African American Midwives in the South," in *The American Way of Birth*, 273–291, and Holmes, *'Listen to Me Good'* (Columbus: Ohio State University Press, 1996); Sharon Robinson, "A Historical Development of Midwifery in the Black Community, 1600–1940," *Journal of Nurse Midwifery* 29 (July/August 1984): 247–254. Gertrude Fraser, "Modern Bodies, Modern Minds: Midwifery and Reproductive Change in the African American Community," in Faye Ginsburg and Rayna Rapp, eds., *Conceiving the New World Order: The Global Politics of Reproduction* (Berkeley: University of California Press, 1995), 42–58. Ariska Razak, "Toward a Womanist Analysis of Birth," in Irene Diamond and Gloria Feman Orenstein, eds., *Reweaving the World: The Emergence of Ecofeminism* (San Francisco: Sierra Club Books, 1990), 165–172. Two oral histories, in addition to *"Listen to Me Good,"* are Debra Anne Susie, *In the Way of Our Grandmothers: A Cultural View of Twentieth-Century Midwifery in Florida* (Athens: University of Georgia Press, 1988), and Onnie Lee Logan as told to Katherine Clark, *Motherwit: An Alabama Midwife's Story* (New York: E. P. Dutton, 1989).

17. See Marie Jenkins Schwartz, "'At Noon, Oh How I Ran': Breastfeeding and Weaning on Plantation and Farm in Antebellum Virginia and Alabama," in Patricia Morton, ed., *Discovering the Women in Slavery: Emancipating Perspectives on the American Past* (Athens: University of Georgia Press, 1996), 241–259; Elliot J. Gorn, "Black Magic," in *Science and Medicine.*

18. See Elizabeth Barnaby Keeney, "Unless Powerful Sick: Domestic Medicine in the Old South," in *Science and Medicine*, 276–294.

19. Fraser, "Modern Bodies, Modern Minds," 45.

20 See, among many others, Cheryl Townsend Gilkes, "Dual Heroisms and Double Burdens: Interpreting Afro-American Women's Experience and History," *Feminist Studies* 15 (Fall 1989): 573–590; Christie Farnham, "Sapphire? The Issue of Dominance in the Slave Family, 1830–1865," in Carol Groneman and Mary Beth Norton, eds., *"To Toil the Livelong Day": America's Women at Work, 1780–*

1980 (Ithaca, N.Y.: Cornell University Press, 1978) 68–83; Hine, King, and Reed, eds., *"We Specialize in the Wholly Impossible"*; Morton, ed., *Discovering the Women in Slavery*; White, *A'r'n't I a Woman*.

21. Harriet A. Jacobs, *Incidents in the Life of a Slave Girl: Written by Herself*, ed. Jean Yellin (Cambridge, Mass.: Harvard University Press, 1987), 77.

22. John Campbell, "Work, Pregnancy and Infant Mortality among Southern Slaves," *Journal of Interdisciplinary History* 14 (Spring 1984): 793–812.

23. Rose, "Look for some others for to 'plenish de earth," manuscript, Slave Narrative Collection, Federal Writers' Project, 1941, vol. 17, Texas Narratives, part 4, pp. 174–178, Library of Congress, Washington D.C. Excerpted in Linda Kerber and Sharon DeHart, *Women's America: Refocusing the Past*, 4th ed. (Oxford: Oxford University Press, 1995), 101.

24. Thomas Affleck, *Southern Medical Reports*, vol. 2 (New Orleans, 1850), quoted in Shryock, *Medicine in America*, 287.

25. Dr. M. Marsh, *New Orleans Medical News* 6 (1860): 930, quoted in Felice Swados, "Negro Health on the AnteBellum Plantations," *Bulletin of the History of Medicine* 10 (1941): 470.

26. Kiple and King, *Another Dimension of the Black Diaspora*, 171–172.

27. See John Duffy, ed., *The Rudolph Matas History of Medicine in Louisiana*, vol. 2 (Baton Rouge: Louisiana State University Press, 1962), 65–71. See also Richard B. Sheridan, *Doctors and Slaves: A Medical and Demographic History of Slavery in the British West Indies, 1680–1834* (Cambridge, U.K.: Cambridge University Press, 1985). See Todd Savitt, "Slave Health and Southern Distinctiveness," in *Disease and Distinctiveness*, 120–153.

28. R. H. Day, *New Orleans Medical and Surgical Journal* 4 (1847): 227, quoted by Walter Fisher, "Physicians and Slavery in the Antebellum Southern Medical Journal," *Journal of the History of Medicine* 23 (1968): 44.

29. William Postell, *The Health of Slaves on Southern Plantations* (Baton Rouge: Louisiana State University Press, 1951), 115

30. Savitt, *Medicine and Slavery*, 118, reports on four C-sections done on slave women in the early nineteenth century.

31. See John Duffy, *The Healers: A History of American Medicine* (Champaign-Urbana: University of Illinois Press, 1979), 142. It is interesting to note that while Ephraim McDowell's early ovariotomies (1809 and later) drew great attention, few medical men noticed the use of Caesarian section on slave women.

32. See Theriot, *Mothers and Daughters*.

33. Sometimes slave women themselves were blamed for the deaths of their children. See, for instance, Michael P. Johnson, "Smothered Slave Infants: Were Slave Mothers at Fault?" *Journal of Southern History* 47 (November 1981): 493–520; see also Kiple and King, *Another Dimension of the Black Diaspora*; Todd Savitt, *Medicine and Slavery: The Diseases and Health Care of Blacks in Antebellum Virginia* (Champaign-Urbana: University of Illinois Press, 1978).

34. Kiple and King, *Another Dimension of the Black Diaspora*, 118–119. See also Edward Shorter, *A History of Women's Bodies* (New York: Basic Books, 1982), 22–28, on the prevalence of rickets in the general population of women. Also see Claire E. Fox, "Pregnancy, Childbirth and Early Infancy in Anglo-American

Culture, 1675–1830," Ph.D. diss., University of Pennsylvania, 1966, and the primary sources of William Thompson Lusk, *The Science and Art of Midwifery* (New York: D. Appleton, 1881; 2d ed., 1893), and Charles D. Meigs, *The Philadelphia Practice of Midwifery* (Philadelphia: Jameskan Jin & Bro., 1838).

35. Nicholas Cardell and Mark Hopkins, "The Effect of Milk Intolerance on the Consumption of Milk by Slaves in 1860," *Journal of Interdisciplinary History* 8 (Winter 1978): 507–513.

36. Postell, *The Health of Slaves*, 118.

37. Sims, *Story of My Life*, 226. U.S. Bureau of the Census Population Schedules, U.S. Census of 1840, Montgomery County, Alabama.

38. See Schwartz, "'At Noon, Oh How I Ran.'"

39. Sims, *Story of My Life*, 240.

40. Samuel D. Gross, *Autobiography with Sketches of His Contemporaries*, vol. 2 (Philadelphia: George Barrie, 1887), 148. In these pages, Gross also reported that Lucy and Betsey were each primipara mothers when they contracted vesico-vaginal fistulas.

41. Sims, *Story of My Life*, 230–233.

42. J. Marion Sims, *Silver Sutures in Surgery: The Anniversary Discourse before the New York Academy of Medicine* (New York: Samuel S. Wood, 1858), 47.

43. *Oxford English Dictionary*.

44. See, for instance, T. Gaillard Thomas, "An Address in Obstetrics and Gynecology: Delivered at the First Annual Meeting of the New York State Medical Association, Nov. 19, 1884," reprinted from *The Medical News*, November 22, 1884. See also Ricci, *One Hundred Years*.

45. Sims, *Story of My Life*, chapter 14.

46. On the difficulties of vesico-vaginal fistula surgery, see J. M. Kerr, R. W. Johnstone, and Miles H. Phillips, eds., *Historical Review of British Obstetrics and Gynaecology, 1800–1950* (Edinburgh: E. and S. Livingstone Ltd., 1954).

47. Sims, *Story of My Life*, 234.

48. Sims, *Silver Sutures*, 52.

49. Gross, *Autobiography*, vol. 2, 145–149.

50. Sims, *Story of My Life*, 241.

51. Savitt, *Medicine and Slavery*, 289–290. See also Todd L. Savitt, "The Use of Blacks for Medical Experimentation and Demonstration in the Old South," *Journal of Southern History* 48 (August 1982): 331–348.

52. Sims, *Silver Sutures*, 31.

53. See Pernick, *Calculus of Suffering*.

54. See Sir J. Y. Simpson's Reply to Dr. Jacob Bigelow, "Historical Letter on the Introduction of Anaesthetics in Dentistry and Surgery in America, and on Their First Employment in Midwifery in England," *Boston Medical and Surgical Journal* 5 (February 24, 1870): 137–140.

55. Pernick, *Calculus*. See also Virginia Thatcher, *History of Anesthesia* (New York: J. P. Lippincott, 1953); Harvey Graham, *Surgeons All* (New York: Philosophical Library, 1957); and Alfred Hurwitz and George A. Degenshein, *Milestones in Modern Surgery* (New York: Hoeber-Harper, 1958).

56. See George Hayward, "Cases of Vesico-Vaginal Fistula Treated by Operation,"

Boston Medical and Surgical Journal 44 (April 16, 1851): 220, for a description of a patient on whom he operated and used ether in 1847. H. R. Storer also suggested the use of anesthesia for the operation. See his review, "The Treatment of Vaginal Fistula," *American Journal of the Medical Sciences* 34 (October 1857): 387. In *Woman's Surgeon*, 108–109, Seale Harris discusses the resistance Sims met among white patients. These women refused completion of the surgery, despite its known success, because there was no applied anesthetic and the pain was unbearable.

57. Sims, *Story of My Life*, 243.
58. Ibid.
59. Sims, "Vesico-Vaginal Fistula," 81.
60. Ibid., 80.
61. Ibid.
62. Ibid., 76–77.
63. Ibid., 77.
64. Sims, *Story of My Life*, 238.
65. Ibid.
66. Sims, "Vesico-Vaginal Fistula," 68.
67. Ibid.
68. Conversation in January 1987 with Dr. Dixon N. Burns, Clinical Professor of Obstetrics and Gynecology, University of Oklahoma, Tulsa, concerning the significance of the sigmoid catheter.
69. Manuscript, Sims Collection, Reynolds Historical Library at the University of Alabama at Birmingham.
70. While Sims tells this story most completely in *Story of My Life*, he also becomes fervently enthusiastic in telling the tale of the discovery of silver sutures in *Silver Sutures*.
71. Sims, *Story of My Life*, 245.
72. Conversation in April 1989 with Dr. Robert Bradley, urologist, Philadelphia College of Physicians, concerning the difficulty of performing vesico-vaginal fistula surgery, and the necessity of ongoing, repeated opportunities to practice the technique in order to master it. Sims alludes in *Silver Sutures* to the value of his unlimited opportunity for experimental operations at the Woman's Hospital.
73. Nathan Bozeman, "The Clamp Suture and the Range of its Applicability," *Transactions of the American Gynecological Society* 9 (1884): 357.
74. Marc Columbat, *A Treatise of the Diseases and Special Hygiene of Females*, trans. Charles Meigs (Philadelphia: Lea and Blanchard, 1849), 264.
75. Sewall, "Bountiful Bodies," 121.
76. Fleetwood Churchill, *On the Diseases of Women Including Those of Pregnancy and Childbed* (Philadelphia: Blanchard and Lea, 1852).
77. Charles Meigs, *Woman: Her Diseases and Remedies. A Series of Letters to His Class* (Philadelphia: Blanchard and Lea, 1854), 339.
78. Shryock, *Medicine in America*, 64.
79. Savitt, "The Use of Blacks," and Fisher, "Physicians and Slavery," 36–49.
80. Lucy came from Macon County.

81. See James Jones, "The Tuskegee Syphilis Experiment: A Moral Astigmatism," in Sandra Harding, ed., *The Racial Economy of Science: Toward a Democratic Future* (Bloomington: Indiana University Press, 1993), 275–228, and James Jones, *Bad Blood: The Tuskegee Syphilis Experiment* (New York: Free Press, 1993, new and expanded ed.). See also Allan M. Brandt, "Racism and Research: The Case of the Tuskegee Syphilis Study," in Leavitt and Numbers, *Sickness and Health*, 331–343.

82. Savitt, "The Use of Blacks"; F. N. Boney, "Slaves as Guinea Pigs: Georgia and Alabama Episodes," *Alabama Review* 37 (1984): 5–51. See also Diana E. Axelson, "Women as Victims of Medical Experimentation: J. Marion Sims' Surgery on Slave Women, 1845–1850," in Darlene Clark Hine, ed., *Black Women in United States History*, vol. 1 (Brooklyn: Carlson Publishing, 1990), 51–60.

83. Historical research looks for definitions and premises of action in the context of the past. See Noel Ignatiev, *How the Irish Became White* (New York: Routledge, 1995).

84. See, for instance, Charles E. Rosenberg, "The Therapeutic Revolution: Medicine, Meaning and Social Change in Nineteenth-Century America," in Morris J. Vogel and Charles E. Rosenberg, eds., *The Therapeutic Revolution: Essays in the Social History of American Medicine* (Philadelphia: University of Pennsylvania Press, 1979), 3–25.

85. Sims, *Story of My Life*, 229.

86. Gross, *Autobiography*, vol. 2, 148.

87. Nell Irvin Painter, *Sojourner Truth: A Life, A Symbol* (New York: W. W. Norton, 1996), 17.

88. Sims, "Vesico-Vaginal Fistula," 82.

89. See Eric Homberger, *The Historical Atlas of New York City: A Visual Celebration of Nearly 400 Years of New York City's History* (New York: Henry Holt, 1994), 83.

90. Richard Shryock, "Medical Practice in the Old South," 173. Shryock provides no documentation. Bozeman in 1884 described a slave patient of Sims's who was also his servant. By the time of the 1850 Census, Sims had twelve females (out of a total of seventeen slaves). All but three were either of childbearing age or older, making them possible victims of vesico-vaginal fistulas.

91. Savitt, "The Use of Blacks."

92. Sims, *Silver Sutures*, 55.

93. Nell Irvin Painter, "Sojourner Truth's Defense of the Rights of Women" (as reported in 1851; rewritten in 1863), *Women's America*, 215–217.

94. Sims, *Silver Sutures*, 60.

95. Ibid., 52.

96. See Virginia Drachman, "The Loomis Trial: Social Mores and Obstetrics in the Mid-Nineteenth Century," in Susan Reverby and David Rosner, eds., *Health Care in America: Essays in Social History* (Philadelphia: Temple University Press, 1979), 67–83.

97. J. Marion Sims, "Removal of the Superior Maxilla for a Tumour of the Antrum; Apparent Cure. Return of the Disease. Second Operation. Sequel," *Journal of*

the American Medical Sciences (April 1847): 310–314; "Osteo-Sarcoma of the Lower Jaw," *American Journal of the Medical Sciences* 11 (1846): 128–132.

98. Savitt, "Use of Blacks." See also Elbert, "Good Times on the Cross: A Marxian Review," *Review of Radical Political Economics* 7 (Fall 1975): 55–66.

99. See Pernick, *Calculus of Suffering*, and Savitt, "Use of Blacks." See also Ronald L. Numbers, "William Beaumont and the Ethics of Human Experimentation," *Journal of the History of Biology* 12 (Spring 1979): 113–135, and John J. Young, "Moral Problems Related to Research and Experimentation: A Survey," in Dennis Robbins and Allen Dyer, eds., *Ethical Dimensions of Clinical Medicine* (Springfield, Ill.: Charles C. Thomas, 1981), 3–15; Boney, "Slaves as Guinea Pigs."

100. John P. Mettauer, "On Vesico-Vaginal Fistula," *American Journal of the Medical Sciences* (July 1847): 117–121. See also Savitt, *Medicine and Slavery*, Fisher, "Physicians and Slavery," and Duffy, *Healers*, 134–142.

101. Nathan Bozeman, "Remarks on Vesico-Vaginal Fistule, with an Account of a New Mode of Suture, and Seven Successful Operations," *Louisville Review* 1 (1856): 339.

102. Bozeman, "The Clamp Suture."

103. Nathan Bozeman, "Remarks on Vesico-Vaginal Fistule," 339.

104. Schuppert, *A Treatise*;. C. S. Fenner, "Vesico-Vaginal Fistula," *American Journal of the Medical Sciences* 37–38 (October 1859): 353–355.

105. David Hayes Agnew, *Lacerations of the Female Perineum and Vesico-Vaginal Fistula: Their History and Treatment* (Philadelphia: Lindsay and Blakiston, 1873).

106. Agnew, *Lacerations*, 112–113.

107. Bozeman, "Vesico-Vaginal Fistule," 339.

108. Nathan Bozeman, "Urethro-Vaginal, Vesico-Vaginal and Recto-Vaginal Fistules; General Remarks; Report of Cases Successfully Treated with the Button-Suture," *New Orleans Medical and Surgical Journal* 17 (1860): 185; "The Clamp Suture," 361.

109. Bozeman, "The Clamp Suture," 361.

110. Review Essay, "Silver Sutures in Surgery," *North American Medico-Chirurgic Review* 2 (July 1858): 635–653.

111. Sims, *Silver Sutures*, 51.

112. Stephen Jay Gould, *The Panda's Thumb: More Reflections in Natural History* (New York: W. W. Norton, 1980), 30.

113. See Stanley Joel Reiser, *Medicine and the Reign of Technology* (Cambridge, U.K.: Cambridge University Press, 1978), and Audrey Davis, *Medicine and Its Technology: An Introduction to the History of Medical Instrumentation* (Westport, Conn.: Greenwood, 1981).

114. Bozeman, "Urethro-Vaginal," 348.

115. Valentine Mott, *First Anniversary Woman's Hospital Report* (New York: Miller and Holman, 1856), 18.

116. See Columbat, *Treatise,* 242.

117. Agnew, *Lacerations*, 10.

118. James Y. Simpson, *Clinical Lectures on Diseases of Women* (Philadelphia: Blanchard and Lea, 1863), 23. The date of the lecture is 1859.
119. Ibid., 24. H. Levert of Alabama also experimented on pigs to compare metallic versus silk sutures in this same time period.

CHAPTER 3   *Missions and Medicine*

1. Report of the Committee on Charitable and Religious Societies on Memorial of the Woman's Hospital, for an appropriation, State of New York, February 28, 1856, Senate, no. 52.
2. Ibid.
3. Thomas Addis Emmet, *Twelfth Annual Report of the Woman's Hospital of the State of New York*, 1867.
4. James Pratt Marr, *James Marion Sims: Founder of the Woman's Hospital in the State of New York.*
5. See Charles Rosenberg, "The Practice of Medicine in New York a Century Ago," *Bulletin of the History of Medicine* 41 (1967): 223–253.
6. 9th Annual Report of the Woman's Hospital Association (1864), 13.
7. See Charles E. Rosenberg and Carroll Smith-Rosenberg, "Pietism and the Origins of the American Public Health Movement: A Note on John H. Griscom and Robert M. Hartley," in *Sickness and Health,* 2d ed., rev., 385–398.
8. Dr. Sims on a Hospital for Females, *New York Daily Times* May 19, 1854, 1, quoting John Griscom.
9. See Gerald Grob, "Class, Ethnicity, and Race in American Mental Hospitals, 1830–1875," in Gert Brieger, ed., *Theory and Practice in American Medicine: Historical Studies from the Journal of the History of Medicine and Allied Sciences* (New York: Science History Publications, 1976), 227–249.
10. Carroll Smith-Rosenberg and Charles Rosenberg, "The Female Animal: Medical and Biological Views of Woman and Her Role in Nineteenth-Century America," in Judith Walzer Leavitt, ed., *Women and Health in America: Historical Readings* (Madison: University of Wisconsin Press, 1984), 12–27. See also Russett, *Sexual Science.*
11. See Wendy Mitchinson, *The Nature of Their Bodies: Women and Their Doctors in Victorian Canada* (Toronto: University of Toronto Press, 1991), 50–52.
12. Catherine Beecher, *Letters to the People on Health and Happiness* (New York: Harper and Bros., 1855; reprinted by Arno Press, 1972), 120–131.
13. Rosenberg and Smith-Rosenberg, "Pietism."
14. Ibid., 386.
15. Smith, "The Emergence of Organized Clinical Instruction." This thesis offers a wealth of information.
16. See Jane E. Mottus, *New York Nightingales: The Emergence of the Nursing Profession at Bellevue and New York Hospital, 1850–1920* (Ann Arbor: UMI Research Press, 1981), 1–12. See also Charles Rosenberg, *The Care of Strangers: The Rise of America's Hospital System* (New York: Basic Books, 1987), and Rosenberg, "New York City a Century Ago."
17. See Morantz-Sanchez, *Sympathy and Science,* and Barbara Berg, *The Remembered Gate: Origins of American Feminism* (New York: Oxford University Press, 1978).

18. See Morantz-Sanchez, *Sympathy and Science*.
19. The Women's Medical College in Philadelphia and the New England Hospital for Women and Children in Boston were established soon after the Woman's Hospital. See Morantz-Sanchez, *Sympathy and Science*.
20. See Moscucci, *The Science of Woman*, 86. See Jane Sewall, "Bountiful Bodies," 90.
21. Article III, Constitution of the Woman's Hospital, *First Anniversary of the Woman's Hospital* (New York: Miller and Holman, 1856), 29.
22. Mary Putnam Jacobi, "Woman in Medicine," in Annie Nathan Meyer, ed., *Woman's Work in America* (New York: Henry Holt, 1891), 169.
23. New York State Document No. 52, February 28, 1856.
24. Ibid., 2.
25. Ryan, *Cradle of the Middle Class*; Barbara Epstein, *The Politics of Domesticity: Women, Evangelism, and Temperance in Nineteenth-Century America* (Middletown, Conn.: Wesleyan University Press, 1981); Cott, *Bonds of Womanhood*.
26. Margaret Fuller, *Woman in the Nineteenth Century* (New York: W. W. Norton, Norton Library ed., 1971); Ellen Dubois, commentator and ed., *Elizabeth Cady Stanton/Susan B. Anthony: Correspondence, Writings, Speeches* (New York: Schocken Press, 1981).
27. Sims, *Story of My Life*, 292.
28. See Morantz-Sanchez, *Sympathy and Science*, 47–49; Walsh, *Doctors Wanted*; Virginia Drachman, "Female Solidarity and Professional Success: The Dilemma of Women Doctors in Late Nineteenth-Century America," *Journal of Social History* 15 (Winter 1982): 607–619; and Gloria Moldow, *Women Doctors in Gilded Age Washington: Race, Gender and Professionalization* (Champaign-Urbana: University of Illinois Press, 1987).
29. See Nancy Hewitt, *Women's Activism and Social Change: Rochester, New York, 1822–1872* (Ithaca, N.Y.: Cornell University Press, 1984), for a framework with which to analyze women and reform. See Virginia Drachman, *Hospital with a Heart: Women Doctors and the Paradox of Separatism at the New England Hospital (1862–1969)* (Ithaca, N.Y.: Cornell University Press, 1983), for a different kind of hospital run by women.
30. E. H. Clarke, *Sex in Education: A Fair Chance for Girls* (Boston: James R. Osgood and Co., 1873; New York: Arno Press Reprint, 1972).
31. Mary Putnam Jacobi's *The Question of Rest for Women during Menstruation* (New York, 1877) was her answer to Clarke. It won the Boylston Prize from Harvard. See Morantz-Sanchez, *Sympathy and Science*, 55.
32. Woman's Hospital of the State of New York, *Reports, 1856–1869*.
33. See Sims, *Story of My Life*, 457.
34. See Eric Homberger, *Scenes from the Life of a City: Corruption and Conscience in Old New York* (New Haven, Conn.: Yale University Press, 1994); Ryan, *Women in Public*.
35. Ryan, *Women in Public*.
36. Homberger, *Scenes*; Eric Homberger, *The Historical Atlas of New York City: A Visual Celebration of Nearly 400 Years of New York City's History* (New York: Henry Holt, 1994), 84.
37. Rothman, *The Discovery of the Asylum*.

38. David Rosner, Introduction, in Rosner, ed., *Hives of Sickness: Public Health and Epidemics in New York City* (New Brunswick, N.J.: Rutgers University Press, 1995), 3.
39. Ryan, *Women in Public*, 39, and Homberger, *Atlas*.
40. Ryan, *Women in Public*, 68.
41. Harry F. Dowling, *City Hospitals: The Undercare of the Underprivileged* (Cambridge, Mass.: Harvard University Press, 1982).
42. Michael B. Katz, *In the Shadow of the Poorhouse: A Social History of Welfare in America* (New York: Basic Books, 1986).
43. Casebooks of the Woman's Hospital of the State of New York; Annual Reports of the Woman's Hospital.
44. Daniel M. Fox, *Power and Illness: The Failure and Future of American Health Policy* (Berkeley: University of California Press, 1993); Rosenberg, *Care*; Morris Vogel, *The Invention of the Modern Hospital: Boston, 1870–1930* (Chicago: University of Chicago Press, 1980); David Rosner, *A Once Charitable Enterprise* (New York: Cambridge University Press, 1982).
45. Other hospitals carried a similar structure which allowed lay personnel to participate in the admission of certain patients. See Rosenberg, *Care*, and Mottus, *New York Nightingales*.
46. See Rosner, *A Once Charitable*; Vogel, *Invention*; Starr, *Transformation*; Drachman, *Hospital*; Rosenberg, *Care*; see also Regina Morantz and Sue Zschoche, "A Comparative Study of Nineteenth-Century Medical Therapeutics," *Journal of American History* 67 (December 1980): 568–588.
47. Barbara G. Rosenkrantz, "The Search for Professional Order in 19th-Century American Medicine," *Proceedings of the 14th International Congress of the History of Science* (Tokyo Science Council of Japan, 1975), no. 4, 113–124. Leavitt, Warner, and Rosenberg have all contributed significant revisions to our understanding of the history of medicine and hospitals. See Warner, *Therapeutic Perspective*; Leavitt, *Brought to Bed*; Rosenberg, "The Therapeutic Revolution," and *Care*.
48. Kenneth A. Scherzer, *The Unbounded Community: Neighborhood Life and Social Structure in New York City, 1830–1875* (Durham, N.C.: Duke University Press, 1992).
49. Scherzer, *Unbounded*; Steven Thernstrom, *Poverty and Progress in the American City* (Cambridge, Mass.: Harvard University Press, 1964), and *The Other Bostonians: Poverty and Progress in the American City* (Cambridge, Mass.: Harvard University Press, 1973). See also Stephen Thernstrom and Richard Sennett, eds., *Nineteenth Century Cities: Essays in the New Urban History* (New Haven: Yale University Press, 1969), and Clyde and Sally Griffen, *Natives and Newcomers: The Ordering of Opportunity in Mid-Nineteenth-Century Poughkeepsie* (Cambridge, Mass.: Harvard University Press, 1978).
50. Citizens' Association of New York, *Sanitary Condition of the City: Report of the Council of Hygiene and Public Health of the Citizens' Association of New York* (New York: D. Appleton, 1865; repr., New York: Arno Press, 1970), part 2, VI, no. 15, on the twelfth sanitation inspection district.
51. Scherzer, *Unbounded*; Citizens' Association, *Sanitary Condition*.

52. Thomas Addis Emmet, "Reminiscences of the Founders of the Woman's Hospital Association" (New York: Reprint of the *American Gynecological and Obstetrical Journal*, April 1899, 1).
53. Citizens' Association, *Sanitary Condition*, 277.
54. Robert J. Carlisle, ed., *An Account of Bellevue Hospital with a Catalogue of the Medical and Surgical Staff from 1736 to 1894* (New York: Bellevue Hospital, 1893); repr., New York: Bellevue Hospital, 1986), 107.
55. Thomas A. Emmet, "A Memoir of James Marion Sims," *New York Medical Journal*, January 5, 1884, 2.
56. Fordyce Barker in the *Annual Report* of the Woman's Hospital of the State of New York (New York: Bradstreet, 1868), 22.
57. Theresa Sims also bore nine children. There is no description of her health or any consequences of repeated pregnancies.
58. Caroline Thompson (1857) quoted in the *Annual Reports, 1856–1869: Woman's Hospital of the State of New York* (private copy of Margaret Sage).
59. Quote from Mrs. E. C. Benedict, Manager, Constitution and *Fourth Annual Report of the Woman's Hospital Association*, 23.
60. Dr. John Francis, "Address," *First Anniversary of the Woman's Hospital* (New York: Miller and Holman, 1856), 9.
61. Ibid., 13.
62. Letter from Laura Bellows, Chairman of the Committee from the Board of Supervisors to Revise the Bylaws of the Constitution, to James Beekman and the Board of Governors, March 24, 1868. There is a possibility that Laura Bellows was either the daughter or daughter-in-law of Henry Bellows, minister and co-leader of the Sanitary Commission. Clinton Scott, *These Live Tomorrow: Twenty Unitarian Universalist Biographies* (Boston: Beacon Press, 1964).
63. Ibid.
64. *First Anniversary*, 30.
65. Constitution and *Third Annual Report of the Woman's Hospital Association* (New York: Daniel Fonshaw, 1857), 15–16.
66. William Leach, *True Love and Perfect Union: The Feminist Reform of Sex and Society* (New York: Basic Books, 1980); Regina Markell Morantz, "Nineteenth-Century Health Reform and Women: A Program of Self-Help," in *Medicine without Doctors*, 73–94; and Morantz, "Making Women Modern: Middle-Class Women and Health Reform in Nineteenth-Century America," *Journal of Social History* 10 (1977): 490–507; Donegan, *Hydropathic Highway*; Cayleff, *Wash and Be Healed*; Kathyrn Kish Sklar, *Catherine Beecher: Study in American Domesticity* (New York: W. W. Norton and Co., 1976).
67. Barbara Berg, *The Remembered Gate: Origins of American Feminism: The Woman and the City, 1800–1860* (New York: Oxford University Press, 1978).
68. Iver Bernstein, *The New York City Draft Riots: Their Significance for American Society and Politics in the Age of the Civil War* (New York: Oxford University, 1990). Minturn was a member of the Union League and its first head.
69. Emmet, "Reminiscences of the Founders," 6.
70. Thomas Emmet, *Incidents of My Life—Profession-Literary-Social with Services in the Cause of Ireland* (New York: Knickerbocker Press, 1911), 197.

71. Patricia Hill, *The World Their Household: The American Woman's Foreign Mission Movement and Cultural Transformation, 1870–1920* (Ann Arbor: University of Michigan Press, 1985), 45.
72. Edward James, Janet Wilson James, and Paul Boyer, eds., *Notable American Women, 1607–1950: A Biographical Dictionary* (Cambridge, Mass.: Belknap Press, 1971), 500–501; Berg, *Remembered Gate*; Estelle Freedman, *Their Sisters' Keepers: Women's Prison Reform in America, 1830–1930* (Ann Arbor: University of Michigan Press, 1981).
73. See Thomas Bender, *Toward an Urban Vision: Ideas and Institutions in Nineteenth-Century America* (Lexington: University of Kentucky Press, 1975); Paul S. Boyer, *Urban Masses and Moral Order in America, 1820–1920* (Cambridge, Mass.: Harvard University Press, 1978); Christine Stansell, *City of Women: Sex and Class in New York, 1789–1860* (New York: Alfred A. Knopf, 1986).
74. Berg, *Remembered Gate*, 36. See also Virginia Quiroga, "Poor Mothers and Babies: A Social History of Childbirth and Child Care Institutions in Nineteenth-Century New York City," Ph.D. diss., SUNY-Stony Brook, 1985; Janet Golden, *A Social History of Wet Nursing in America: From Breast to Bottle* (Cambridge, U.K.: Cambridge University Press, 1996).
75. Golden, *Wet Nursing*, and Quiroga, "Poor Mothers."
76. Records of the women managers, Lying-In Asylum; Golden, *Wet Nursing*.
77. Quiroga, "Poor Mothers"; records of the Lying-In Asylum, Cornell Medical School Archives, New York Hospital.
78. Hill, *World*.
79. J. Marion Sims, "Anniversary Address," Woman's Hospital (New York: Baker and Godwin, 1868), 4.
80. *National Cyclopedia of American Biography* (New York: James T. White and Co., 1904), 12, 58; James W. Beekman, "Centenary Address," Society of the New York Hospital (New York: Society of the New York Hospital, 1871), and W. Gill Wylie, *Hospitals: Their Organization, and Construction* (New York: D. Appleton, 1877), on ventilation and the construction of hospitals. Wylie was Sims's son-in-law and a resident physician of the Woman's Hospital in 1872.
81. Hill, *World*.
82. Demas Malone, ed., *Dictionary of American Biography* 16 (New York: Charles Scribner's Sons, 1935), 292–293.
83. Lori Ginzburg, *Women and the Work of Benevolence: Morality, Politics, and Class in the Nineteenth-Century United States* (New Haven: Yale University Press), 142. Mottus, *New York Nightingales*, 30.
84. Homberger, *Scenes*, 162.
85. Matthew 25: 40.
86. Hewitt, *Women's Activism*.
87. See Bernstein, *Draft Riots*.
88. James H. Smylie, "The Reformed Tradition," in Ronald L. Numbers and Darrel W. Amundsen, eds., *Caring and Curing: Health and Medicine in the Western Religious Traditions* (New York: Macmillan, 1986), 204–239.
89. Steven Mintz, *Moralizers and Modernizers: America's Pre-Civil War Reformers* (Baltimore: Johns Hopkins University Press, 1995).

90. Sims, *Silver Sutures*, 52.
91. Ibid., 54.
92. Ibid., 52.
93. Emmet, "Reminiscences," 1.
94. Sims, *Story of My Life*, 268.
95. J. Marion Sims, letter to Theresa Sims, January 25, 1855.
96. Sims, *Silver Sutures*, 47.
97. Ernest Trice Thompson, *Presbyterians in the South*, vol. 1 (Richmond, Va.: John Knox Press, 1963), provides a history for the years 1607–1861; John B. Boles, ed., *Masters and Slaves in the House of the Lord: Race and Religion in the American South, 1740–1870* (Lexington: University of Kentucky, 1988), contains several useful interpretive essays.
98. J. Marion Sims, letter to Theresa Sims, December 31, 1854.
99. See letters in the appendix of Sims's *Story of My Life* from J. Marion to Theresa concerning the names of slaves and correspondence about their desire not to be sold. Some of them had been part of Sims's medical experiments.
100. J. Marion Sims, letter to John Sims, August 8, 1855.
101. Ibid.
102. J. Marion Sims, letter to Theresa Sims, December 29, 1854.
103. Sims, *Story of My Life*, 83. See also *Silver Sutures*, 61.
104. Steven Stowe, "Religion, Science and the Culture of Medical Practice in the American South, 1800–1870," Gilbert, Gilman, Scott and Scott, eds., *The Mythmaking Frame of Mind*.
105. Article 16, Constitution of the Woman's Hospital, *First Anniversary*, 30.
106. Deborah Kuhn McGregor, "Marie Elizabeth Zakrzewska (1829–1902)," in Lois Magner, ed., *Doctors, Nurses, and Medical Practitioners: A Bio-Bibliographical Sourcebook* (Westport, Conn.: Greenwood Press, 1997), 320–325.
107. Marie Zakrzewska, *A Woman's Quest: The Life of Marie E. Zakrzewska, M.D.*, ed. Agnes Vietor (rept., New York: Arno Press, 1972), 225.
108. Drachman, *Hospital with a Heart*.
109. Jacobi, "Women in Medicine," 154–155.
110. Linda Goldstein, "Emily Blackwell," in Lois Magner, ed., *Doctors, Nurses, and Medical Practitioners: A Bio-Bibliographical Source Book* (Westport, Conn.: Greenwood, 1997), 19.
111. *Second Anniversary Report of the Woman's Hospital Association* (New York: Daniel Fonshaw, 1857), 7.
112. Thomas Addis Emmet, *Memoirs of Thomas Addis and Robert Emmet*, vol. 1 (New York: Emmet Press, 1915), 474–475; Kelly, *Cyclopedia of American Medical Biography*, 285.
113. Kerby A. Miller, *Emigrants and Exiles: Ireland and the Irish Exodus to North America* (New York: Oxford University Press, 1985); Walter J. Walsh, "Religion, Ethnicity, and History: Clues to the Cultural Construction of Law," in *The New York Irish*, 48–69.
114. Walsh, "Religion, Ethnicity and History: Clues to the Cultural Construction of the Law," in *The New York Irish*, 64.
115. Kirby, *Emigrants*, 186.

116. See Walsh, "Religion and Ethnicity," and Emmet, *Memoirs*, vol. 1.
117. Emmet, *Incidents*; *Memoirs*, vol. 1.
118. The awkwardness of repeated names across generations is representative of a different time when names were used to keep the dead alive, so to speak, and to renew the patriarchy of a family structure. The Emmet name itself was also variously spelled—again reflecting an earlier time—as Emmet as well as Emmett. The confusion of names and prominence of individuals involved, particularly in New York City, confounds the problems of researching individual activities, particularly when women are factored in their genealogical heritage masked by patronyms.
119. In addition to family histories and an essay on the Battle of Harlem Heights, Emmet published *Ireland under English Rule* (New York: G. P. Putnam's Sons, 1907) and "Irish Emigration during the Seventeenth and Eighteenth Centuries" (New York, 1899) reprinted from the *Journal of the American Irish Historical Society*, vol. 11.
120. Hasia Diner, *Erin's Daughters in America: Irish Immigrant Women in the Nineteenth Century* (Baltimore: Johns Hopkins University Press, 1983), 31. Emmet, "Reminiscences," 18.
121. See Emmet, *Incidents*, 140–146, on the voyage, and *Ireland under England*, 47–48, for information on the immigration experience.
122. F. E. Hyde, "The Hospitals of the City of New York," *The Sanitarian* 1 (November 1873): 344. See also Emmet, "Reminiscences."
123. Homberger, *Scenes*.
124. See Alan M. Kraut, "Illness and Medical Care among Irish Immigrants in Antebellum New York City," in Ronald Bayor and Timothy Meagher, eds., *The New York Irish* (Baltimore: Johns Hopkins University Press, 1996), 153–168; Noel Ignatiev, *How the Irish Became White* (New York: Routledge, 1995).
125. See Emmet, *Incidents*.
126. Kerber, "Separate Spheres, Female Worlds," 183.

CHAPTER 4   *Patients and Practice*

1. Emmet in "Reminiscences," 19, suggests he has operated on more than four hundred vesico-vaginal fistula patients by 1878.
2. Diner, "The Great Migration," 91. See also Stansell, *City of Women*.
3. See Diner, "Great Migration," 90.
4. Cormac Ó Gráda, *The Great Irish Famine* (Cambridge, U.K.: Cambridge University Press, 1989), 26. See also Thomas Malthus, *Occasional Papers of T. R. Malthus*, ed. Bernard Semmel (New York: Burt Franklin, 1973), for his earlier predictions on Ireland's future—predictions that did not include a great famine.
5. See Cecil Woodham-Smith, *The Great Hunger: Ireland 1845–1849* (New York: Old Town Books, 1962).
6. See Ó Gráda, *Famine*, 41, and Diner, "Great Migration." As is common with massive deaths, there is dispute among scholars about the actual numbers.
7. Scherzer, *Unbounded Community*; Diner, *Erin's Daughters*; Carol Groneman,

"Working-Class Immigrant Women in Mid-Nineteenth-Century New York: The Irish Woman's Experience," *Journal of Urban History* 4 (May 1978): 255–273.

8. Golden, *Wet Nursing*; Scherzer, *Unbounded Community*; Stansell, *City of Women*; Groneman, "Working-Class Immigrant."

9. Mary Smith, 1854, Casebook, Bolling Medical Library, St. Lukes-Roosevelt Hospital Center in New York City.

10. Sue Fisher, *In the Patient's Best Interest: Women and the Politics of Medical Decisions* (New Brunswick, N.J.: Rutgers University Press, 1986).

11. Emmet, "Reminiscences," 4.

12. Ibid., 5.

13. Ibid.

14. Wm. Thompson Lusk, *The Science and Art of Midwifery* (New York: D. Appleton, 1893), 466.

15. Ó Gráda, *Famine*.

16. See Harold Speert, *Obstetric and Gynecologic Milestones: Essays in Eponymy* (New York: Macmillan, 1958), 145. See Jean-Louis Baudelocque, *L'Art des Accouchements* (Paris: Mequignon, 1781), as cited in Speert, *Milestones*.

17. Dixon Burns and Lisa Calache, "An Evaluation of Some Early Obstetrical Instruments," *Caduceus* 3 (Spring 1987): 32–39.

18. Speert, *Milestones*, 152–158.

19. See Franz Carl Naegele, *The Obliquely Contracted Pelvis* (Mainz, Germany: Victor von Zabern; New York: Centennial Edition, 1993), and Speert, *Milestones*, 174–178.

20. Charles D. Meigs, *The Philadelphia Practice of Midwifery* (James Kan Jun and Bros., 1838).

21. The character of the Schoolteacher in Toni Morrison's novel *Beloved* demonstrates the cultural bias and prejudice implicit in the use of measurements. See *Beloved* (New York: New American Library, 1987), 191.

22. See Moscucci, *The Science of Woman*, 36–38. See also Schiebinger, *Nature's Body*, 156–158.

23. Naegele, *The Obliquely Contracted Pelvis*, 55.

24. Kilkelomo Bello, "Vesicovaginal Fistula (VVF): Only to a Woman Accursed," *Health Care Provider* (cited 1/30/97) http://www.idrc.ca/books/focus/773/bello.html; and "Women Find God's Love at Fistula Hospital," *Christian Internet Sources* (cited 1/30/97) at http://www.xir.com: 80/SIM/013sim.shtml; "Ethiopia's Fistula Hospital Offers Hope to Desperate Women," *New York Times*, November 6, 1984. Thanks to Bert Hansen for showing me this article. J. Chassar Moir, a British surgeon and the foremost contemporary authority on vesico-vaginal fistula, gained his experience in India. See J. C. Moir, *The Vesico-Vaginal Fistula*; "Personal Experiences in the Treatment of Vesico-Vaginal Fistula," and "J. Marion Sims and the Vesico-Vaginal Fistula: Then and Now," *British Medical Journal* 2 (1940). See J. M. Kerr, R. W. Johnstone, and Miles H. Phillips, eds., *Historical Review of British Obstetrics and Gynecology, 1800–1950* (Edinburgh: E. and S. Livingstone, 1954). See Andrew Appleby, "Disease, Diet, and History," *Journal of Interdisciplinary History* 8 (Spring 1978): 725–735, for an overview of the debates concerning nutrition, disease, and the history of medicine.

See also Kiple and King, *Another Dimension*, and Edward Shorter, *A History of Women's Bodies* (New York: Basic Books, 1982).

25. Churchill, *Midwifery*, 468.
26. Thomas Addis Emmet, *Vesico-Vaginal Fistula from Parturition and Other Causes with Cases of Recto-Vaginal Fistula* (New York: Wm. Wood and Co., 1868), in the introduction.
27. Emmet, "Reminiscences," 19.
28. Schuppert, *Treatise*; Bozeman, "The Clamp Suture."
29. See Fleetwood Churchill, *On the Theory and Practice of Midwifery* (Philadelphia: Lea and Blanchard, 1848), 468.
30. New York State Senate Document 52.
31. See Adrian Wilson, *The Making of Man-Midwifery: Childbirth in England, 1660–1770* (London: UCL Press, 1995). See Davis-Floyd, ed., *Authoritative Knowledge*.
32. Emmet, "Reminiscences," 18–19.
33. Quiroga, "Poor Mothers and Babies," 60–61.
34. Alan M. Kraut, "Illness and Medical Care among Irish Immigrants in Antebellum New York," in *New York Irish*, 163.
35. Judith Walzer Leavitt and Whitney Walton, "'Down to Death's Door': Women's Perceptions of Childbirth in America," in Leavitt, ed., *Women and Health in America*, 155–165.
36. Ulrich, *A Midwife's Tale*, 192.
37. See Theriot, *Mothers and Daughters*, 51.
38. See, for instance, David Hayes Agnew, M.D., *Lacerations of the Female Perineum and Vesico-Vaginal Fistula: Their History and Treatment* (Philadelphia: Lindsay and Blakiston, 1873).
39. Thomas A. Emmet, *Principles and Practice of Gynecology* (Philadelphia: Henry C. Lea, 1869), 663.
40. Churchill, *On the Theory and Practice*; Francis Ramsbotham, *The Principles and Practice of Obstetric Medicine and Surgery, in Reference to the Process of Parturition*, 6th ed. (Philadelphia: Blanchard and Lea, 1851); William DeWees, *A Compendious System of Midwifery, Chiefly Designed to Facilitate the Inquiries of Those Who May Be Pursuing This Branch of Study*, 5th ed. (Philadelphia: Carey and Lea, 1832).
41. Emmet, *Principles and Practice*, 669; idem, "The Necessity for Early Delivery, as Demonstrated by the Analysis of One Hundred and Sixty-One Cases of Vesico-Vaginal Fistula," *Transactions of the American Gynecological Society* 3 (1878): 114–134.
42. Churchill, *Theory and Practice*.
43. Dr. Victoria Nichols-Johnson, a gynecologist and obstetrician at Memorial Medical Center in Springfield, Illinois, described the possible benefits of exercise during labor at a luncheon at the University of Illinois at Springfield, fall, 1986.
44. See Ulrich, *Midwife's Tale*.
45. Janet Bogdan, "The Transformation of American Birth," Ph.D. diss., Syracuse University, 1986.
46. Churchill, *Theory and Practice*, 468; Ramsbotham, *Principles and Practice*,

183–186; J. Ashhurst, *Principles and Practice of Surgery,* 6th ed. (Philadelphia: Lea Bros., 1893), and Agnew, *Lacerations,* all list direct injury and use of instruments as possibly culpable for fistulas.

47. D. Hayes Agnew, *Principles and Practice of Surgery* 2 (Philadelphia: J. B. Lippincott Co., 1881), 742.

48. J. Marion Sims, letter to Fordyce Barker, *Transactions of the Medical Society of New York* (1858), 130.

49. Emmet, *Principles and Practice,* 669.

50. Emmet, *Incidents,* 232.

51. Virginia Drachman, "The Loomis Trial: Social Mores and Obstetrics in the Mid-Nineteenth Century," in *Healthcare in America,* ed. Reverby and Rosner, 166–174.

52. Emmet, "The Necessity for Early Delivery." In a footnote to his section on vesico-vaginal fistula, Edward Shorter in *Women's Bodies* inaccurately attributes a statement concerning the absolute contribution of forceps to the end of vesico-vaginal fistula to Emmet, when in fact the statement was made by a Dr. Smith. See Emmet, "The Necessity for Early Delivery," 124.

53. Mary Jordan Finley, "A Thesis on Vesico-Vaginal Fistula," dissertation for the Doctorate of Medicine, Women's Medical College of Pennsylvania, Philadelphia, 1880–1881), 12.

54. Ibid.

55. See Wilson, *Man-Midwifery.*

56. Carolyn Merchant, *Ecological Revolutions: Nature, Gender, and Science in New England* (Chapel Hill: University of North Carolina Press, 1989).

57. Schiebinger, *Nature's Body.*

58. See Arisika Rasak, "Toward a Womanist Analysis of Birth," in Irene Diamond and Gloria Feman Orenstein, eds., *Reweaving the World: The Emergence of Ecofeminism* (San Francisco: Sierra Club Books, 1990), 165–172. Entry, October 24, 1799, in the *The Diary of Elizabeth Drinker: The Life Cycle of an Eighteenth-Century Woman,* edited and abridged by Elaine Forman Crane (Boston: Northeastern University Press, 1994), 216.

59. Michel Odent, *Birth Reborn* (New York: Pantheon Books, 1984). See Davis-Floyd, *Birth.*

60. Thomas Addis Emmet, "The Necessity for Early Delivery, as Demonstrated by the Analysis of One Hundred and Sixty-One Cases of Vesico-Vaginal Fistula," *Transactions of the American Gynecological Society* 3 (1878): 118.

61. See Bert Hansen's "Medical Education in New York City in 1866–1867: A Student's Notebook of Professor Budd's Lectures on Obstetrics at New York University," *New York State Journal of Medicine* 85, part 1 (August 1985): 488–498, for valuable information regarding the use of ergot and other interventionist techniques used by medical professionals as well as midwives. Edward Shorter, *Health of Women,* believes only midwives employed violent doses of ergot. There is ample evidence that physicians also experimented with the drug. See Janet Bogdan, "Aggressive Intervention and Mortality," in Pamela Eakins, ed., *The American Way of Birth* (Philadelphia: Temple University Press, 1986), 60–103.

62. For more on the use of obstetrical instruments, see Longo, "Obstetrics and

Gynecology"; Virginia Drachman, "Gynecological Instruments and Surgical De-
cisions at a Hospital in the Late Nineteenth-Century America," *Journal of Ameri-
can Culture* 3 (1980): 660–672. See Judith W. Leavitt, "'Science' Enters the
Birthing Room: Obstetrics since the Eighteenth Century," *Journal of American
History* 70 (September 1983): 281–304. See also Audrey B. Davis, *Medicine
and Its Technology: An Introduction to the History of Medical Instrumentation*
(Westport, Conn.: Greenwood, 1981), and Stanley J. Reiser, *Medicine and the
Reign of Technology* (Cambridge, U.K.: Cambridge University Press, 1978).

63. Stansell, *City of Women*, 199. See Michael R. Haines, "Mortality in Nineteenth-
    Century America: Estimates from New York and Pennsylvania Census Data,
    1865 and 1900," *Demography* 14 (August 1977): 311–331.
64. For mortality statistics in New York City for the first half of the nineteenth cen-
    tury, see appendixes in John Duffy, *A History of Public Health in New York City,
    1625–1866* (New York: Russell Sage Foundation, 1968).
65. Emmet, *Vesico-Vaginal Fistula.*

CHAPTER 5   *A School for Gynecologists*

1. See Margaret Washington Creel, *"A Peculiar People": Slave Religion and
   Community-Culture among the Gullahs* (New York: New York University Press,
   1988); Charles Joyner, *Down by the Riverside: A South Carolina Slave Community* (Champaign-Urbana: University of Illinois Press, 1984); Willie Lee Rose,
   Rehearsal for Reconstruction: The Port Royal Experiment (Indianapolis: Bobbs-
   Merrill, 1964).
2. Joseph I. Waring, *A History of Medicine in South Carolina, 1825–1900*, vol. 2
   (South Carolina Medical Association, 1967).
3. Marr, *Pioneer*,124–127.
4. Bonner, *Becoming.*
5. F. E. Hyde, "Hospitals of the City," 339.
6. Smith, "The Emergence of Organized Clinical Instruction," 266.
7. Dale Smith, "The Emergence of Organized Clinical Instruction," 156–158. See
   also Carlisle, *Bellevue Hospital.*
8. Bogdan, "Transformation," 385.
9. Notebook of Thomas Savage, "Friday Afternoon Clinic (1872–1873)," a
   student's notes from the lectures of T. Gaillard Thomas, held in Special Collections of the August C. Long Health Sciences Library, Columbia University Libraries, New York City.
10. See Rosenberg, "Rise of the Dispensary," and "New York City a Century Ago."
11. See Rosenberg, "New York City a Century Ago," and Mottus, *New York Night-
    ingales.*
12. T. Gaillard Thomas, *A Practical Treatise on the Diseases of Women*, 2d ed.,
    (Philadelphia: Henry C. Lea, 1869).
13. Deborah Jean Warner, "The Campaign for Medical Microscopy in Antebellum
    America," *Bulletin of the History of Medicine* 69 (1995): 375.
14. Marr, *Pioneer*, 109.
15. Rosenberg, "New York City: A Century," 238.

16. Kelly, *Cyclopedia of American Medical Biography*.

17. Augustus Gardner, "Amputation of the Cervix Uteri," *Bulletin of the New York Academy of Medicine* 1 (1862): 440–461.

18. Marr, *Pioneer* 41

19. Ibid., 40.

20. John W. Francis, quoted by the Board of Managers in the *Constitution and Fourth Annual Report of the Woman's Hospital Association* (New York: Daniel Fonshaw, 1859), 19.

21. Thomas A. Emmet, quoted in the *Twelfth Annual Report of the Woman's Hospital Association* (New York: Bradstreet Press, 1867), 31–32.

22. Emmet, *Incidents*, 204.

23. T. Gaillard Thomas, quoted in *Sixteenth Annual Report of the Board of Governors and Board of Lady Supervisors of the Woman's Hospital of the State of New York* (New York: Russells' Am. Steam Printing, 1871), 34.

24. T. Gaillard Thomas, quoted in the *Seventeenth Annual Report of the Board of Governors and Board of Lady Supervisors of the Woman's Hospital of the State of New York* (New York: Evening Post Steam Presses, 1872), 334.

25. E. R. Peaslee, quoted in ibid., 37.

26. E. R. Peaslee, "On the Treatment of Uterine Disease," *Bulletin of the New York Academy of Medicine* 1 (1862): 79–90.

27. Margaret Marsh and Wanda Ronner, *The Empty Cradle: Infertility in America from Colonial Times to the Present* (Baltimore: Johns Hopkins University Press, 1996); Brodie, *Abortion and Contraception*; Ricci, *One Hundred Years*, 24. See, for instance, Augustus Gardner, *Conjugal Sins against the Laws of Life and Health and Their Effects upon the Father, Mother and Child* (New York: J. S. Redfield, 1870).

28. Peaslee, "On the Treatment of Uterine Diseases."

29. Augustus Gardner, "Amputation of the Cervix Uteri," *Bulletin of the New York Academy of Medicine* 1 (1862): 441.

30. Emmet, *Principles and Practice*, 224. See also J. Marion Sims, "Amputation of the Cervix Uteri," *Transactions of the New York State Medical Society* (1861): 367–371. See also Sims's comments following Gardner's article, "Amputation of the Cervix Uteri," in *Bulletin of the New York Academy of Medicine* 1 (1862): 440–461.

31. Poovey, *Uneven Developments*, 36–37. See also Edward Shorter on reflex theory, *From Paralysis to Fatigue: A History of Psychosomatic Illness in the Modern Era* (New York: Free Press, 1992).

32. Laqueur, *Making Sex*, 187.

33. Augustus Gardner, "Case of Supposed Consumption—Vicarious Menstruation Dependent upon Stricture of Cervix Uteri Cured by Incision of the Cervix," *Bulletin of the New York Academy of Medicine* 1 (1862): 134–137.

34. See Vern Bullough and Martha Voght, "Women, Menstruation, and Nineteenth-Century Medicine," *Bulletin of the History of Medicine* 47 (1973): 66–82.

35. W. Gill Wylie, "Menstruation and Its Disorders" in Matthew Mann, ed., *A System of Gynecology by American Authors*, vol. 1 (Philadelphia: Lea Bros., 1887), 413.

36. James Y. Simpson, *Obstetric Memoirs and Contributions*, ed., W. O. Priestley and H. R. Storer (Philadelphia: J. B. Lippincott, 1855), 34.

37. Donegan, *Hydropathic Highway*.
38. See particularly Ulrich, *Midwife's Tale*, for an outstanding appendix on the herbs of midwives.
39. Leslie Reagan, *When Abortion Was a Crime: Women, Medicine and Law in the United States, 1867–1973* (Berkeley: University of California Press, 1997), 14.
40. See Barbara Duden, *Disembodying Women: Perspectives on Pregnancy and the Unborn*, trans. Lee Hoinacki (Cambridge, Mass.: Harvard University Press, 1993).
41. On the history of abortion, see Reagan, *When Abortion Was a Crime*; Kristin Luker, *Abortion and the Politics of Motherhood* (Berkeley: University of California Press, 1984); James Mohr, *Abortion in America: The Origins and Evolution of National Policy, 1800–1900* (New York: Oxford University Press, 1978); Smith-Rosenberg, *Disorderly Conduct*; Rosalind Pollack Petchesky, *Abortion and Woman's Choice: The State, Sexuality, and Reproductive Freedom* (Boston: Northeastern University Press, 1984).
42. Charles West, *Lectures on the Diseases of Women* (Philadelphia: Blanchard and Lea, 1857).
43. See A.J.C. Skene, *Treatise on the Diseases of Women* (New York: D. Appleton, 1889), and Paul F. Mundé, *Minor Surgical Gynecology and the Lesser Technicalities of Gynecological Practice* (New York: William Wood and Co., 1880).
44. For example, see John Eberle, *A Treatise on the Practice of Medicine*, vol. 2, 2d ed. (Philadelphia: John Grigg, 1831), 539.
45. Charles D. Meigs, "On Acute and Chronic Diseases of the Neck of the Uterus," *Transactions of the American Medical Association* 6 (1853): 365–418; Gunning S. Bedford, *Clinical Lectures on the Diseases of Women and Children* (New York: William Wood and Co., 1872).
46. Emmet, "A Memoir of James Marion Sims," 3.
47. Thomas A. Emmet, "The Etiology of Uterine Flexures, with the Proper Mode of Treatment Indicated," *Transactions of the American Gynecological Society* 1 (1876): 48–90; E. R. Peaslee, "Incision and Discission," *Transactions of the New York Academy of Medicine* (1876): 408–437; J. Marion Sims, "On the Surgical Treatment of Stenosis of the Cervix Uteri," *Transactions of the American Gynecological Society* 3 (1878): 54–100.
48. See J. Y. Simpson, *Memoirs*; see also J. Y. Simpson, *Clinical Lectures on Diseases of Women* (Philadelphia: Blanchard and Lea, 1863). See the comments of Fordyce Barker following Sims's article, "Stenosis of the Cervix," and Peaslee, "Incision and Discission."
49. Emmet, *Incidents*.
50. J. Marion Sims, letter to the editor, *Lancet*, July 8, 1865, 42. All quotes in this period used in the text of articles, not letters, from *Lancet* can also be found in J. Marion Sims, *Clinical Notes on Uterine Surgery with Special Reference to the Management of the Sterile Condition* (New York: William Wood and Co., 1866). Sims wrote the book originally for *Lancet* of London. He became embroiled in a dispute with others during the publication there. He rearranged and edited the material for publication as a book.
51. Meigs, "On Acute and Chronic Diseases."

52. Gardner, "Amputation."

53. Meigs, "On Acute and Chronic Diseases," 25.

54. Sims, *Clinical Notes*, 55–57.

55. Ibid., 142.

56. Schiebinger, *The Mind Has No Sex*; Laqueur, *Making Sex*.

57. Marr, *Pioneer*, 129.

58. Sims, *Clinical Notes*, 141.

59. Ibid., 142.

60. J. Marion Sims, "Painful Menstruation," *Lancet*, April 1, 1865, 339.

61. Case Records, 1858, Woman's Hospital, Archives of Bolling Medical Library.

62. On the Isaac Baker Brown controversy, see Pat Jalland and John Hooper, eds., *Women from Birth to Death: The Female Life Cycle in Britain, 1830–1914* (Atlantic Highlands, N.J.: Humanities Press, 1986), 350–365. Primary sources include Isaac Baker Brown's letter to the editor, *Lancet*, December 1866, 325–326. Also, "Proposition of the Council for the Removal of Mr. I. B. Brown," *British Medical Journal*, April 6, 1867, 395–410.

63. T. Gaillard Thomas, *Abortion and Its Treatment, from the Standpoint of Practical Experience* (New York: D. Appleton, 1893). See Luker, *Abortion*; Mohr, *Abortion in America*; Cassedy, *Medicine and American Growth*.

64. Simpson, *Memoirs*, 265.

65. Quoted from the records of a patient hospitalized from January 6 through May 8, 1869. The author has not used the names of any patients in research or writing (except in two or three cases where doctors had already publicized the treatment).

66. See Bullough and Voght, "Women, Menstruation, and Nineteenth-Century Medicine."

67. See discussion following Barker's reading of Sims's paper, "Stenosis of the Cervix."

68. Meigs, "On Acute and Chronic Diseases."

69. See Emmet, "Etiology," in *Transactions of the American Gynecological Society* 1 (1876); Peaslee, "Incision and Discission"; Sims, "Stenosis of the Cervix Uteri."

70. See Marsh and Ronner, *Empty Cradle*.

71. *Twenty-Second Annual Report of the Woman's Hospital in the State of New York Including a Tabular Statement of all the Cases Treated in the Hospital from Its Foundation* (New York: Evening Post Steam Presses, 1877).

72. Emmet, "Etiology." Emmet, "The Necessity for Early Delivery, as Demonstrated by the Analysis of One Hundred and Sixty-One Cases of Vesico-Vaginal Fistula," *Transactions of the American Gynecological Society* 3 (1878): 114–134. Emmet also uses statistics extensively in his books, *Vesico-Vaginal Fistula* and *Principles and Practice*.

73. J. Marion Sims, "Painful Menstruation," *Lancet*, March 4, 1865, 225.

74. Thomas A. Emmet, "On the Treatment of Dysmenorrhoea and Sterility, Resulting from Anteflexion of the Uterus," *New York Medical Journal* 1 (June 1865): 209.

75. Simpson, *Memoirs*, vol. 1, 264–66.

76. Warner, *Therapeutic Perspective*, offers a stimulating exploration of the

intellectual underpinnings of heroic medicine. See also Charles Rosenberg, "The Therapeutic Revolution"; Eberle, *Treatise*; Berman, "The Heroic Approach."

77. Skene, *Treatise.*
78. Emmet, *Principles and Practice*, 131.
79. Thomas, *On the Diseases of Women.*
80. Thomas A. Emmet, "Surgery of the Cervix in Connection with Treatment of Certain Uterine Diseases," *American Journal of Obstetrics and Diseases of Women* 1 (1869): 340. Paul Mundé edited this journal.
81. Edward J. Tilt, *A Handbook of Uterine Therapeutics and of Diseases of Women*, 4th ed. (New York: William Wood and Co., 1881), 40.
82. Review, *New York Medical Journal* 8 (October-March, 1868–1869): 528.
83. J. Marion Sims, letter to the editor, *Lancet*, July 8, 1865, 42.
84. Henry Bennet, letter to the editor, *Lancet*, June 24, 1865, 673.
85. J. Marion Sims, letter, *Lancet*, July 8, 1865, 42.
86. T. Spencer Wells, letter to the editor, "Dr. Sims on Hysterotomy," *Lancet,* May 7, 1865, 42.
87. G. T. Gream, "Dilation or Division?" *Lancet*, April 8, 1865, 381.
88. J. Marion Sims, "Pregnancy-Vomiting," reprint from *Archives of Medicine* 3 (June 1880).
89. J. Marion Sims, "Painful Menstruation," *Lancet,* June 3, 1865, 588.
90. Augustus Gardner, *The Causes and Curative Treatment of Sterility with a Preliminary Statement of the Physiology of Generation* (New York: DeWitt and Davenport, 1856), 78.
91. See Howard Kelly, *Medical Gynecology* (New York: D. Appleton, 1909). See Sims, "On Vaginismus."
92. Sims, "Pregnancy-Vomiting," 5.
93. Sims, *Clinical Notes*, 115.
94. Sims, "Pregnancy-Vomiting."
95. See Thomas, *Abortion*, for further elaboration of this condition, including the death of Charlotte Bronte.
96. Sims, *Clinical Notes*, 331–336.
97. Emmet, "Reminiscences," 5.
98. Sims, *Clinical Notes*, 193.
99. See Elaine Tyler May, *Barren in the Promised Land: Childless Americans and the Pursuit of Happiness* (Cambridge, Mass.: Harvard University Press, 1995), 65–66. See also Harris, *Woman's Surgeon.*
100. Marsh and Ronner, *Empty Cradle*, 286, n. 65. Harry Sims changed his name to carry on his father's reputation as Harry Marion-Sims.
101. Review, *Clinical Notes on Uterine Surgery*, in *Medical Times and Gazette*, February 10, 1866, 151.
102. Foucault, *History of Sexuality.*
103. Sims, "On Vaginismus," 429.
104. Sims, *Clinical Notes*, 369.
105. Emmet, "A Memoir of Dr. James Marion Sims," 4.
106. See Marsh and Ronner, *Empty Cradle*. Sims's text suggests he was in many ways oblivious to the patient and not concerned with her perspective.

107. Review, *Medical Times and Gazette.*

108. D. Warren Brickell, "Review of *Clinical Notes on Uterine Surgery*," *Southern Journal of Medical Sciences* 1 (1886): 300.

109. Sims, *Clinical Notes,* 372–373. See Ben Barker-Benfield, "The Spermatic Economy: A Nineteenth-Century View of Sexuality," *Feminist Studies* 1 (Summer 1972): 45–74.

110. Sims, *Clinical Notes*, 372–373.

111. Ibid., 359.

112. Ibid., 360.

113. See Laqueur, *Making Sex.*

114. Sims, *Clinical Notes*, 361.

115. Edmund R. Peaslee, *Ovarian Tumors: Their Pathology, Diagnosis, and Treatment, Especially by Ovariotomy* (New York: D. Appleton, 1872).

116. Kelly, "History of Gynecology," and Thomas, "An Address in Obstetrics and Gynecology."

117. James V. Ricci, *The Development of Gynaecological Surgery and Instruments* (Philadelphia: Blakiston, 1949), 279. Kate Hurd-Mead suggests oophorectomy was performed as early as the sixteenth century in the American colonies by midwives. See her *A History of Women in Medicine* (Boston: Milford House, 1938). See Robert W. Ikard, "Surgical Operation on James K. Polk by Ephraim McDowell of the Search for Polk's Gallstone," *Tennessee Historical Quarterly* 43 (Summer 1984): 121–131.

118. Peaslee, *Ovarian Tumors*, 278.

119. See Jane Sewall, "Bountiful Bodies"; Ricci, *Development*; Longo, "Obstetrics and Gynecology"; John A. Shepherd, *Lawson Tait: The Rebellious Surgeon* (Lawrence, Kans.: Coronado Press, 1980).

120. See Peaslee, *Ovarian Tumors*; Washington L. Atlee, *A Retrospect of the Struggles and Triumph of Ovariotomy in Philadelphia* (Philadelphia: Philadelphia County Medical Society, 1875). See also Duffy, *Healers.*

121. Simpson, *Clinical Lectures*, 313.

122. David Hayes Agnew, *Principles and Practice of Surgery* (Philadelphia: Lea Bros., 1881), 799.

123. Peaslee, *Ovarian Tumors* 340.

124. Christopher Lawrence, "Democratic, Divine and Heroic: The History and Historiography of Surgery," in Christopher Lawrence, ed., *Medical Theory, Surgical Practice: Studies in the History of Surgery* (London: Routledge, 1992), 1–47; Christopher Lawrence and Richard Dixey, "Practising on Principle: Joseph Lister and the Germ Theories of Disease," in *Medical Theory*, 153–215. See Curt Proskauer, "Development and Use of the Rubber Glove in Surgery and Gynecology," in Gert Brieger, ed., *Theory and Practice in American Medicine* (New York: Science History Publications, 1976), 203–211. See Phyllis Richmond, "American Attitudes toward the Germ Theory," in *Theory and Practice*, 58–84.

125. Peaslee included cleanliness as part of surgical procedure in his *Ovarian Tumors.*

126. See Morantz-Sanchez, "Making It in a Man's World," and forthcoming book, for the history of Mary Dixon Jones. She was a practicing gynecologist and

ovariotomist in Brooklyn during the later seventies and eighties and an example of a woman practitioner. See also *Sympathy and Science*.

127. Emmet, "Memoir of James Marion Sims," 11.
128. *Bulletin of the New York Academy of Medicine* (1862): 439, 461.
129. *Annual Report of the Board of Governors, Board of Lady Supervisors, and Medical Board of the Woman's Hospital in the State of New York* (New York: Evening Post Presses, 1874), 41.
130. Ibid., 37.
131. Dr. Charles Budd, quoted in the *Annual Report of the Board of Governors and Board of Lady Supervisors of the Woman's Hospital of the State of New York* (New York: Bradstreet Press, 1870), 31.
132. J. Marion Sims, "On the Microscope, as an Aid in the Diagnosis and Treatment of Sterility," *New York Medical Journal* 8 (1868): 393–413; Reiser, *Reign of Technology*.
133. Bonner, *Becoming*.
134. Lawrence and Dixey, "The Germ Theories of Disease."
135. Ruth Abram, "Will There Be a Monument? Six Pioneer Women Doctors Tell Their Own Stories," in Abram, ed., *"Send Us a Lady Physician": Women Doctors in America, 1835–1920* (New York: W. W. Norton), 81.
136. Letter from J. Marion Sims, "Professor Lister's Introductory: Antiseptic Surgery," under "Correspondence" in the *British Medical Journal*, October 27, 1877, 608–609, and response under "Surgical Memoranda" in *The British Medical Journal*, November 10, 1877, 664.
137. See Rosenberg, *Care*, 127–137.
138. John Harley Warner, *Therapeutic Perspective*.

CHAPTER 6   *Power, Politics, and Profession*

1. James Pratt Marr, *James Marion Sims: Founder of the Woman's Hospital in the State of New York* (privately published pamphlet).
2. Herman Melville, *Moby-Dick or, The Whale* (1851) (New York: W. W. Norton, 1976).
3. Letter from Sarah Doremus to the Board of Governors of the Woman's Hospital, December 26, 1862, from the Bolling Medical Library Collection at St. Luke's-Roosevelt Hospital, New York.
4. E. R. Peaslee, *Seventeenth Annual Report of the Board of Governors and Board of Lady Supervisors of the Woman's Hospital of the State of New York* (New York: Evening Post Steam Presses, 1872), 36–37.
5. Emmet, *Incidents*.
6. Marr, *Sims*; Marr, *Pioneer Surgeons*; J. Riddle Goffe, "The Woman's Hospital in the State of New York, Founded in 1855," *The American Journal of Obstetrics and Diseases of Women and Children* 77 (April 1918): 530–543; Wylie, *Hospitals;* Emmet, *Incidents*, and "Reminiscences"; Sims, *Story of My Life*. See also Kelly, "History of Gynecology."
7. Letter from Sarah Doremus to Joseph B. Collins, August 14, 1865, Bolling Medical Library Collection.

8. Letter from James Beekman to Joseph B. Collins, March 27, 1867, in the Bolling Medical Library Collection.
9. Women's Hospital of the State of New York, *Annual Report* of 1868.
10. Wetmore was a member of the City Tract Society and involved in evangelical revivals during the antebellum period. See Bernstein, *Draft Riots,* 178–179.
11. Letter from Sarah Doremus to the assistant treasurer of the building fund, December 26, 1862, in the archives of the Bolling Medical Library.
12. J. Riddle Goffe, "The Woman's Hospital," 534.
13. Hayes Martin, Harry Ehrlich, and Francelia Butler, "J. Marion Sims, Pioneer Cancer Protagonist," *Cancer,* March 1950, 187–204. See Harris, *Woman's Surgeon.*
14. Letter from Sims to James Sparkman, December 28, 1868, from the South Caroliniana Library at the University of South Carolina. Thanks to Herbert Hartsook for bringing this letter to my attention.
15. Samuel D. Gross, "A Century of American Medicine: II, Surgery," *American Journal of the Medical Sciences* 71 (1876): 431–484.
16. Sims, "Stenosis of the Cervix Uteri," 78.
17. *American Journal of Obstetrics and Diseases of Women and Children*, vol. 2 (1870).
18. Emmet, *Incidents*, 200–220. See Reginald Horsman, *Josiah Nott of Mobile* (Baton Rouge: Louisiana State University Press, 1987), and Harris, *Woman's Surgeon.*
19. Thomas, *Treatise*, 58
20. Ann Stoler, *Race and the Education of Desire: Foucault's History of Sexuality and the Colonial Order of Things* (Durham, N.C.: Duke University Press, 1995); Bernstein, *Draft Riots.*
21. Emmet, *Incidents.*
22. Harris, *Woman's Surgeon.* See also Marr, *Pioneer Surgeons.*
23. J. Marion Sims, "The Woman's Hospital Anniversary Address" (New York: Baker and Godwin, 1868), 1.
24. Kenneth DeVille, *Medical Malpractice in Nineteenth-Century America* (New York: New York University Press, 1990); James C. Mohr, *Doctors and the Law: Medical Jurisprudence in Nineteenth-Century America* (New York: Oxford University Press, 1993).
25. Harris, *Woman's Surgeon*, 272–277. Joseph Leach, *Bright Particular Star: The Life and Times of Charlotte Cushman* (New Haven: Yale University Press, 1970); Edward James et al., *Notable American Women: A Biographical Dictionary*, vol. 1 (Cambridge, Mass.: Belknap, 1980).
26. Leach, *Star.*
27. Susan Sontag, *Illness as Metaphor* (New York: Vintage Press, 1977).
28. Closely tied to the Woman's Hospital was the Nursery and Child's Hospital, where Mary Dubois and Sarah Doremus were executive officers. Mary Dubois in 1870 dismissed Abraham Jacobi, a pediatrician and well-established New York physician, from his practice at the institution. The issues involved wet nursing and the care of foundlings—what concerned Jacobi was the exceedingly high rate of infant mortality and the role of urban asylums as a cause. The bone of

contention was a more specific confrontation between Jacobi and a patient. See Janet Golden, *Wet Nursing*; also Golden, ed., *Infant Asylums and Children's Hospitals: Medical Dilemmas and Developments, 1850–1920* (New York: Garland, 1989). See Quiroga, "Poor Mothers."

29. Sims, *Silver Sutures*, 37.
30. Marilyn Yalom, *A History of the Breast* (New York: Alfred Knopf, 1997), 229.
31. Thomas, *Treatise*.
32. Ludmilla Jordanova, *Sexual Visions: Images of Gender in Science and Medicine between the Eighteenth and Twentieth Centuries* (Madison: University of Wisconsin Press, 1989). Yalom, *The Breast*. See Francis Burney, "A Mastectomy," in David Rothman, Steven Marcus, and Stephanie Kiceluk, eds., *Medicine and Western Civilization* (New Brunswick, N.J.: Rutgers University Press, 1995) 383–389.
33. J. Marion Sims, letter to the *New York Times*, and personal letter of defense to Committee on Ethics of the New York Academy of Medicine, April 4, 1870, and W. E. Johnston's letter in defense of Sims, Southern Historical Collection, New York Academy of Medicine Committee on Ethics Scrapbook at the New York Academy of Medicine. See also Leach, *Star*, 344–346; Harris, *Woman's Surgeon*.
34. *New York Daily Times*, October 3, 1869.
35. Letter from Thomas Finnell, N.Y.A.M. Committee on Ethics Scrapbook.
36. Ibid.
37. Ibid.
38. See Drachman, "Loomis Trial"; Rosenkrantz, "The Search for Professional Order"; Starr, *Social Transformation*.
39. Leach, *Particular Star*, 325.
40. Sims's holograph address, July 4, 1871, reprinted in *Story of My Life*, 420.
41. "Fighting Physicians: Two American Medical Men in Court," *New York Times*, Sunday, September 10, 1871, front page.
42. Emmet, *Incidents*, 235.
43. Gert H. Brieger, "From Conservative to Radical Surgery in Late Nineteenth-Century America," in Laurence, ed., *Medical Theory*, 217–221.
44. *Annual Report of the Board of Governors and Lady Supervisors of the Woman's Hospital* (New York: Russell's American Steam Printing House, 1871), and Emmet, *Incidents*.
45. Mattus, *New York Nightingales*, 33.
46. James Beekman, "Centenary Address Delivered before the Society of the New York Hospital" (New York: New York Hospital Society, 1871).
47. Kristie Ross, "Arranging a Doll's House: Refined Women as Union Nurses," in Catherine Clinton and Nina Silber, eds., *Divided Houses: Gender and the Civil War* (New York: Oxford University Press, 1992), 98.
48. Elizabeth Leonard, *Yankee Women: Gender Battles in the Civil War* (New York: W. W. Norton, 1994), 10–11.
49. See, for instance, George Fredrickson, *The Inner Civil War: Northern Intellectuals and the Crisis of the Union* (New York: Harper and Row, 1965).
50. See Ross, "Union Nurses."

51. Susan Reverby, *Ordered to Care: The Dilemma of American Nursing, 1850–1945* (Cambridge, U.K.: Cambridge University Press, 1987), 41–42.
52. Regina Morantz-Sanchez, forthcoming publication on the career of Mary Dixon-Jones.
53. Carroll Smith-Rosenberg, "The Abortion Movement and the A.M.A., 1850–1880," in *Disorderly Conduct*, 217–244. Reagan, *When Abortion Was a Crime*, 13.
54. Brodie, *Abortion and Contraception*. Also see Homberger, *Scenes*, on Mme Restell and Anthony Comstock.
55. Emmet, "Etiology."
56. Thomas Savage, student notes.
57. Mottus, *New York Nightingales,* 41.
58. Ibid., table 6 and 7.
59. Emmet, "Reminiscences" and *Incidents*.
60. Minutes of the Board of Lady Supervisors, Mary Jay Edwards, Secretary, April 12, 1875.
61. *Annual Report of the Board of Governors and Board of Lady Supervisors of the Woman's Hospital of the State of New York* (New York: Bradstreet Press, 1870).
62. The hospital rules were listed every year in the annual report. See also archives of the Lying-In Asylum, and Quiroga, "Poor Mothers," and Reverby, *Ordered to Care*.
63. See Robert Battey, "Normal Ovariotomy-Case," *Atlanta Medical and Surgical Journal* 10 (1872/3): 321–329; "Normal Ovariotomy," *Atlanta Medical and Surgical Journal* 11 (April 1873): 1–84; J. Marion Sims, "Remarks on Battey's Operation," *British Medical Journal*, December 8, 1877, 916–917. See Lawrence D. Longo, "The Rise and Fall of Battey's Operation: A Fashion in Surgery, "*Bulletin of the History of Medicine* 53 (1979): 244–261, and G. J. Barker-Benfield, *Horrors*.
64. Today oophorectomy denotes the surgical removal of the ovaries, and ovariotomy is the removal of an ovarian tumor only.
65. J. Marion Sims, "On Intra-Uterine Fibroids"(New York: D. Appleton, 1874; *New York Medical Journal* 18 (1874): 336–360.
66. Janet Bogdan, "Aggressive Intervention and Mortality," in Pamela Eakins, ed., *The American Way of Birth* (Philadelphia: Temple University Press, 1986), 80.
67. Ibid., 93.
68. Thomas, "Prophylactic Resource in Midwifery," *New York Medical Journal* 10 (April 1870): 449–469.
69. Thomas, "On Obstetrics and Gynecology."
70. Thomas Addis Emmet, "In Memoriam: Edmund Randolph Peaslee," *American Journal of Obstetrics and Diseases of Women and Children* 11 (October 1878): 390–393. Marr, *Pioneer*, 109.
71. Mottus, *New York Nightingales*, 57.
72. Society of the New York Hospital, *Report on Enquiry into Practicability of Extending the Hospital*, 8–9, 12. Quoted in Mottus, *New York Nightingales*, 56.
73. W. Gill Wylie, *Memorial Sketch of the Life of J. Marion Sims* (New York: D.

Appleton, 1884; repr. of an article in *New York Medical Journal*, April 12, 1884), 18.

74. See Minutes of the Woman's Hospital Association for January 7, 1870, and January 4, 1862.
75. Inspecting Committee Notes, Board of Lady Supervisors, November 1868.
76. Minutes of the Board of Lady Supervisors, April 20, 1872.
77. Report of the Medical Board to the Board of Governors, November 21, 1872.
78. Minutes of the Board of Lady Supervisors, January 4, 1873.
79. Ibid.
80. Ibid.
81. Ibid., June 3, 1873.
82. Special Report of the Board of Governors, from the Board of Lady Supervisors, December 31, 1873.
83. Ibid.
84. Letter from M. J. Edwards to the Board of Governors, May 31, 1873.
85. Letter to the Board of Lady Supervisors from house surgeon, W. Baker, December 1, 1873.
86. Special Report from the Board of Lady Supervisors, December 31, 1873.
87. Ibid.
88. Report of the Medical Board by T. G. Thomas, *Annual Report of the Board of Governors, Board of Lady Supervisors and Medical Board of the Woman's Hospital of the State of New York* (New York, 1874).
89. Minutes of the Board of Lady Supervisors, February 6, 1874; minutes of the Executive Committee of the Board of Lady Supervisors, January 1874.
90. T. Gaillard Thomas, Report from the Medical Board, *Nineteenth Annual Report of the Woman's Hospital in the State of New York* (New York, 1874).
91. Ibid., 37.
92. "Editorial Interview with Dr. J. Marion Sims," Extra of the *St. Louis Clinical Record* 4, September 1877.
93. James Beekman, quoted in *Nineteenth Annual Report*, 37.
94. Thomas, in ibid.
95. Ibid.
96. Ibid.
97. G. T. Davis, President, Resolution for the Board of Governors, December 1874.
98. Ibid.
99. Letter from the Board of Lady Supervisors to the Board of Governors, December 7, 1874.
100. Ibid.
101. Ibid.
102. Letter from Caroline Lane to the Board of Governors, January 9, 1874.
103. Ibid.
104. Ibid.
105. Letter from M. J. Edwards to the Board of Governors, January 9, 1874.
106. Manuscript, letter from Caroline Lane, December 1870.
107. Histories of hospitals in the United States include Rosner, *A Once Charitable*

Enterprise; Vogel, *The Invention of the Modern Hospital;* Rosenberg, *The Care of Strangers*; Drachman, *Hospital with a Heart*.

108. Notes and records of the Lady Supervisors and the annual reports of the Woman's Hospital of the State of New York provided material for statistics on the hospital accounts.

109. Martin J. Burke, *The Conundrum of Class: Public Discourse on the Social Order in America* (Chicago: University of Chicago Press, 1990).

110. See, for example, Mary H. Blewett, *Men, Women, and Work: Class, Gender, and Protest in the New England Shoe Industry, 1780–1910* (Urbana: University of Illinois Press, 1990); Ginzburg, *Women and the Work of Benevolence*; and Jean Boydston, *Home and Work: Housework, Wages, and the Ideology of Labor in the Early Republic* (New York: Oxford University Press, 1990).

111. *First Anniversary of the Woman's Hospital* (New York: Miller and Homan, 1856), 8.

112. Ibid., 23.

113. Ibid.

114. Agnew, *Lacerations*, 10.

115. T. A. Emmet, in *Tenth Annual Report* (New York: J. M. Bradstreet, 1865).

116. See T. Gaillard Thomas, quoted in *Nineteenth Annual Report of the Woman's Hospital in the State of New York* (New York: Evening Post Steam Presses, 1875), and letter from Caroline Lane to the Board of Governors, January 13, 1874, Archives, Bolling Medical Library, St. Luke's Hospital. See Ginzburg, *Women and the Work of Benevolence*.

117. J. Marion Sims, *The Woman's Hospital: Anniversary Address*, pamphlet (New York: Baker and Godwin, 1868), 6–7.

118. See Blewett, *Men, Women and Work*; see also Stansell, *City of Women*.

119. Emmet, *Incidents*, 335.

120. Sims, "Painful Menstruation," 253.

121. Sims, "Stenosis of the Cervix Uteri," 66.

122. Savage's notebook on Thomas's clinic.

123. Emmet, "Necessity for Early Delivery," 120.

124. See, for instance, Augustus Gardner, "The Physical Decline of American Women," an appendix to Gardner, *The Conjugal Sins*.

125. See Elaine Showalter, *The Female Malady: Women, Madness, and English Culture, 1830–1980* (New York: Pantheon Books, 1985). See Carroll Smith-Rosenberg, "Sex as Symbol in Victorian Purity: An Ethnohistorical Analysis of Jacksonian America," *American Journal of Sociology* (suppl.) 84 (1978): 212–247.

126. See John Eberle, *Treatise*, for an early description of chlorosis. Emmet and Thomas both discuss chlorosis in their texts. See Joan Jacobs Brumberg, "Chlorotic Girls, 1870–1920: A Historical Perspective on Female Adolescence," in *Women and Health*.

127. Thomas Savage's notebook on T. Gaillard Thomas's Clinic.

128. Ibid. See Lawrence Longo, "Electrotherapy in Gynecology: The American Experience," *Bulletin of the History of Medicine* 60 (Fall 1986): 343–366.

129. Emmet, *Incidents*, 208.

130. Ibid., 209.
131. Ibid., 210.
132. Emmet, *Principles and Practice*; Emmet, "Etiology."
133. Sewall, "Bountiful Bodies."
134. Agnew, *Principles and Practice of Surgery*, vol. 3 (Philadelphia: J. B. Lippincott Co., 1881), 577–578.
135. Emmet, "Etiology of Uterine Flexures," *Transactions of the American Gynecological Society* (1876): 48–90.
136. Emmet, "Etiology," 49.
137. See Virginia Drachman, "The Loomis Trial," in Rosner and Reverby, eds., *Health Care in America.*
138. James Platt White, Comments, *Transactions of the American Medical Association* 28 (1877): 315.
139. Emmet, *Principles and Practice*, 144–145.
140. Ibid., 145.
141. See Sims, "Stenosis of the Cervix Uteri," 78.
142. See obituary for J. Marion Sims, *New York Medical Journal*, November 17, 1883; James White, "On Cervical Incision," *Transactions of the American Medical Association* 28 (1877): 315–317; and Sims, "Editorial Interview," *St. Louis Clinical Record* (June 1877), 74–75.
143. Obituary for J. Marion Sims, *New York Medical Journal*, November 17, 1883, 550–551.
144. Sims, "Editorial Interview," *St. Louis Clinical Record* (June 1877): 74–75.
145. E. R. Peaslee, T. Gaillard Thomas, and Thomas A. Emmet, "To the Medical Profession. Statements Respecting the Separation of Dr. J. Marion Sims from the Woman's Hospital, New York," circular dated May 5, 1877; *Reply to Dr. J. Marion Sims' Pamphlet, entitled "The Woman's Hospital in 1874"* (New York: Trow's Printing, 1877). J. Marion Sims, *The Woman's Hospital in 1874*, pamphlet, New York, June 1877.
146. Sims, "Editorial Interview," *St. Louis Medical Record.*
147. Peaslee, Thomas, and Emmet, "Reply," 13. See also *Twenty-Second Annual Report of the Woman's Hospital of the State of New York Including a Tabular Statement of All the Cases Treated in the Hospital from Its Foundation* (New York: Evening Post Steam Presses, 1877).
148. Ibid., 5–6. See also John Haller, *Medicine in Transition*, 261.
149. Sims, "The Woman's Hospital in 1874."
150. Emmet, *Principles and Practice.*
151. Atlee, "A Retrospective," 20–21.
152. Wylie, *Hospitals.*
153. Thomas, "On Obstetrics and Gynecology."
154. Sims, *Story of My Life*, 304.
155. Longo, "Obstetrics and Gynecology," 215.
156. Marr, *Pioneer Surgeons.*
157. *The Modern Hospital*, October 1925, 171–175.

Conclusion

1. Nancy M. Theriot, "Women's Voices in Nineteenth-Century Medical Discourse: A Step toward Deconstructing Science,"in Barbara Laslett, Sally Gregory Kohlstedt, Helen Longino, and Evelynn Hammonds, eds., *Gender and Scientific Authority* (Chicago: University of Chicago Press, 1996), 124–154. This excellent essay includes a discussion of the patient's perspective.
2. J. Marion Sims, "On Ovariotomy," *New York Medical Record* 17 (1873): 377.
3. Ibid., 378.
4. The abortions may or may not have indicated what we today distinguish as miscarriages. See Carroll Smith-Rosenberg on the etiology of "abortion" in her *Disorderly Conduct*, 219. The *Oxford English Dictionary* substantiates her argument. Note that despite the ambiguity of the term, physicians by the 1870s were vociferously condemning the practice of abortion. By the mid-1870s there were several who used the term "criminal abortion."
5. See Sewall, "Bountiful Bodies"; see also Peaslee, *Ovarian Tumors.*
6. Sewall, in "Bountiful Bodies," 274, describes the central issues in ovariotomy among surgeons: whether to externalize the pedicle or how to prevent peritonitis. Here Sims instead made a special case of addressing septicemia.
7. Sims, "On Ovariotomy," 377.
8. J. Marion Sims in discussion, *Transactions of the American Medical Association* 25 (1874): 199.
9. Sims, "On Ovariotomy."
10. James Burke on nineteenth-century surgery in *The Day the Universe Changed* (Boston: Little, Brown, 1985), 220.
11. Sewall, "Bountiful Bodies," 313. See also Dale Smith, "A Historical Overview of the Recognition of Appendicitis," *New York State Journal of Medicine* 86 (1986): 571–583, 639–647.
12. Ibid., 378.
13. See Mottus, *New York Nightingales*, on hospitalism.
14. Emmet, "Reminiscences of the Founders of the Woman's Hospital Association," *American Gynecological and Obstetrical Journal* 15 (1899): 379. Emmet estimated that by 1878 he had treated at least four hundred cases of vesico-vaginal fistulas.
15. Houston Everett, M.D., and Richard Mattingly, "Vesicovaginal Fistula," *American Journal of Obstetrics and Gynecology* 72 (1956): 712–724; Moir, *Vesico-Vaginal Fistula*. See Louis E. Phaneuf, "Genital Fistulas in Women," *American Journal of Surgery* 64 (April 1944): 3–27, on the occurrence of surgical tears. See George Rosen, "Fees and Fee Bills: Some Economic Aspects of Medical Practice in Nineteenth-Century America," *Bulletin of the History of Medicine* 16 (1946), (suppl.), and Virginia Drachman, "Gynecological Instruments and Surgical Decision," for some sketchy evidence on the waxing and waning of the operation for vesico-vaginal fistulas.
16. Nancy Stepan and Sander Gilman, "Appropriating the Idioms of Science: The Rejection of Scientific Racism," in Dominick LaCapra, *The Bounds of Race: Perspectives on Hegemony and Resistance* (Ithaca. N.Y.: Cornell University Press, 1991), 72–103; Emily Martin, *The Woman in the Body: A Cultural Analysis*

of Reproduction (Boston: Beacon Press, 1992), offers an outstanding model of textual analysis in the language of medicine. Excellent also on metaphor is Nancy Leys Stepan, "Race and Gender: The Role of Analogy in Science," in Evelyn Fox Keller and Helen Longino, eds., *Feminism and Science* (Oxford: Oxford University Press, 1996), 121–136.

17. Thomas, "An Address in Obstetrics and Gynecology"; John Harley Warner, "Ideals of Science and Their Discontents in Late Nineteenth-Century American Medicine," *Isis* 82 (1991): 454–478.

18. Sims to Protheroe Smith, *The British Gynecological Journal* 1 (1886): 202. As quoted in Sewall, *Bountiful Bodies*.

19. Gert Brieger, "Surgery," in Ronald L. Numbers, ed., *The Education of American Physicians*, 175–204.

20. Diana Scully, *Men Who Control Women's Health: The Mis-Education of Obstetrician-Gynecologists* (New York: Teachers College Press, 1994). Leslie Laurence and Beth Weinhouse, *Outrageous Practices: The Alarming Truth about How Medicine Mistreats Women* (New York: Fawcett Columbine, 1994). See Sue V. Rosser, *Women's Health—Missing from U.S. Medicine* (Bloomington: Indiana University Press, 1994).

21. See Richard Gillam and Barton Bernstein, "Doing Harm: The DES Tragedy and Modern American Medicine," *Public Historian* 9 (Winter 1987): 57–82.

22. Angela Davis, *Women, Race and Class* (New York: Random House, 1981).

23. Sue Fisher, *In the Patient's Best Interest: Women and the Politics of Medical Decisions* (New Brunswick, N.J.: Rutgers University Press, 1986).

24. Helen Bequaert Holmes and Laura M. Purdy, eds., *Feminist Perspectives in Medical Ethics* (Bloomington: Indiana University Press, 1992); "Special Issue: Feminist Ethics and Medicine," *Hypatia* 4 (Summer 1989). See also Barbara Katz Rothman, *The Tentative Pregnancy: Prenatal Diagnosis and the Future of Motherhood* (New York: Viking Press, 1986).

25. Susan Sherwin, *No Longer Patient: Feminist Ethics and Health Care* (Philadelphia: Temple University Press, 1992)

26. Takaki, *Iron Cages*.

27. Ross, "Union Nurses," 373, n. 11.

28. Nancy Krieger and Elizabeth Fee, "Man-Made Medicine and Women's Health: The Biopolitics of Sex/Gender and Race/Ethnicity," in Elizabeth Fee and Nancy Krieger, *Women's Health, Politics, and Power: Essays on Sex/Gender, Medicine, and Public Health* (Amityville, N.Y.: Baywood, 1994), 11–29

INDEX

medicine (*continued*)
98, 134; clinical, 13, 19, 21, 55, 162;
craft of, 24, 31, 48; empirical, 13;
ethics of, 7, 56, 177–179, 205–206,
219–220; rise of modern, 4, 13, 161–
162, 165; sectarian, 13, 14, 172, 205,
208; women practicing, 75, 76, 96, 99,
103, 171, 184, 195, 205; women's,
122, 199. *See also* experimentation;
heroic medicine
Meigs, Charles, 21, 54, 44, 67, 111, 112,
134, 139, 143
Memorial (New York State Legislature),
69, 167
menorrhagia, *see under* menstruation
menstruation, 76, 137, 138, 141, 142, 145,
152, 155, 158, 202; ammenorhea, 140,
142; and adolescence, 148, 201;
dysmennorhea, 139, 140, 141, 144,
145, 147, 148, 149, 150, 151, 152,
201, 206, 207; menorrhagia, 140, 142,
143; and surgery, 142, 144, 145. *See
also* pain
Metcalfe, John T., 129, 130, 163
metritis, 49, 150, 151
Mettauer, John, 48, 53, 62
Mexican-American War, 59
Michaelis, Gustav Adolphus, 110–111
micrococci, 164
microscope, 131, 156, 162, 163, 190, 218
midwifery, midwives, 5, 29, 35, 36, 38,
39, 42, 43, 45–46, 87, 107, 108, 113,
117, 118, 119, 123, 138, 154; African
American, 38, 39–41, 232*n*16; and
cosmology, 117; Irish, 117; and
medicine, 6, 35, 185, 188
Minturn, Mrs. Robert, 88
Minturn, Robert, 88, 92
Missionary Crumbs, 91
Mitchell, S. Weir, 21
Moby Dick (Melville), 167
monogeny, 12
Montgomery, Alabama, 26, 30 *fig.*, 95,
96, 97, 155, 219; experiments in, 43–
54, 44 *fig.*, 56, 58, 60, 61, 62, 63, 67
Moore, Charles, 175–176
mortality, 29, 78, 159, 166, 175, 180, 186,

197, 209, 210, 210 *table,* 218, 220;
child, 28, 31, 34, 123; infant, 29, 34,
38, 41, 78, 90, 124 *table*; maternal, 35,
37, 38, 187, 188. *See also* death
Morton, William, 50
motherhood, 34–35, 66, 67, 74, 76, 85,
90, 104, 175
Mott, Valentine, 66, 70, 73, 76, 83, 86,
136

Naegele, Carl, 111, 112
Native Americans, 56, 173
neonatal tetanus, 29, 31, 32, 41
New England Hospital for Women and
Children, 99
New Orleans, 57, 63, 113, 173
New York Academy of Medicine, 66, 95,
126, 131, 132, 134, 137, 163, 174,
177, 178, 206; Committee on Ethics,
174, 176–179; Sims's "Silver Sutures"
Anniversary Address (1858), 65, 174.
*See also Bulletin of the New York
Academy of Medicine*
New York Almshouse, 72, 78, 80
New York Cancer Hospital, 212
New York City, 5, 9, 60, 65, 105, 112,
116, 123, 131, 139, 159, 165, 177,
178, 179, 181, 187, 198, 211;
Brooklyn, 74; and Civil War, 102–103,
181–184; Draft Riots in, 84, 102;
ethnicity in, 102; founding the
Woman's Hospital in, 69–104; history
of, 77–79, 101–103, 126, 129, 130;
Manhattan, 59, 69, 76, 77, 84, 88, 101,
129, 131; new hospital buildings in,
170–173; Old New York, 92, 94; and
Tweed Ring, 179–180. *See also*
medical education, in New York City
New York City Tract and Mission Society,
90, 93
New York County Medical Society, 71,
207
New York Daily Times, 176
New York Dispensary, 92, 180
New York Emigrant Hospital, *see*
Emigrant's Refuge Hospital
New York Hospital, 73, 74, 91, 92, 180

Thomas, T. Gaillard (*continued*)
  conflict with Sims, 200–210; and
  Caesarian section, 151; and gynecology, 133, 188; and Woman's Hospital,
  126, 133, 166, 180, 191, 193, 195,
  196. *See also* Bellevue Hospital;
  obstetrics
Thompson, Caroline, 85
Thomsonian medicine, 14
Thornwell, James, 22–24, 72, 229*n*76
Tilt, Edward, 151
Tombs (New York City), 77, 78, 90
traction, 114–115 *fig.*, 123
trismus nascentium, 28–32, 46, 48. *See
  also* neonatal tetanus; slavery, trismus
  nascentium and
trocar, 161
Truth, Sojourner, 61
tuberculosis, 10, 137, 140, 175, 231*n*5
tumors, 140, 142, 189, 190, 196; of the
  jaw, 26, 27; ovarian, 55, 160, 161, 190,
  214–216
Tuskegee Study of Syphilis, 56. *See also*
  experimentation
typhoid fever, 17, 77, 105
typhus, 78, 101, 162

Union League (New York City), 92, 181
United Irishmen, 100
United States Sanitary Commission, 178,
  181–184
uterine cancer, 176, 191, 209, 213
uterine prolapse, 43, 85, 134, 140, 201
uterine sound, 138, 144, 145, 147, 150
uterus, 34, 36, 37, 43, 48, 118, 132, 134
  fig., 135 *fig.*, 136, 137, 142, 143, 144,
  145, 146, 147, 150, 188, 202, 203,
  204, 206, 207; anteflexion of, 144,
  145, 147, 148, 149, 204; displacement
  of, 135, 148; retroversion of, 143, 148,
  150. *See also* uterine cancer; uterine
  prolapse

vagina, 2, 33, 34, 44, 46, 47, 64, 109, 113,
  118, 134 *fig.*, 135 *fig.*, 144, 148, 156,
  160, 188, 203. *See also* speculum
vaginismus, 1–2, 5, 7, 127, 154, 155

Van Buren, John, 80
Velpeau (French surgeon), 27, 62
vesico-vaginal fistula, 6, 33, 43, 44, 45,
  47, 49, 53, 55, 58, 59, 61, 62, 74, 76,
  85, 86, 94, 96, 97, 106 *fig.*, 108, 114–
  115 *fig.*, 124 *table*, 133, 140, 143, 144,
  151, 156, 161, 171, 172, 187, 188,
  199, 217, 218; and class, 51; defined,
  33–35; and Irish women, 105–125;
  origins of, 33–35, 42–43, 109–125;
  and slave women, 33–68; success of
  surgery for, 63–67. *See also* Emmet,
  Thomas Addis; experimentation
Vesico-Vaginal Fistula (Emmet), 113, 124,
  124 *table*
Victorian culture, 4, 49, 71, 87, 103, 104,
  156, 158, 159, 183, 202, 203. *See also*
  sex, and Victorian culture
Virginia Medical Monthly, 208

Walker, W. T., 214, 215, 216
water cures, 14, 103, 180
Welch, William, 190
Wells, Spencer, 55, 74, 106, 152, 160,
  161, 210, 219
West, Charles, 139
Wetmore, Appollos R., 170
Wetmore Pavilion (Women's Hospital),
  80, 167, 168 *fig.*, 169 *fig.*, 169, 170,
  171, 172, 181, 185, 194, 194 *fig.*, 197,
  218
wetnurses, 90, 91, 96, 107, 175
White, James Platt, 121, 206–207
womanhood, 75, 85, 94, 104, 152, 163,
  178, 183, 184, 199
Woman's Hospital Association, 69, 71, 76,
  77, 79, 81, 85, 86, 88, 92, 94, 133,
  168, 198; logo, 87 *fig.*
Woman's Hospital of the State of New
  York, 73 *fig.*, 168 *fig.*, 169 *fig.*, 194
  fig., 213 *fig.*; architecture of, 165,
  193–195, 194 *fig.*; founding of, 69–
  104; medical practice at, 126–166; and
  patients, 105–125, 214, 220; in
  postwar years, 167–214. *See also*
  Baldwin Pavilion; Outdoor Department; Wetmore Pavilion; Woman's

ABOUT THE AUTHOR

Deborah Kuhn McGregor is an associate professor of history and women's studies at the University of Illinois at Springfield. She has a Ph.D. in history from
Binghamton University. Recently her essay, "'Childbirth-Travells' and 'Spiritual Estates': Anne Hutchinson and Colonial Boston, 1634–1638," was published
in *Midwifery Theory and Practice*, edited by Philip K. Wilson. In addition to
teaching, she is currently researching and writing a history of midwifery and
childbirth in South and Central Illinois.